THE PRACTICE OF
NURSING

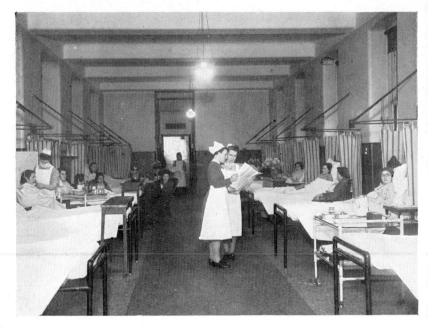

A hospital ward

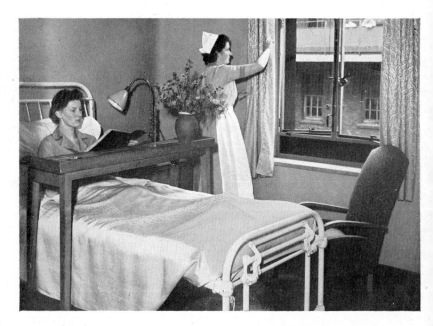

A side ward

THE PRACTICE OF NURSING

by

HILDA M. GRATION

S.R.N., S.C.M., D.N. (Lond.)

Sister Tutor, Guy's Hospital: Examiner in Nursing for the General Nursing Council of England and Wales

FABER AND FABER LTD

24 Russell Square

London

1944

First published in Mcmxliv
by Faber and Faber Limited
24 Russell Square London W.C.1
Second impression February Mcmxlv
Printed in Great Britain by
Latimer Trend & Co Ltd Plymouth

FOREWORD

by Sir Herbert L. Eason
C.B., C.M.G., M.D., M.S.

One often hears the phrase 'a born nurse' and it is true. To be a born nurse one must have a deep-rooted affection for one's fellow-creatures and an instinctive desire to help them in their sufferings. But a born nurse cannot do her best unless she is properly trained, and with the complexities of modern medicine and surgery that training is long and arduous.

Miss Hilda Gration has been the senior Sister Tutor at Guy's Hospital for many years and this book represents the teaching she has given and is giving. It is individual, as all good text-books should be, characteristic of her and of the Guy's tradition in practical nursing. The spirit of the book is, I think, summed up in the phrase on page forty-three, 'The aim of bedmaking is to make the patient comfortable, and not to make the bed tidy.'

That the comfort and well-being of the patient override all other considerations and customs, is the essential of good nursing. Miss Gration has always in mind the importance of training and efficiency to this end.

Herbert L. Eason

PREFACE

The practice of nursing cannot be taught in the classroom or from a textbook. It is learnt by experience and example. Hence the daily contact with patients, working with and supervised by a good sister, is the real method by which the student nurse learns her art. This simple book aims at putting the patient in the centre of the picture, emphasizing the right method of approach and describing the various nursing techniques. It seems best that student nurses should learn one way of doing treatments and learn that way thoroughly; later, when they see other equally good methods used, they can modify details, provided that they understand underlying principles.

It is expected that nurses will study medical and surgical text-books together with this *Practice of Nursing* which does not claim to be a comprehensive guide to the whole nursing field.

The tables of food values and vitamins have been compiled from *Food Values at a Glance* by permission of Mrs. V. G. Plimmer and Messrs. Longmans Green & Co., Ltd. The hospital diets and instructions in chapters 5 and 18 are those drawn up by the Medical Committee of Guy's Hospital and acknowledgment is made to the Governors of the Hospital for permission to use them. My thanks are due to the Ward and Departmental Sisters of Guy's Hospital, whose help has been a great encouragement, also to members of the Medical Staff for corrections of detail. It would be invidious to mention any by name, when so many have contributed to the result. I should also like to thank Mr. C. W. Stewart of Messrs. Faber and Faber for his patience and help throughout.

H. M. GRATION

CONTENTS

PLATES

Chapter One

THE PATIENT'S DAY

The time when the patient wakes and begins the daily routine naturally varies according to her condition and the administration of the hospital or home in which she is being nursed. Other factors have also to be considered. For instance, if the hospital is situated in a large city, one has to consider at what time the markets open and the street noises are likely to disturb the patient. This explains why in some city hospitals it is more restful for the patients to settle down early for their night's sleep, when traffic is quiet, to be awakened as early as six a.m. when the streets are busy again.

We may take as an example a seriously ill patient who, having required drugs to make her sleep, wakes at about seven-thirty a.m. The nurse should pull back the curtains and then offer the patient a bedpan. She sponges her face and hands, gives her a mouthwash and dentures (if any), and arranges her comfortably for breakfast. She should open the windows to freshen the room and wash her own hands preparatory to bringing in the breakfast tray. The latter is laid by the night nurse, and the tea or coffee and any food required to be cooked, should be just ready at the right moment. The nurse should give the cook ten or fifteen minutes' warning so that there is no waste of time and the patient is not kept waiting. The nurse pours out the tea, butters the toast and helps the patient in any way required. She should remember that the patient is ill and will probably refuse breakfast if it is just put in front of her, but if small amounts are presented in an attractive way with a good cup of tea or coffee the patient will probably feel better for it. The nurse should always try to adapt her attitude to the patient's mood in the early morning, and not be too brisk and irritatingly cheerful when the patient is bound to feel heavy and depressed as a result of her illness and sleeping draughts. It is important for the nurse to think out the above details so that the patient has not to ask for anything. If the nurse does not attend to her she will probably be too tired and ill to ask.

THE TOILET OF THE PATIENT

This comes next in the day's routine. An interval of not more than half an hour should elapse after breakfast, during which the patient may feel well

9

enough to look at her letters if they are opened for her, or she may glance at the headlines of the newspaper.

Before beginning to wash the patient the nurse should: (1) Take the temperature, pulse, and respiration. (2) Close the windows. (3) Give a bedpan.

Whilst the patient is using the bedpan the requirements for the bath are collected. The bedpan is then removed and emptied and the nurse washes her own hands. She then strips the bed and gives a complete bath between blankets. She attends to the patient's back and pressure points and helps her to clean her teeth. She puts on a clean nightgown and bed jacket if required and arranges the patient's hair. Dressings and appliances such as splints and bandages, should be readjusted and the bed thoroughly made, giving clean linen if necessary. Help may be required at some stages in the toilet; for lifting the patient on and off the bedpan, and for treating the pressure points, and it is certainly more satisfactory for two nurses to make the bed. Medicines are given at the times prescribed, and if there is a dressing to be done, it is usually better to leave it until later in the morning when the patient has recovered from the exertion of the blanket bath and bed making. By this time it is usually 9—10 a.m., and the patient will need a cup of milk or other suitable drink. It should be remembered that an ill patient usually eats so little at mealtimes that regular intermediate feeds are absolutely necessary. After having the drink, the patient will probably like to have a short sleep and in many cases will be almost oblivious of the sweeping, dusting, and general clearing up which must be done about this time of day. If necessary, she may be screened to ensure less disturbance.

The routine above described becomes very familiar to the nurse, but it is not as easy as might appear to bathe and settle up an ill patient, thoroughly and expeditiously. The best nurses know that it is not a case of doing it once or twice, but that it will take years of experience to learn to handle all types of patients with confidence and skill. The whole procedure should be made as little irksome as possible for the patient and this depends not only on the methods taught in the classroom and wards, but much more upon the nurse's personality and tact. Either the patient likes being bathed by a certain nurse or she does not; the human element counts most in the intimate care of the sick. During the morning the doctor usually visits the patient and the nurse must be prepared for any treatment or dressings which he may wish to do, having all apparatus, etc., ready. The temperature charts and records must be at hand together with any recent X-ray or pathological reports. She must have given some thought to the problems presented by the case, and have decided what observations she should make to the doctor on her patient's progress. She should also draw his attention to any medicines or drugs for which prescriptions may be required. A good nurse is prepared for the visit in all these respects, and it shows lack of forethought and method to have to ring up the doctor unnecessarily later in the day.

Midday. Before lunch is served the nurse should see that her patient is comfortable and not in immediate need of a bedpan; if this is necessary it should be given. The pillows should be readjusted and the patient arranged as comfortably as possible for the meal. Again as at breakfast, the nurse should give all the necessary help so that the patient eats the maximum of food with the minimum of effort. Drinks are given as required, unless the patient is on a special diet. The patient is allowed at least half-an-hour's interval after dinner. The nurse should then take her temperature, pulse, and respirations, give any medicines which are due, again offer a bedpan, sponge the hands and give a mouthwash and do any other treatment prescribed. She makes the patient comfortable, refilling a hot water bottle if necessary. Probably the patient will like to change her position at this time of day and lie with only one or two pillows if allowed. The curtains should be drawn, windows opened or shut as seems most suitable and the patient left to rest for 1—1½ hours. This afternoon rest should invariably be arranged for and it must be clearly understood that no visitors or interruptions of any kind should spoil it. Outsiders forget that although the patient is in bed, her day can be a very tiring one with treatments, bedpans, meals, and doctor's visits and unless the afternoon rest is enforced she may be thoroughly exhausted by the evening. Even in a busy ward it is possible to create a quiet and peaceful atmosphere for an hour in the afternoon. At about 3.30 p.m., or before if the patient is restless, the nurse should draw the curtains, offer the bedpan and sit her up comfortably. The face and hands should be sponged and the hair brushed, and the patient made to look as attractive as possible as this is often the time when visitors are allowed. The psychological effect of paying attention to the personal appearance is not to be neglected, even with a very ill patient provided that it is not so overdone as to tire her. Tea is then served and the patient may feel well enough to chat with relatives or possibly with a convalescent patient whose acquaintance she has made if she is in a general ward.

Evening. By 6 p.m. it is time for the temperature, pulse, and respirations to be taken again, the evening toilet performed and possibly for treatment to be given. The evening wash varies with the condition of the patient, but the minimum that must be done is hands, face, and back. The nightgown should be changed, the undersheet tightened and drawsheet changed or turned. If the patient is well enough she may like the bed completely stripped and re-made as in the morning, but for a seriously ill patient this may be unnecessarily exhausting. It may be that a patient with a high temperature or one who is perspiring freely may benefit very much from

11

a complete sponge down with warm water. It may soothe her restlessness and prove more refreshing than exhausting. In deciding how much toilet treatment should be done for any individual patient it is for the nurse to use her observation and judgment; no hard and fast rules can be made.

A light supper should be served at about 6.30 p.m., and it is found that after this the patient appreciates a short chat with her day nurse, before the latter goes off duty. A good nurse will always try to make time for this and she herself will look forward to a friendly talk with her patient as one of the pleasures of her nursing day. She will not be satisfied to say good night to her patient in a hurried and casual way. At this point one may emphasize the advantage held by the nurse whose interests are wide and cultured and who can find something of interest to talk about to most types of patient. This is particularly important in the case of patients who are in bed for a long time and cared for by the same nurses. Without being tiring a conversation of this kind can be stimulating and refreshing to the patient who is depressed. This few minutes' conversation often gives the patient an opportunity to talk of her home and any worries or fears she may have in connection with it or herself. It is often a great relief to find that she can confide in a sympathetic nurse who she knows will not gossip amongst relations and neighbours. Many a lasting friendship has sprung up in this way between patient and nurse.

As a result of experience it is found that a good proportion of hospital patients appreciate an evening hymn and prayer and it is customary in some hospitals for a five to ten minutes' service to be conducted by the chaplain or ward sister.

The End of the Day. Later on the patient must be settled for sleep and the night nurse is likely to be on duty in time to do this. She should tidy the undersheets, readjust pillows, refill the hot water bottles, take the temperature, pulse, and respirations and do any treatment which is due. She should then give the patient a hot drink and any hypnotic drug which may have been ordered. The light should be removed or shaded, windows and blinds attended to. After this, if the patient wakes during the night, no conversation should be encouraged unless she is really alert and wakeful. Probably she will sleep for some hours and as a rule is not wakened for treatment unless it is of vital importance. The pulse and respiration may be taken while she sleeps and the temperature is taken when she wakes. If treatment has to be done, everything should be in readiness to do it as expeditiously as possible when the patient wakes. Nothing so thoroughly rouses the patient as having to wait ten minutes for a fomentation or other application to be prepared. She may want a bedpan and this should be given without delay and then a refilled bottle, warm blanket and hot drink to follow. The nurse should note the time and report accurately any long periods of wakefulness, pain or unusual symptoms. The patient may then sleep until early morning. If there is still an hour or two before breakfast a good cup of tea will be appreciated, after which she may drop off to sleep again until another day's routine begins.

This broad outline of a day in the life of a patient, allows of readjustment if the patient is one in a busy ward, but it is an axiom of good hospital treatment that detailed nursing treatment is not a matter of money, but of the requirements of the patient. Hence a patient in a general ward if seriously ill should be nursed as described. In order to get through the work in a busy ward of thirty to forty patients there is necessarily a definite ward routine in which meals, bedpan rounds, bed making and dressings follow each other in sequence. Most patients in their convalescence can fit into this routine, without much inconvenience, and they do so cheerfully, knowing that when they themselves require special care and treatment they will have the detailed attention which they see the critical cases receive.

Receiving a New Patient. The first impression a patient receives of the ward and the nurses in it goes a long way towards putting her at ease and giving her confidence. The nurse should be cheerful and welcoming in her manner and should not suggest that she is too busy or rushed to give her every attention. The bed is prepared and the patient if well enough, undresses in the bathroom, has a bath, and then is put to bed. The relatives are interviewed by the sister and may wait to take the clothes and valuables home with them if they wish, leaving just what is required, handkerchiefs, toothbrush, soap, flannels, hairbrush and comb and a little money for daily paper, etc. If the patient comes from a poor home, gowns and washing materials are provided. If the clothes are not taken home, a list is made of them before they are put in store. Valuables and money are listed and checked by a second nurse and handed over for safe keeping to the ward sister. Before the relatives leave they should be taken to see the patient. The sister tells them all she can about the hospital arrangements, possibility of operation, etc. She tells them when next to visit or inquire, and which articles would be most appreciated as gifts when they next visit the patient. The nurse who is to look after the patient should introduce herself and the relatives should leave feeling satisfied that she is in good hands. All particulars of the patient are taken as described below. They are obtained either from the patient herself, or from the relatives. The writing and spelling must be clear and accurate so that information could be given without delay to the family in case of emergency. A good deal of careful questioning may be required in some cases to ensure that the correct name and address of the nearest relative or whoever is responsible is obtained. If the patient is under twenty-one years of age, and is likely to have an operation, the written consent of the parent or guardian should be obtained.

It may be necessary in some cases for the nurse to take a *history of the case* though usually it is the doctor (or senior medical student) who does this. Good headings for the nurse to use if she has to take details are the following:

1. *Condition on arrival*, e.g. walking, chair, or stretcher case. Temperature, pulse, and respiration; observations on general condition, e.g. breathing, colour, paralysis, delirium, coma, etc.

2. *Family history*, number of family alive or dead, illnesses, etc.

3. *History of previous disease of patient*, illnesses, operations, name of doctor, etc.

4. *History of present illness with all relevant details.*

If the case is an emergency 'take-in' e.g. an accident, or a patient for immediate operation, the relatives or police must not be allowed to leave until all relevant details have been taken. Orderlies or dressers usually undress a male patient and the nurses attend to females and children. The house physician or surgeon must always be notified without delay of the arrival of any new patient. It shows poor administration if a patient is some hours in hospital before being visited by the doctor who is to take charge of him.

ADMISSION SLIP

WARD—BRIGHT—		2—7—1943
Bed 32		DR. CLARKE
Sister:	JONES, David Peter	Sex—Male (Single)
MRS. SMITH,	97 Sweet Road,	Religion—C. of E.
Same address	Wallington,	Age—27 yrs.
(6 p.m.—8 a.m.)	Surrey	Occupation—Clerk
Phone WAL. 1936		
(next door) or		
Police Station WAL. 1682		T. 99°
		P 110
		R 20
Business Address		
(9 a.m.—5 p.m.)		
Brown's, Ltd.	Diagnosis—Gastritis	
High St., Wallington.		
Tel. WAL. 1431		

Chapter Two

TEMPERATURE, PULSE, AND RESPIRATION

The normal temperature of the body is usually taken as 98·4 degrees Fahrenheit, or 37 degrees Centigrade, but in health there is variation during the twenty-four hours according to the rate of metabolism. The temperature is taken with a clinical thermometer and for the Fahrenheit scale it is usually marked from 95—110 degrees. For ward use the thermometers are kept in a jar of disinfectant such as dettol 25 per cent. Carbolic lotion tends to obliterate the markings. Small pieces of lint cut to size are placed at the bottom of the jars to prevent the ends of the thermometers from being broken.

METHOD OF TAKING THE TEMPERATURE

A tray containing the following is required :
1. Thermometers in disinfectant.
2. Jar of small lint or gauze squares.
3. Jar of swabs in water.
4. Jar for receiving soiled swabs.
5. Watch with second hand or pulsometer.
6. Red and black ink and pens.

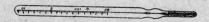

FIG. 1. Clinical Thermometer

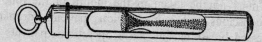

FIG. 2. Pulsometer

In the mouth. The thermometer is taken in the right hand and the mercury is shaken down to the 95° mark. It is wiped with a dry lint square, and placed under the patient's tongue ; he is told to close his lips. It is left in position for the time indicated on the thermometer—a half to three minutes. It is wiser to leave it in position for the full three minutes if an accurate reading is specially important, as in cases of phthisis. On removing the thermometer from the mouth, the nurse reads the temperature and wipes the thermometer with a wet swab. The swab is then discarded, the

15

mercury shaken down and the thermometer replaced in its own jar. The temperature is marked on the chart with a clear, round, neat dot and, if abnormal, it is entered in the book provided for the purpose. A nurse must always report a raised temperature or one abnormally low.

The following patients should have thermometers kept separate for their own use: phthisis; malignant diseases of the tongue; all cases with infected mouths or throats; all infectious diseases.

About six thermometers are kept for general use in a ward of thirty beds.

In the axilla. The axilla is carefully dried with a towel to remove any sweat which would interfere with the correct reading. The thermometer is laid deeply in the axillary fold. The patient's arm is put across the chest and the thermometer is kept in place for double the time that it would be in the mouth. It is then removed, read and dealt with as above.

In the groin. The groin is thoroughly dried and the thermometer is laid in the fold. One leg is then crossed over the abdomen to hold the thermometer in position. It is kept there for twice the length of time it would remain in the mouth.

In the rectum. Rectal thermometers are sometimes marked by a little sealing wax at the top end so that there is no risk of them being confused with those used for taking mouth temperatures, or it may be possible to obtain them of a slightly different pattern. The patient is turned on to the left side, the thermometer is wiped with a lint square and lubricated with vaseline. It is then carefully inserted for a distance of one inch into the anus and held in position for the time indicated. On removal the nurse wipes off the vaseline, notes the recording and then cleans it thoroughly before putting it back into the jar of disinfectant. Temperatures taken rectally are usually recorded in red ink.

Notes. 1. *Mouth temperatures.* Half an hour must elapse before the temperature is taken in the mouth if the patient has had food or drink. Temperature must not be taken in the mouth in the following cases: Children, unconscious and semi-conscious patients, drunken patients, cases of distressed breathing and nasal operations, patients with mental illness. In these cases the axilla or the groin will be the alternative.

2. *Rectal temperature.* The temperature of children is taken in the rectum; also this method is used when a very accurate reading is required for diagnostic purposes as for phthisis and early heart disease, in which a slight deviation might not be detected if the temperature were taken in the mouth. Temperatures taken in the rectum are usually one degree higher than those taken in the mouth.

3. Temperatures are taken twice daily, in the early morning, and after tea, but patients whose temperature is above normal have it recorded every four hours.

4. If there is an unexpected rise in temperature or if for any reason the reading is in doubt, it should be taken again using a different thermometer.

5. In the case of neurotic patients the nurse should stand by the patient all the time and, if the temperature is being taken in the axilla, rectum or groin, the hot water bottle should have been previously removed from the proximity of the patient.

Heat is produced in the body by metabolic activity of cells especially in the muscles and glands. Heat is lost chiefly from the skin and lungs and to a small extent by the urine and faeces. The regulation of heat production and loss is controlled by the heat regulating centre in the cerebrum, and is influenced by such factors as food, clothing, and exercise. Hence it is understood that what is called normal temperature may be variable in a healthy human being. A baby's temperature is very easily upset as its heat regulating mechanism has not developed stability as in the adult. In old age, when metabolic activity is lower, temperature tends to be somewhat subnormal. Apart from these extremes, the normal temperature of individuals varies and it is commonly observed that the average temperature in certain people may range between 97° F. and 99° F. It is also noticed that during the early hours of the morning in all individuals the temperature falls to its lowest point during the twenty-four hours. There is usually a slight rise in women during the few days previous to menstruation.

RANGE OF TEMPERATURE

Pyrexia. Temperature 99°—102° F.

Hyperpyrexia. 102°—105° F. These conditions are usually associated with fever due to (1) bacterial infections; and (2) cerebral conditions in which the heat regulating centre is disturbed in its function as in some cases of cerebral haemorrhage, and head accidents involving the brain; also in sun and heatstroke.

Subnormal temperature. This is below 97° F. and is associated with:

1. Shock and collapse.
2. Haemorrhage.
3. Senility and severe cases of malnutrition in which the body processes are not sufficiently active to maintain a normal temperature.
4. Metabolic disturbances, e.g. myxœdema.

Pyrexia may be of the following varieties:

1. *Continuous.* The temperature is maintained at a high level throughout the day, with very little remission. This may be seen during the acute stage of lobar pneumonia (unless influenced by the action of drugs), also during the second and third weeks of typhoid fever.

2. *Intermittent.* The temperature is high in the evening but falls to normal or below in the early morning. This type of chart is seen in phthisi-

cal patients and if the evening temperature reaches 103° or 104° and the morning temperature falls to as low as 97° F., the patient usually sweats profusely. This condition is sometimes described as hectic fever. Apart from this typical example one sees many less striking examples of intermittent temperature. An intermittence of more than 2° is considered of serious significance.

3. *Remittent.* The temperature is high in the evening and falls during the early hours of the day but never comes within the limits of the normal. This is the 'swinging' temperature seen in many conditions such as septic infections, broncho-pneumonia, and relapsing fever.

4. *Inverse.* In rare cases the temperature reaches a higher level in the morning than in the evening. It is occasionally seen in some cases of phthisis.

The following terms should also be understood:

Crisis. A sudden fall of temperature within twenty-four hours accompanied by a corresponding decrease in the pulse and respiration with a dramatic improvement in the patient's condition. Classical cases of lobar pneumonia untreated by chemotherapy, most often showed this phenomenon in the past as resolution took place in the lungs. Since the introduction of treatment by the sulphonamide group of drugs a crisis is seldom seen in pneumonia. It is often seen at the end of the first week of measles. If a true crisis does occur in an illness it is, as the name implies, a critical time for the patient. It usually happens in the night and the nurse should watch the patient's condition carefully. The patient falls into a deep and peaceful sleep and the forehead will be damp with perspiration. The pulse should be taken at frequent intervals without disturbing her, and it will be found to be gradually decreasing and becoming more steady. If the perspiration is profuse it is necessary to rub the patient down with a warm towel and put on a warm dry gown, to turn the pillows, and give a warm blanket and fresh hot water bottles. This opportunity should be taken for taking the temperature, after which the patient should be given a warm drink. If this nursing attention is quickly and expertly done the patient should drop off to sleep again almost immediately. It would be extremely bad nursing to let the patient get cold and find that her temperature had fallen too suddenly. The nursing treatment should be directed to counteract any collapse during the crisis.

Pseudo crisis. Sudden fall in temperature without corresponding decrease in pulse and respiration and without any improvement in the patient's condition. This is sometimes seen twenty-four hours before a true crisis.

Lysis. A gradual fall of temperature, pulse, and respiration accompanied by a gradual improvement in the patient's condition. The chart may show lysis lasting several days. It is seen in many conditions of bacterial infections; perhaps broncho-pneumonia and typhoid fever are the best ex-

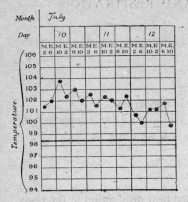

FIG. 3. Continuous pyrexia

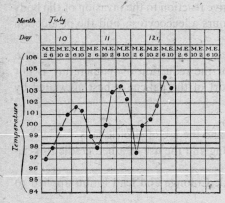

FIG. 4. Intermittent pyrexia

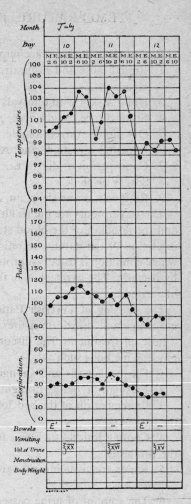

FIG. 6. Pseudo-crisis and crisis

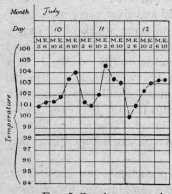

FIG. 5. Remittent pyrexia

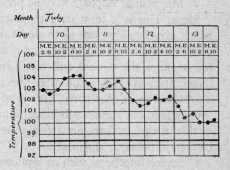

FIG. 7. Lysis

FEVER

Rise of temperature is accompanied by characteristic febrile symptoms:

1. Raised pulse and respiration rate.
2. Headache.
3. Hot dry skin with intervals of sweating.
4. Flushed face, bright eyes: or pale toxic appearance.
5. Dry mouth, furred tongue, sordes on the lips and sometimes herpes.
6. Impaired digestion, anorexia, nausea and vomiting.
7. Constipation or diarrhœa.
8. Scanty urine.
9. Restlessness and delirium.

These symptoms are the result of increased heat production in the body and the flooding of the blood stream by bacterial toxins. The heat causes inhibition of the natural secretions and this explains the symptoms. The whole condition is usually a protective reaction to the invasion of the body by bacteria. The pyrexial state favours a leucocytosis and the production of anti-bodies.

The Nursing of Feverish Patients. It follows from the above that to use drugs and drastic measures for the reduction of temperature is not a rational treatment. The discomfort of the patient is best alleviated by physical methods such as:

1. Frequent baths and sponging.
2. Fresh air (avoiding draughts) and the use of electric fans.
3. By regulation of the bedclothing and the use of a bed cradle to keep the patient cool.
4. Cooling lotions such as eau-de-Colonge and lead lotion applied to the forehead.
5. Fluids are given in abundance especially fruit drinks of all kinds with glucose.
6. The amount of urine passed should be measured.
7. Magnesium sulphate may be prescribed and given every morning.

Rigor. This is a term used to describe an acute attack of shivering, which may be so violent as to shake the bed. The patient feels very cold yet when the temperature is taken it is found to be 104° to 105° F. In a few minutes the patient will break into a heavy sweat, and when the temperature is taken again after fifteen minutes, it will have dropped to its original level. A rigor is always of serious import. It is caused by a sudden influx of certain substances into the blood. These may be bacteria or their toxins, or foreign material usually of a protein nature. Rigors may be seen in the early stages of:

1. Severe infections such as septicæmia, pneumonia, and scarlet fever.
2. After blood transfusions in which there is some incompatible element in the blood.

3. Malaria—as the larvæ of the parasite emerge from the red cells into the blood stream.

Treatment. When the patient complains of feeling cold apply a hot blanket and give a hot drink. During the stage of sweating rub the patient down with hot towels and put on a clean warm gown and another hot blanket. Take the pulse every five minutes and the temperature every fifteen minutes (in the axilla). Record in red ink on the temperature chart the highest degree reached. The doctor should be informed.

TAKING THE PULSE

Pulse is the beat of the heart transmitted along the walls of the arteries as a wave of expansion followed by an elastic recoil. This may be felt wherever the artery comes to the surface of the body and crosses a bone. It may be felt at the following places:

1. Radial artery at the wrist.
2. The temporal artery an inch in front of and above the ear.
3. Facial artery (the anæsthetist feels this pulse constantly while the patient is under an anæsthetic) an inch in front of and under the angle of the jaw.
4. Dorsalis pedis artery between the great and second toe.
5. Posterior tibial behind the internal malleolus.
6. Over the anterior fontanelle in infants.

Method of taking the radial pulse. The arm should be placed in a relaxed position either across the patient's chest or on a pillow. Three fingers of the right hand should be placed lightly on the radial artery with support from the thumb underneath the wrist. The general character of the pulse should first be noted and then the rate is counted for one minute, using a watch with a second hand or a pulsometer.

When the nurse has had experience, she may count the pulse for thirty seconds and multiply the result by two, except in the case of seriously ill patients, when it should always be counted for a full minute. It is best to count for two consecutive half minutes and if they are the same, add them together. If there is a difference, another count should be made. In taking the pulse of a patient for the first time, both radial arteries should be felt and the results compared. There is sometimes a difference in the rate, as in cases of aortic aneurysm and growths of the thorax. In the case of babies and restless patients, the pulse should be taken when the patient is asleep. In an out-patient department the patient should lie down or sit still for a few minutes before the pulse is taken: convalescent patients should also be sitting quietly before the pulse is taken.

Observations should be made as to:

1. Rate.
2. Rhythm.

3. Quality of the pulse.

Rate. Normal pulse rates are as follows:

1. Infants—100 to 120 per minute.
2. Children 6 to 10 years of age—80 to 100 per minute.
3. Adults—70 to 80 per minute.
4. Old age—56 to 70 per minute.

Rapid pulse or tachycardia. Increased frequency is found in the following conditions: Fevers, hæmorrhage, some heart conditions, exophthalmic goitre, nervousness, excitement and over-exertion.

Slow pulse or bradycardia. A decrease in the pulse rate is found in conditions of: heart block, where it may only register 30 or 40 beats per minute; some cases of shock and some cerebral diseases.

Rhythm. The disturbance of rhythm may be of several types:

a. *Regular intermittent* in which a beat is dropped at regular intervals, e.g. after every second or third beat.

b. *Irregular intermittent* in which there is a total irregularity of the pulse, both in the rate and rhythm. This is typically seen in a case of auricular fibrillation and it may occur in other heart conditions and in cases of extreme collapse.

c. *Pulsus bigeminus.* Coupled beats are felt followed by a pause. It occurs in cases of digitalis accumulation.

d. *Pulsus alternans*, in which large and small beats alternate, is a serious but uncommon condition.

e. *Dicrotic.* In this case an echo of a beat may be felt, so that unless the nurse is very discriminating she might record the pulse as double the true figure. It is observed in cases of extreme muscular relaxation, when the closure of the aortic valve is felt as a feeble wave following the true expansion wave. In these cases the radial pulse should be compared with the apex beat to verify the count.

f. *Waterhammer pulse (Corrigan's)* is characteristic of incompetence of the aortic valve. The left ventricle contracts, the blood is driven through the open valve. If the valve is unable to close properly owing to disease, some of the blood regurgitates into the ventricle, and the pressure in the artery is not maintained. In the radial pulse this is felt as a strong wave of expansion which suddenly collapses under the fingers.

Quality. There are three distinct observations to be made on the quality of the pulse.

a. *Volume.* A nurse judges this by estimating the amount of blood in the artery. If the feel of the pulse can be described as small or soft, the volume of blood in the artery is low. This type of pulse is found in cases of hæmorrhage, collapse, extreme weakness and dehydration. It is due to the weak contraction of the heart and poor tone of the muscular walls of the arteries as well as to lack of circulating blood. If on the other hand the pulse is described as full and bounding it means that the volume of the blood is high. This is seen in cases of high blood pressure (hyperpiesis or hypertension) and congestive heart failure.

b. *Tension.* This is judged by the compressibility of the artery. If it is felt to be tense and it is not easy to obliterate by the fingers it indicates a high blood pressure. If, however, slight pressure by the fingers is sufficient to stop the pulse the condition is one of low blood pressure.

Hyperpiesis or hypertension.—Hyperpiesis is found in cases of arteriosclerosis and chronic kidney disease. Hypotension, the opposite condition, is seen in weakness, typhoid fever and Addison's disease.

c. *State of the artery walls.* When arteries deteriorate as in old age and diseases associated with high blood pressure the middle muscular coat becomes infiltrated by calcium salts; it is then felt, when rolled under the fingers, as a hard resistant vessel. The nurse may describe this as a wiry or 'whipcord' pulse. In extreme deterioration the arteries may be of the 'pipe stem' variety, the wall being very hard and thick and the lumen small. Calcified arteries are visible under X-ray.

The opposite condition of a very soft and relaxed wall is found in some cases of extreme malnutrition and weakness.

To Take the Apex Beat. A nurse is sometimes required to count the apex beat of the heart in order to compare it with the beat in the radial pulse. The fingers are placed over the apex in the left fifth intercostal space which is $3\frac{1}{2}$ inches from the midline at nipple level in the normal individual. It may be felt several inches beyond the nipple line if the heart is displaced.

The nurse is sometimes asked to use a stethoscope for taking the apex beat and she should practise doing this when the opportunity occurs. The apex beat is usually charted in red ink in order to show quite clearly when the beats approximate to those counted at the pulse.

The Use of the Sphygmomanometer. Nurses should know how to estimate the systolic blood pressure by this instrument. Midwives always have to use it in their routine examination of the patient in the ante-natal clinic. The rubber bag is placed round the arm and inflated by pressure on a rubber bulb. The observer feels carefully the normal rhythm of the pulse at the wrist, and then slowly inflates the bag until the pressure on the

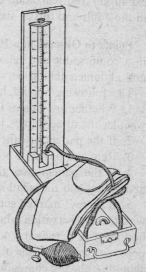

Fig. 8. Sphygmomanometer

brachial artery is sufficient to obliterate the pulse at the wrist, or at the elbow (when listening through a stethoscope). The reading of the level of the mercury in the vertical tube should be taken at the exact moment of the disappearance of the pulse. In normal healthy adults the mercury will be found to have risen to 140 mms. A reading of 160—220 may be considered abnormal according to the age of the patient. Blood pressure usually rises with advancing age.

Exercise Tests. In a cardiac case the nurse may find the patient being submitted to certain standard tests. For instance, stepping on and off a stool of given height twenty times, or walking up a certain flight of stairs so many times. The pulse is taken before the exercise and immediately after, and again after one minute and two minutes. A healthy heart with a good reserve should register a normal pulse after two minutes, following a standard exercise.

RESPIRATION

Respiration means breathing and consists of inspiration and expiration. Inspiration is the taking in of air through the respiratory passages into the lungs. The diaphragm contracts and is flattened. The intercostal muscles raise the ribs and thus expand the thorax from side to side and from front to back, and the air is taken in to the spongy tissue of the lungs by suction. The gaseous interchange takes place in the alveoli of the lungs and the accumulation of carbon dioxide from the tissues act on the nerve centres in the medulla, stimulating the muscles of respiration. The rhythmical expansion and relaxation takes place sixteen to twenty times per minute in the adult and forty—sixty times in infants.

Points to Observe in a Patient's Breathing. The patient should lie or sit in a comfortable and relaxed position, and the rise and fall of the chest and abdomen should be watched.

The following should be particularly noted:

1. Whether one side of the chest moves more freely than the other, and whether the upper (apical) or lower (diaphragmatic) lobes are used most.

2. If the patient breathes through the mouth or nose or both.

3. Rate and depth of breathing.

4. If the patient uses the accessory muscles of breathing, e.g. neck, abdominal and the small muscles in the nostrils (alae nasi).

5. If there is marked sucking in of the ribs in the case of babies. Along with these observations should go a careful note of the colour of the face, lips, and tips of the ears. A blue tinge is described as cyanosis and indicates poor oxygenation of the blood (anoxæmia). It is important that the patient should not be too conscious of the nurse's scrutiny, as he may become self-conscious and the rhythm and method of respiration may change. Hence

24

it is usual to watch and count the respirations after taking the pulse, and if the arm is placed across the chest and the wrist held in that position the nurse can not only see the chest movements, but can also feel them. She should count for a full minute before recording the result.

Rapid breathing occurs in heart and lung cases, and after exertion and emotion. A slight rise in the rate occurs in conjunction with the rise of temperature and pulse in febrile conditions and is one sign of the general increase in the metabolic rate.

Slow breathing is found:

1. In some cases of shock owing to severe depression of the nerve centres.

2. In brain injury and disease.

3. As a result of the depressing influence of morphia and other drugs on the medullary control.

Shallow breathing, in which the upper lobes of the lungs only are used; this is sometimes called thoracic breathing as the abdominal muscles do not come into play. It is found in cases of (1) shock; (2) after heavy doses of morphia; (3) after avertin (bromethol) anæsthesia. In these cases the cause is depression of the respiratory centre in the medulla. Other causes for the lower lobes not being used are: (1) hypostatic congestion of the lungs in elderly patients, and those who are kept lying flat for too long; (2) in cases where the bases are collapsed due to obstruction in the bronchioles by mucus; (3) air in the pleural cavity from various causes (accidents and rupture of tubercular cavities into the pleura); (4) abdominal conditions with peritonitis in which the abdominal muscles including the diaphragm go into spasm as a protective measure.

Sighing respirations. This is a sign of air hunger and is seen in cases of hæmorrhage when the loss of red corpuscles has been so great that the tissues are lacking oxygen. It is a serious sign of exhaustion.

Dyspnœa. This is distressed breathing and occurs in chest and heart diseases, e.g. asthma, pneumonia, pleurisy and congestive heart failure. It also occurs in accidents involving the chest wall.

Orthopnœa. This is the term used to indicate such distress that the patient cannot breathe unless he sits in an upright position. It occurs in the same diseases as above in their more advanced stages.

Apnœa. This term indicates cessation of breathing. There is always a period of apnœa between one act of respiration and the next, sometimes, however, it is markedly prolonged in certain cases of shock, toxæmia and brain conditions.

Cheyne-Stokes breathing. This is a type of respiration characteristic of the later stages of almost any fatal illness, but most often seen in uræmia and cerebral diseases. The rhythm follows a definite course and the respirations are at first shallow and quiet, then become deeper and more and more laboured. They then become quieter again until the patient hardly appears to breathe at all. The period of apnœa between the sequences may be alarmingly prolonged, and eventually the respirations stop altogether.

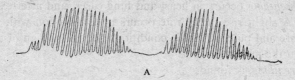

A

Fig. 9. Cheyne-Stokes Rhythm. A =Apnœa

Stridor. This is a noisy crowing respiration which is heard when the larynx is obstructed by a growth or foreign body. Laryngeal stridor due to obstruction by a diphtheritic membrane is sometimes called 'croup'.

Sinus arrhythmia. This is a physiological phenomenon observed in childhood and during convalescence. There is a rhythmical increase and decrease in the pulse rate corresponding to the rhythm of respiration.

Chapter Three

THE TOILET OF THE PATIENT

This is a most important part of a nurse's work. It needs much practice to perform every detail of the daily bath skilfully and thoroughly.

Preparation

1. Temperature, pulse, and respiration are taken and recorded.
2. Windows and doors are shut, and screens placed in position.
3. The bed is partially stripped.
4. A bedpan is given.

Requirements for bathing a patient in bed (see plate 1):

1. Bed mackintosh.
2. Two bath blankets.
3. Jugs of hot and cold water.
4. Pail.
5. Bowl.
6. Soap and two flannels, nail brush.
7. Spirit (methylated or eau-de-Cologne) talcum powder.
8. Two towels (face and bath).
9. Clean night gown and bed linen as required.
10. Toothbrush and mouthwash bowls.
11. Hairbrush and comb and accessories.
12. Nail scissors.
13. Warm blanket.

Method. The warmed mackintosh and one bath blanket are rolled under the patient, and unnecessary pillows and apparatus are removed. The towel is placed in position under the parts to be washed. The patient is kept covered by a second bath blanket, or by a large warm bath towel.

The patient's body is washed all over in the following order:

1. The face, paying special attention to the nose, eyes, and around the mouth.
2. The neck and ears; every corner and fissure behind the latter must be thoroughly washed and dried.
3. Each arm in turn, paying special attention to the axillæ, which should be powdered as they are dried.

Begin to use the second flannel: add more hot water.

4. Chest and abdomen, with special attention to the umbilicus, and to the folds under the breasts in women; the folds should be powdered.

Add more hot water to the bowl. The water must be very hot all the time.

5. Wash and dry each leg in turn. Dry particularly well between the toes and sprinkle with a little powder.

Add more hot water or change if necessary.

Turn the patient on to her side, if possible, and get help if necessary.

6. Wash the whole back from the nape of the neck to the buttocks and dry with good friction.

7. Soap the flannel very well, raise the upper leg, wash very thoroughly between the legs. Dry and powder carefully, especially the fold of the groins and the fold between the buttocks.

8. Soap the hand well, and massage the areas of pressure with firm circular movements. Dry off the surplus soap, then rub thoroughly with spirit and dust with talcum powder. The areas to be treated thus are: buttocks, sacrum, shoulder blades, heels, ankles and hips, and in some cases the hip bones and the occiput. The treatment of pressure areas should be done after the full washing is completed as a definite treatment to prevent sores. If spirit is not available it is of no great import: soap may be used instead. What is important is the amount of friction and energy used in the rubbing.

As soon as the bath is finished a clean warm gown is put on. A towel is placed round the patient's neck and the patient helped into such a position that she can do her teeth and rinse out her mouth; if she is unable to do this, the mouth toilet must be done by the nurse. The bath blankets are then removed and the patient's own blanket is put next to her; this may be removed later if desired. The hair is brushed and combed and arranged as conveniently and attractively as possible. The hair at the back of the head must not be allowed to get into a bad condition; nails must be kept short and clean.

The next thing to do is to make the bed. Help should be obtained if available and clean linen inserted if necessary and the patient made comfortable in whatever position she is to be nursed. Other little details should be thought of before the toilet is considered complete, a clean handkerchief, eau-de-Cologne, etc. It may be suitable to give the patient her hand mirror, so that she can attend to the details of her appearance herself. On the other hand it might be depressing for her to see herself in the mirror.

Clearing away. Bowls, tooth mugs, etc., should all be cleaned with Vim or some such cleansing agent, rinsed thoroughly and dried. Flannels should be rinsed under the tap, wrung dry and hung up. The toothbrush should be rinsed under cold water and left exposed to the air. All hairs are re-

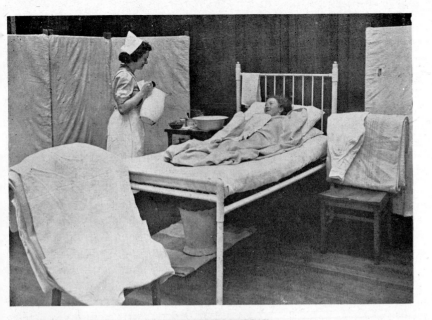

Plate 1 (above).
Giving a blanket bath.
See page 227

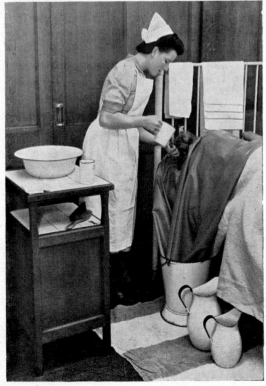

Plate 2. Washing hair
of patient. See page 36

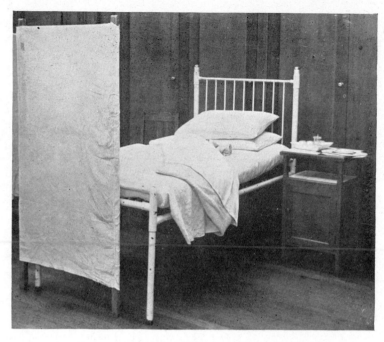

Plate 3. Bed prepared for a new patient. See page 44

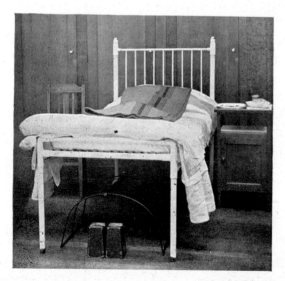

Plate 4. Bed prepared for an emergency case.
See page 44

moved from the hairbrush and comb, which should be washed frequently. The towels and bath blankets are dried. The patient's bedside locker and table are cleaned, flowers arranged, fruit put on a clean dish and all unnecessary articles put away tidily. The patient's morning toilet should not be considered complete until all her surroundings have been tidied.

The toilet as described above is a daily procedure. When, however, a new patient is admitted to the ward and a nurse gives the first bath, she should consider it a good opportunity for careful observation to enable her to give a report on the patient.

Her *observations* should be on the following lines:

1. *General Condition*—well nourished, emaciated, neglected.

2. *Skin*—dry and scaly, perspiring. (Note particularly palms of hands, soles of feet. Cracks and fissures, corners of mouth, behind the ears, between the toes.)

3. *Nails*—brittle, ridged; clubbed fingers.

4. *Hair*—clean, good or poor condition; presence of vermin or nits. (The latter particularly in the nape of the neck and behind the ears); unhealthy scalp conditions with scabs and patches of short deformed hairs as in impetigo and with ringworm; dandruff or patches of baldness (alopecia).

5. *Mouth*—condition of teeth, odour of breath (sweet smell of acetone in acidosis, diabetes, and starvation; urinary odour in uræmia; smell of stale blood in hæmatemesis; characteristic odour in intestinal complaints). Appearance of tongue, gums and lips—cracked, dry or unusually pale.

6. *Presence of scars and their position*, indicating previous accidents or operations.

7. *Deformity*, such as clubfoot, harelip, paralysis, etc.

8. *Discharges* of the ear (otorrhœa), nose (rhinorrhœa), vagina (leucorrhœa).

9. *Position or attitude in bed.* (a) Relaxed and inert, with head to one side, knees slightly flexed (severe toxæmic conditions such as typhoid fever and diphtheria). (b) Knees drawn up (acute abdominal pain). (c) Hand over the ear (children with earache).

10. *Mental condition.* Drowsiness, restlessness, twitching of the muscles, depression and unwillingness to talk, over-excitability, anxiety, etc.

The trained nurse will make it her practice to observe such details as these, not only during the first bath but all the time the patient is under her care. She must report them carefully at once. The surgeon or physician is dependent upon those who are with the patient during the twenty-four hours of the day for these significant observations.

It is to be remembered that the patient's first bath in bed, in a hospital or wherever it may be, is not infrequently the patient's first experience of what trained nursing can mean in illness. The patient has probably been at home with little attention for several days, feeling ill and miserable, and to have a skilled and experienced nurse making her comfortable, with the use of pillows, cradles, air cushions and whatever appliances are needed, must give her much confidence and comfort. Clean linen and bodily cleanliness are unfortunately unknown to some of the poorer members of the population.

1. **Notes.** Every patient ill in bed should wash or be washed all over every day. Nothing less satisfies a good nurse, whether her patient is in a hospital ward or a private room.

2. It is seldom possible in a hospital ward for each patient to have two bath blankets for her exclusive use. The correct procedure to meet this difficulty is to use the top blanket off the patient's bed as a bath blanket. It should be the oldest and thinnest on the bed and should always be used as the topmost one. When the patient is discharged it is sent to the laundry. In no case must the same blanket be used for washing different patients.

3. A thorough daily blanket bath given to a neglected, poor or ignorant patient during a prolonged stay in hospital often instils into her habits of cleanliness and hygiene which will be carried back to the home. The nurse should keep this in mind and use every opportunity for talking about rules of healthy living, giving simple reasons as she carries out her duties. She should regard herself not only as a nurse who bathes and treats patients when they are ill, but as a teacher of health.

BATHING A PATIENT IN THE BATHROOM

When the patient is well enough to bathe herself in the bathroom the nurse must make all the preparations and help her as much as is necessary. The following rules should be observed:

1. The windows should be shut.

2. A screen is placed round the end of the bath.

3. Bath mat and chair are put in readiness.

4. The bath is then prepared. The cold water is run in first and hot water added until the temperature of the bath is 100° F., tested with a bath thermometer.

It should not be possible for the door to be locked on the inside. The key should be removed if necessary. There is always a risk in allowing an ill or convalescent patient to be shut up in a bathroom. The nurse, although not necessarily with the patient all the time, should never be far away and should inquire frequently if all is well. The patient may suddenly feel faint or tired, and the nurse should be prepared for this and have a wheel chair at hand to take her back to bed. While the patient is in the bathroom, the windows of her room should be opened, the bed stripped and remade, and the mattress turned. The top bedclothes should be turned down and a hot water bottle put in the bed for the patient's return. A warm blanket may also be necessary in cold weather. The windows should then be closed until the patient is warm in bed. All these details give finish to a nurse's work.

Case Assignment Method of Training Nurses

This means that in a ward each nurse has certain patients assigned to her as her special responsibility. She should do everything for these patients when on duty, washings, treatments, special feeds, etc. Even the most junior nurse in the ward should have one patient delegated to her care, and the staff nurse supervises and teaches her exactly what to do and how to do it.

Advantages of this method of training

1. It trains nurses to take responsibility from the earliest days of training. This is most important, for a woman who is not prepared to assume her responsibilities and take the initiative is of no use when dealing with sick and helpless people.

2. The nurse's interest is stimulated by what she may feel at first to be a difficult task. If she is intelligent and keen she will rise to her responsibilities and learn all she can about the case, alike by reading, listening and inquiring. It gives her a sense of satisfaction to think of a particular person as 'my patient'.

3. From the patient's point of view the method nearly always succeeds. The patient likes to feel that one particular nurse is particularly interested in her. The nurse will interest herself in the relatives and friends and will look out for and recognize them when they visit, and tell them little details of her patient's wants, worries, and progress. It is while doing the daily bath and treatment that the nurse is expected to acquaint herself with the patient's family and background as much as possible. With this method of training, however, much careful supervision is required, for if the nurse is unconscientious or careless the patient will suffer unless the staff nurse steps in to see that this cannot happen. Many ward sisters agree that this method of training nurses is the ideal one, but it undoubtedly entails more trouble and supervision on their part. It trains the intelligent and keen nurse to be adaptable and responsible and gives her plenty of scope to use her initiative. It is important, however, that the junior nurse should be made to feel that the staff and head nurses are there to help and advise her. She should feel no compunction in approaching them when she meets with difficulties and is not quite sure what to do.

PRESSURE SORES

These arise in patients in the following circumstances:

1. *Certain types of patients:*
a. Old age.
b. Very thin patients in whom the bones are not well covered, or very

fat patients who lie heavily in the same position and cannot move themselves.

   c. Restless, fidgety patients, e.g. chorea.

   d. Badly nourished patients.

  2. *Certain conditions:*

   a. Cases of paralysis, as in spinal injury, hemiplegia, etc.

   b. Incontinence of urine and fæces.

   c. Severe toxæmia such as typhoid, infective endocarditis, etc.

  3. *Faulty nursing care:*

   a. Bedmaking (crumbs and creases in the bed. Uncomfortable position of the patient; patches and seams in the linen; damp and dirty drawsheets.)

   b. Careless lifting on to stretchers, bedpans, etc.; bedpans left wet after disinfection.

   c. Ill-fitting splints and plasters.

N.B. Burns from hot water bottles should also be guarded against, particularly in the case of infants and unconscious and helpless patients; and although these injuries are not pressure sores they also arise from carelessness in nursing.

Prevention of Pressure Sores

  1. The *routine care*, as described in the daily toilet of the patient, is, of course, of first importance. In connection with this, emphasis is again laid upon the use of friction to stimulate the circulation. Poor circulation is the root cause of most pressure sores.

  2. *Careful bedmaking.* The bedclothes beneath the patient must be kept in good condition, pulled very tight and kept perfectly dry and clean. If a drawsheet has been repaired, care should be taken that the patient does not lie on the seam or patch. Every use should be made of accessories such as air beds and cushions; water beds, heel and elbow rings; soft pillows and bed cradles, as required.

The patient's position should be changed as often as possible, in cases where bed sores are likely to form. In long illnesses the nurse should insist upon having a comfortable mattress for her patient. A hair mattress on a bed with good springs, or a spring mattress of the Vi-spring type, or a rubber mattress, such as a Dunlopillo, are all very comfortable. Hospital mattresses are usually of horsehair. They should not be allowed to get thin in the middle, but must be remade at intervals. The springs of the bed frame should be tightened from time to time.

The lifting of patients by orderlies and porters should be supervised as far as possible by the nurse, who can thus help to train them in the correct handling of patients.

A well-balanced diet with the required vitamins and plenty of fresh air is certainly an important factor in prevention of bed sores in long and exhausting illnesses.

PRESSURE SORES

The first signs of redness over a pressure point must be reported at once to the sister in charge.

1. *An incipient sore* (the area is red). (a) Treat the area by rubbing with spirit and powder at least four-hourly, in addition to thorough treatment when the patient is bathed.

(b) Keep the area dry.

(c) Consider whether it is possible to change the patient's position, or make use of extra pillows, air ring or pad.

(d) See that all the nurses in the ward are aware that a sore may develop, so that responsibility for preventing it is shared by all, when the patient's own nurse is 'off duty'.

2. *If there is an abrasion of the skin*, continue the above treatment unless the area becomes very raw and sore. It is worth trying to heal a very superficial abrasion by the use of spirit. If, however, it continues to develop, the following applications may be tried: compound tincture of benzoin; zinc and eucalyptus ointment; gentian violet; emolkelœt or Fuller's earth powder.

3. *A deep ulcerated sore* may be treated by the use of eusol packs, which will help to clear away the slough. When this has been done, the cavity may be packed with lotio rubra to stimulate granulation. Alternative methods for treating a sloughing bed sore are:

a. Application of a charcoal poultice.

b. Syringing with hydrogen peroxide.

c. Hot fomentations or antiphlogistine poultice.

Whichever application is chosen it is often beneficial to change from one treatment to another, after a few days. The principle which guides the choice is first to use a cleansing agent to remove the slough or septic material, and then to follow this with a stimulating antiseptic, of which there are many. Every nurse, in her experience, will learn to recognize the types of sores and what treatment is likely to be successful.

4. *Septic spots on the buttocks.* The spots may be treated with liquor iodi 2 per cent. If they come to a head, the pus should be gently squeezed out, using a sterile swab, and the areas again painted. The whole surrounding area should be treated vigorously with spirit and kept very dry. The spots will spread if the area is allowed to become sodden by moist applications; the staphylococcus, the organism present in the pustules, thrives under these conditions.

Notes. 1. If dressings are required, for example, on the back, they may be kept in position by a T-bandage or by strapping. If the latter is used, it should be affixed as far as possible from the area of soreness.

2. In cases of incontinence, the skin area, including the groins, may be rubbed with an ointment, such as ung. zinc and eucalyptus, to keep the skin waterproof.

c

3. Elastoplast, as a dressing, should never be used in incontinent cases.

CARE OF THE MOUTH

In many cases of illness the mouth becomes very dry and dirty and needs special nursing care and attention. Cases in which this is likely to happen are:

1. Fevers.
2. Patients who are being fed artificially.
3. Patients on a milk diet.
4. Patients with alimentary diseases.

The following details should be observed:

1. *The tongue*
   a. White and coated in patients with gastric conditions.
   b. Brown and furred, as in intestinal obstruction and uræmia.
   c. Cracked and glazed, in pernicious anæmia.
   d. Raw and 'beefy', in typhoid fever.
   e. Red with white spots, i.e. 'strawberry tongue', in scarlet fever.

2. *The gums*
   a. Pale in anæmia.
   b. Inflamed and receding from the teeth in pyorrhœa.
   c. Swollen and bleeding as in scurvy, or swollen in mercurial poisoning.
   d. Exhibiting a blue line at the margins of the gums in lead poisoning.
   e. Ulcerated, in conditions of debility or in patients with ill-fitting dentures. Gross ulceration is seen in cases of Ludwig's Angina.

3. *The teeth*
   a. Septic, with swollen, receding gums, e.g. pyorrhœa alveolaris.
   b. Notched, as in congenital syphilis (Hutchinson's teeth).

4. *Mucous membrane of the cheeks*
   a. Koplik's spots, i.e. white spots with red centres opposite molar teeth, as in measles.
   b. White furry growth, possibly extending to the uvula, in thrush, a parasitic condition in babies, caused by the fungus oidium albicans.
   c. A whitish exudate across the fauces, in secondary syphilis; this is called a 'snail-track' ulcer.

5. *Tonsils*
   a. Large and swollen.
   b. Swollen and covered with yellow patches, as in follicular tonsillitis (septic throat).
   c. Greyish membrane, characteristic of diphtheria.

6. *Lips*. May be dry and cracked and mucus may form in tough scales or flakes (sordes). These should be cut off with sterile scissors if necessary and the lips should be kept moist with glycerine. Cracks may be painted with silver nitrate stick. Herpes often form on the lips in colds and fevers.

They begin as swellings of the mucous membrane. Fluid appears and then dries up, forming a yellow scab. Treat by swabbing with methylated spirit and apply zinc powder.

7. *Odour of Breath.* Offensive, as in alimentary disturbances; sweet, smelling of acetone, as in diabetes and starvation and acidosis; smelling of urine as in uræmia.

When making observations on the mouth, the nurse should feel if the glands of the neck are enlarged.

Treatment of the Mouth. The use of the toothbrush and frequent mouth washes is to be encouraged in every patient. The nurse herself must attend to the mouths of seriously ill or helpless patients. Patients on a low diet often get a very parched mouth, though not necessarily sore as described above. Attempts should be made to stimulate the salivary glands to further action, by giving the patient rusks to chew, even if they cannot be swallowed, or chewing gum. Pieces of raw pineapple are very refreshing and sometimes the mouth can be swabbed with ice-cold water, containing vinegar. All good and experienced nurses will have found out for themselves different methods of dealing with difficult mouth conditions. The above suggestions are only a few of many.

Requisites for cleaning the mouth. Tray containing:

1. Forceps.
2. Squares of soft old linen.
3. Cleansing agent, e.g. glycerine boracis and lemon juice in equal parts; glycothymoline.
4. Pot for receiving dirty swabs.
5. Mackintosh and towel.
6. Gag and tongue forceps, for unconscious patients.

Method. The structures are cleaned in the following order:

1. The teeth. Clean between and in a vertical direction as well as horizontally.
2. The gums.
3. Mucous membrane of the cheeks.
4. The tongue.
5. The palate.

Swabs must be thoroughly moistened and as many clean ones used for each part as is necessary. The mucous membrane should be treated very gently or more harm than good may be done. Some very dirty cases may be treated successfully with hydrogen peroxide $2\frac{1}{2}$ volume strength followed by glycothymoline. In the case of babies with thrush, the mouth is very gently cleaned with sodium bicarbonate, $\mathfrak{Z}$i to Oi water. In this case, scrupulous care must be taken with bottles and teats. They must always be boiled after use and kept quite separate. A swab sent to the laboratory will confirm the presence of the organism.

Ulcers in the mouth may be treated with alum, $\mathfrak{Z}$i to Oi water. The ulcer may be touched up with silver nitrate stick and the dentures should be attended to if necessary.

A sore mouth interferes with the patient's appetite.

Treatment of the gums. These may give the patient trouble and the soreness is likely to increase rather than recover unless treated. Vitamin B is likely to help in restoring a healthy condition, and it is often found in anæmic patients with sores and cracks in the mouth that they are relieved with a course of iron.

Avitaminosis is a recognized cause of sore mouths. The diet should be revised and extra vitamins given.

CARE OF THE HAIR

The condition of the patient's hair deteriorates in illness and good detailed nursing is often reflected in the appearance of the hair. The hair should be brushed thoroughly every day and combed. It should be frequently washed and in long-standing cases of illness, this must be done as often as convenient.

Washing the hair in bed. Arrangement of patient (see plate 2).

a. The mattress may be pulled down on the bed frame if this is possible. A mackintosh is arranged under the head and over the springs of the bed, and a bowl of water stands on the springs. Pillows are removed and the floor protected if necessary.

b. The patient may be turned on to her side, and the bowl arranged on a chair, protected by a mackintosh at the side of the bed.

c. If a patient can only be nursed in a sitting position, as in some heart and lung conditions, the bowl must be put on a bed-table in front of the patient and the whole bed protected.

Requirements:

1. Mackintoshes.
2. Small jug containing a shampoo, which need only be a simple soap solution.
3. Large jugs of water, temperature 100° F.
4. Pail.
5. Face towel and warm towels for drying the hair. Clean comb and brush.

Method. First drape the patient's bath towel securely round her neck. Arrange one mackintosh in front of the patient, tucking it round her neck and shoulders, making a roll at the end to prevent the water from running into the bed. Have a second mackintosh behind the patient's head, well tucked into the neck with the end falling into a pail. Fold the face towel into a pad to protect the eyes. Pour a little warm water over the head and follow with the shampoo.

Rub the scalp gently, but vigorously, with the tips of the fingers, particularly the nape of the neck and behind the ears. Rinse by pouring warm water from the small jug. Rinsing should be thorough. The hair is then dried with warm towels or an electric drier, if available. The nurse needs considerable skill to do this expertly without tiring the patient. The method here outlined must be adapted to the particular patient and the type of bed in which she is being nursed (see illustration, page 28).

Pediculosis

1. *Of the head* (capitis). This is a verminous condition found in dirty and neglected people. They are not so common as hitherto in this country, owing to the regular inspection in schools. Pediculi live on the scalp and lay their eggs near the roots of the hair, especially behind the ears, and in the nape of the neck. The eggs are glued to the hairs by gelatinous material which makes them difficult to detach. To clean a head it is necessary to comb out the pediculi and to get rid of every nit.

Requirements for treatment:

1. Mackintosh cape.
2. Comb and brush, tooth comb and carbolic lotion, 1—40.
3. Lint or rag, large double piece of lint, the size of the scalp, gutta percha tissue of the same size, bandage and vaseline.

Method. Thoroughly comb the hair with a tooth comb, getting down to the scalp. Wipe the dirt and pediculi off the comb each time with a swab soaked in carbolic. Then take a swab soaked in carbolic and apply the lotion to the roots of the hairs, separating the hair well to get to every portion of the scalp. Apply vaseline at the margin of the hair, round the forehead, nape of neck, and behind the ears. Soak the large piece of lint in lotion and put all the hair underneath it. Cover with gutta percha tissue and fix in position with a capeline or triangular bandage. Leave the compress in position for twelve to twenty-four hours, then remove and comb the head once more. Finally, wash the hair thoroughly with soap solution and disinfect the comb and brush. The hair should be combed with a fine tooth comb twice daily for another ten to fourteen days, until every nit has disappeared. Eggs take fourteen days to hatch and if one escapes, the head may become verminous again. Sometimes the nits can be pulled off individual hairs with the fingers, if they are very adherent.

Alternative lotions:

1. Sassafras oil.
2. Acetic acid 2 per cent.
3. Warm vinegar and water in equal parts.   4. Turpentine.
5. Binn's solution (a mixture of soft soap and boric lotion).

N.B. Turpentine is very irritating and too strong to use for sick people or children.

Very verminous cases. It is often desirable to cut the hair short. In the case of a child, written permission to do this must be obtained from the parents. Dirty heads are not only a matter to be dealt with from a point of view of hygiene, but they are likely to interfere with the patient's general health. Scratching is often the cause of impetigo of the scalp (due to secondary infection by the staphylococcus or streptococcus) and sometimes it is found that the lymphatic glands which drain the scalp become swollen and painful.

2. *Pediculi of the body* (corporis). These lice cause intolerable itching of the skin. Scratch marks are found particularly over the shoulder blades. It is difficult to see the lice, which hide themselves in the seams of the clothing.

3. *Pediculi pubis* live in the hairy parts of the pubic and axillary regions. In both conditions patients should have the hairy parts shaved and take a hot disinfectant bath in Lysol 1 in 500 and sulphur ointment is rubbed into the skin. Clothing should be fumigated and the seams of heavy garments should be examined and ironed out with a hot flat iron. Any clothes which can be disposed of are better burnt.

CARE OF THE HANDS AND FEET

These are usually dealt with, when the patient has her daily bath as previously described. Some cases, however, are in such a dirty neglected condition that they require special treatment to get them clean. This is especially the nurse's responsibility when they are the site for operation, e.g. hallux valgus, hammer toes, etc.

For foot treatment in these cases the following are required:
1. Mackintosh.
2. Basin and hot water.
3. Liquid ammonia.
4. Soap and nailbrush.
5. Scissors.
6. Vaseline or olive oil.
7. Gauze bandages.
8. Flannel or sponge.

Method. Screen the patient and arrange the requirements at the foot of the bed. Fold the bedclothes back from the feet, arrange the mackintosh on the bed, cover up one foot with a bath towel while the other is treated. Put a teaspoonful of ammonia in the water, then wash the feet and scrub thoroughly with a nail brush. The cracks behind the heels are often ingrained with dirt. Cut and clean the nails with a pair of scissors, as thoroughly as possible. If the latter are hard and horny and impossible to cut satisfactorily, cover them thickly with vaseline and bandage each toe separately with a gauze bandage. Leave the vaseline on for twenty-four hours and then soak the foot again with hot soapy water, and scrub thoroughly. It may be necessary to treat the feet in this way several times before they are really clean. Powder is used freely between the toes. If the big toenail is inclined to grow in, try to cut a V-shaped piece out of the middle of the nail. Other lotions which may be used for cleaning dirty feet and hands are: ether soap (use with great care as it is inflammable and expensive); soda in water; orange stick dressed with wool and dipped in hydrogen peroxide is helpful in cleaning underneath the nails.

The hands sometimes require similar treatment. A nurse caring for a bed-ridden patient for any length of time, keeps the feet and hands of her patient immaculate. Patients who are in hospital for a short stay, become accustomed to having their feet washed daily, and may go home with quite a different standard of cleanliness.

To give a bedpan. Screen the patient. Remove the bed quilt if a heavy one and the patient is weak, and loosen the bedclothes over the top of the patient. Warm the bedpan, either by putting it under the hot tap and drying thoroughly, or it may be that the sluice room has a special cupboard for heating bed pans by steam, so that they are always ready for use. Take the bedpan to the patient covered by a cloth and raise the buttocks by placing the left arm under the sacrum, whilst the bedpan is slipped in position.

When the time comes for removal, it is often necessary for the nurse to complete the toilet by swabbing the anus with tow or paper, or a cheap variety of wool. She uses several swabs, cleaning from front to back. This is particularly important with women patients, so that germs are not carried forward into the genital tract. Sometimes this can conveniently be done by turning the patient on to the side after the bedpan is removed.

In the case of typhoid fever the anal area should be washed with soap and water containing a little disinfectant each time the bowels are opened. The buttocks should be well rubbed and powdered each time.

Disposal. The paper, tow or wool is removed from the bedpan with forceps and put into a pail. The bedpan is emptied, disinfected and dried. There may be special bedpan cleansing apparatus available. The hollow handle of the bedpan, if there is one, must be thoroughly cleaned inside with a mop.

Reservation of specimens. If a stool is to be saved, a lid should be put on the bedpan and the handle stoppered with tow. The specimen should be labelled and put into a special cupboard. If a specimen of the stool is to be sent for pathological examination, urine should not have been passed at the same time as the bowels are opened. A portion of the stool should be scooped with a scoop kept for this purpose only, and a sufficiency of the faecal material put into the specimen pot labelled with the patient's name, ward, number of bed and date. A form is filled in and signed by the doctor to accompany the specimen.

If the case is one of amœbic dysentery, the bedpan and all its contents are sent to the laboratory at once, before the fæces are cold.

Urinals. Glass, china or enamel urinals, used by male patients, are taken to the patient covered with a cloth. When they are emptied they must be thoroughly rinsed in cold water, mopped with disinfectant and again rinsed. They should be boiled up regularly or soaked in hot strong soda

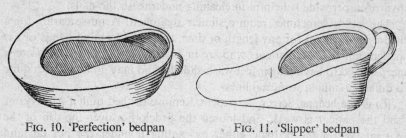

FIG. 10. 'Perfection' bedpan   FIG. 11. 'Slipper' bedpan

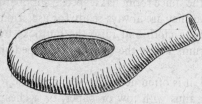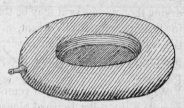

FIG. 12. Round bedpan   FIG. 13. Rubber bedpan

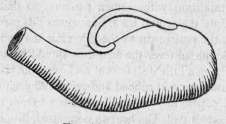

FIG. 14. Male urinal

water and must never be allowed to become coated with deposit on the inside. Perhaps the glass urinals are most satisfactory, as it is easier to see that they are scrupulously clean. Specimens of urine are sent to the pathological laboratory in special bottles for the purpose. If for bacterial examination, a specimen obtained by a catheter is sent in a sterile bottle, otherwise a specimen need not be sterile. Some pathologists require what is known as a mid-stream or interrupted specimen. When the nurse is asked to obtain this, she asks the patient to pass a little urine into a urinal, then gives a second urinal into which the bladder is emptied. The specimen is taken from the second urinal. In this way, organisms congregated at the entrance to the urethra, are not so likely to contaminate the specimen.

Last Offices

After the death of a patient, the following procedure should be followed:

The bed must be efficiently screened. If relatives are present leave them behind the screens for a few minutes with the patient; then take them away from the bedside, offer refreshment and see that they have instructions to come to the hospital for the certificate of death. They should bring with them a clean gown and stockings. The sister-in-charge should be consulted as to the time when they should be told to come. A nurse learns to express her sympathy by kind tactful words.

When they have received the certificate, they are taken to the superintendent's office, where they are given instructions concerning registration of the death and removal of the body.

Two nurses are required to lay out the body of an adult.

Prepare a large enamel tray with wool, forceps, receiver, 5-inch bandage, and small pads of lint wrung out in water. Take to the bedside the soiled linen basket and a sack.

Remove the pillows and strip the bed, leaving the body covered with the top sheet. Remove the night-gown and any rings or other jewellery (these may be given to the relatives before they leave, and they should sign a receipt: or they may be put into an envelope, plainly labelled and handed to the sister of the ward).

False teeth, if they have been removed, should be washed and replaced. Turn the body on to the side and plug the rectum (and vagina, if necessary) with wool, using forceps. Put in a clean drawsheet, and straighten out the body, placing the arms by the side. Close the eyelids and apply wet swabs. Place a firm piece of wool under the chin and on the head and tie up the jaw, taking care not to mark the skin (in some cases a towel rolled up and placed under the chin will be sufficient to keep the jaw in position). The feet may also be tied up if necessary, putting wool between the ankles. Cover the body with a sheet, and leave for one hour while rigor mortis sets in.

Clear everything away as far as possible, leaving only the requirements for washing the body. A shaded light should be left on the locker if it is night time. Be careful not to expose the bed to the rest of the ward. An hour later, wool and bandages are removed and the body is washed, attending carefully to the nails and hair. A gown may be put on. If there is a dressing, remove drainage tubes and apply a double lint carbolic compress (5 per cent). Cover with gutta percha tissue, apply a muslin bandage and sew in position. Cover the face with a square of gauze or lint, or a clean handkerchief. Place the body in a mortuary sheet and fasten with a sufficient number of safety-pins down the middle. Affix the mortuary card, written and signed by the sister-in-charge. Cover the body with a sheet. Clear everything away except the sack to receive the mattress.

Last offices should be performed very quietly and reverently. Every detail of the toilet should be done perfectly. In many cases it is possible for a patient who is seriously ill and likely to die, to be nursed in a side-ward. This is most desirable where it can be arranged.

Children. The hands are placed together with fingers interlaced, holding a white flower. A cotton gown is put on and the body is wrapped in a mortuary sheet and covered with a pall.

Removal. The porters will remove the body on receipt of a removal-slip signed by the sister-in-charge. When they arrive, draw the curtains around or screen the other patients whilst the body is taken from the ward. A senior nurse should be present at the bedside to see the body lifted on to the trolley.

Replace the screens round the bed and finish clearing away.

Personal belongings—to be parcelled and labelled.

Money and valuables—labelled in a separate envelope.

Comb and brush—washed in disinfectant.

Crockery, etc.—boiled.

Mattress and pillows—fumigated. Blankets are fumigated and afterwards sent to the laundry.

Linen, curtains, etc.—sent to the laundry.

Bedstead—washed with disinfectant and covered with clean sheet. Make up the bed as soon as possible.

Jewish patients are usually not touched by the nurses after death. The relatives are consulted beforehand if possible and asked to make their arrangements.

There is usually a mortuary chapel where the relatives may see the body. The sister or a nurse who knew the patient should accompany them.

Chapter Four

BEDMAKING

The aim of bedmaking is to make the patient comfortable and not to make the bed tidy. It follows, however, that an untidy bed usually means an uncomfortable and restless patient; hence apart from actual bedmaking the regular 'tidying' of a hospital ward or sickroom at stated intervals of the day provides an opportunity to shake the pillows and make the patient comfortable.

When the bed has been made the surroundings of the patient should be restored to order—the locker put straight, towels tidied, chair, screen and bed table put in position, and the window reopened, if it has been closed. The patient should be given her book or newspaper. All this routine should become automatic and it should be impossible for a nurse to make a patient's bed without finishing off these details. The patient is the centre of the picture.

A bedpan should be given before the bed is made. As far as the actual bedmaking is concerned the nurse should learn to be neat and quick. There should be a rhythm and precision about the procedure which cuts out all bungling and clumsy movements. It is a pleasure to watch good bedmaking. An essential part of bedmaking is to know how far it is permissible to move the patient, and for this a knowledge of the disease is required.

Every opportunity should be taken to turn the mattress and make the bed when the patient is out of it, whether in the theatre or X-ray department, or out of the ward for special treatment.

Equipment required. Brush, duster, receptacle for soiled linen, clean linen.

The windows are closed.

To make up an empty bed. Brush and turn the mattress, and brush sacking or hessian platform. Dust the bedstead. Cover the mattress with a blanket, tucking in sufficient at the foot, leaving excess at the top. Neat envelope corners are made and the blanket is pulled tightly under the mattress at the sides. Arrange a sheet to cover the blanket in the same way. Put clean pillow cases on two pillows and then a sheet folded back at the foot and two blankets and bedspread. Cover the pillows with a drawsheet.

Empty beds in a hospital ward are generally prepared in this way. Whenever possible, two nurses should make beds together. It is a great saving of time and makes for better bedmaking.

43

2. **To prepare the bed for a new patient.** Take the drawsheet off the pillows and shake it. Turn the top bedclothes down and insert a draw mackintosh and drawsheet across the bed, leaving a sufficiency at one side and excess at the other, so that it may be drawn through when required. Put two hot water bottles in the bed and turn the clothes back cornerwise until the patient is ready to get into bed. Put a gown and blanket on the radiator ready for the patient's arrival. Arrange screens at the foot of the bed and see that clean towels, soap, flannels, toothbrush, hairbrush and comb, temperature charts and bed letters are all in order. A Bible and prayer book are sometimes provided (see plate 3).

3. **Bed for a 'Take-in' case.** Seriously ill patients are admitted to hospital through the casualty department or surgery. They are brought straight to the ward fully dressed and probably in a helpless condition. Examples of such cases are: street accidents, sudden attacks of heart failure, cerebral hæmorrhage.

The bed is made up as follows:

Remove the drawsheet from the empty bed. Fold down the top bedclothes to the foot of the bed. Insert a long mackintosh under the bottom blanket next to the mattress, and place a draw mackintosh and drawsheet in position. Cover the whole bed with a long mackintosh and a dust sheet. Put two bottles in the bed and cover with an 'admission' blanket or rug, and on the radiator a gown and another blanket, ready for the patient's arrival. Screen the bed (see plate 4).

N.B. In a ward into which emergency cases of this kind are admitted a special mackintosh, dust sheet and 'admission' blanket are kept for the purpose only.

Prepare extra equipment according to the type of case to be admitted. (i.e. extra pillows, fracture boards, cradles, vomit bowl, and cloth, pulse chart, bed blocks, resuscitation cradle, etc.)

4. **Daily bedmaking.** This should be done after the patient has been washed. Strip the top bedclothes over the back of a chair at the foot of the bed, folding each article into three folds and turn the end on to the seat of the chair. (Bedding must on no account be allowed to touch the floor.) Leave the patient covered with a blanket. If possible remove all pillows except one and loosen the bottom bedclothes all round. One nurse turns the patient towards her, moving the head pillow with her, and the second nurse rolls the drawsheet and mackintosh under the patient's back. She rolls the bottom sheet and blanket towards the patient, brushes the mattress and then quickly dusts the bed frame, especially at the top. She then pulls the blanket and sheet tight and turns the patient towards her, whilst her partner takes the drawsheet and mackintosh out of the bed. She separates them, gives them a thorough shake, and hangs them over the chair. She then rolls the bottom sheet and blanket on her side of the bed,

dusts the bed frame and brushes the mattress. She pulls the blanket and sheet back over the mattress and brushes out crumbs or debris from under the patient. She then rolls the drawsheet and mackintosh together and inserts them on her side under the patient's back. She takes the patient from her partner, who rolls through the mackintosh and drawsheet. The patient is now on her back. The two nurses will complete the making of the under part of the bed. Beginning at the foot they will pull the bottom blanket straight and tight, and make the corners envelope fashion. They then move up the bed and tighten the blanket under the patient's buttocks, after which it is pulled tight under her head and the top corners finished. Next, the sheet is dealt with in the same way. The draw mackintosh is pulled very tight and both sides are tucked in, and then the drawsheet in the same way. One nurse raises the patient's head while the other one shakes and turns the pillows and makes them comfortable. It gives a tidier appearance if the closed ends of the pillow cases are facing the ward door. The top sheet is put on and the blanket next to the patient is withdrawn from below, avoiding any exposure. The sheet is then adjusted leaving a sufficiency over the patient's shoulders. In hospital, the excess at the foot of the bed will be turned back over the patient's feet, so that the uncreased end may be turned to the top of the bed next day. Each blanket is then placed over the patient, first covering the shoulders well with a single layer. Turning the corners under, the sides are tucked in and the excess drawn to the foot of the bed and secured by envelope corners. Before the bedspread is put on, the clothes over the feet are well loosened. This is important. After the bedspread has been put on, the sheet at the top is turned back. The nurse should then survey the bed to see that the patient is comfortable, and the bed quite tidy. It is very important that the clothes should reach well up into the patient's neck; some patients may prefer the blanket to be folded at the top. With patients, however, who cannot move, it is inadvisable to have a heavy weight of clothes over the chest, as it hampers the movements of the arms still further and is inclined to make breathing shallow. This may be a contributory cause of congestion of the bases of the lung (hypostatic pneumonia) (see plate 7).

Changing the top sheet. (1) When the top part of the sheet is soiled, both nurses take the top corners and turn it to the bottom, drawing the clean bottom fold of the sheet over the shoulders. This is done very quickly without any exposure of the patient.

(2) If a clean top sheet is required, it is placed over the soiled one, which is withdrawn from top to bottom.

Changing the bottom sheet. A clean sheet is rolled lengthways to the middle crease. The patient is rolled over and the soiled one is rolled lengthways to the middle under the patient's back. The clean one is then put in position and as the patient is rolled back, the soiled sheet is removed, gathering it all up together so that crumbs, etc., are not scattered on the floor. The clean sheet is then drawn through. A drawsheet is changed by the same method (see plate 6).

To put a clean pillow case on a pillow. Open the pillow case and free the bottom corners. Fold the pillow lengthways and grip it firmly with the right hand and put it into the pillow case so that the corners coincide.

To Make a Bed when the Patient is Sitting up and cannot be rolled, e.g. *Fowler position.* Strip the bed as before, leaving the patient covered with a blanket. Loosen the bottom bedclothes. One nurse lifts the patient's feet and the second nurse brushes the bottom of the mattress and dusts the bed frame. They then work together tightening the blanket and sheet from the bottom, brushing the sheet and tucking in the corners. The patient may then be lifted down the bed. One nurse supports her, while the other removes the drawsheet and mackintosh, pillows and bed rest. She then loosens the bedclothes at the top of the bed, brushes the mattress, and dusts the bed frame. She replaces the blanket and sheet, pulling them very tight and folding in the corners. She then replaces the mackintosh and drawsheet and arranges the pillows comfortably with the bed rest. Her partner then finishes her side of the bed whilst the patient is supported by the other nurse. The patient is then lifted back in position and the top bedclothes arranged as before (see plate 8).

It is almost essential that the patient should have an air cushion. A bedjacket should be worn and a chest blanket put round the shoulders to keep the patient warm.

Surgical cases nursed in the Fowler position are now allowed, and in fact, encouraged to move more than was formerly the case, and although they are being nursed sitting straight up with four pillows and a knee pillow, all pillows except two may be removed for bedmaking, and the patient rolled over to the side for the making of the under part of the bed. Some surgeons ask the nurse, to whose side the patient is turned, to give her deep breathing exercises while she is on her side and while the second nurse is making her side of the bed. However, with very heavy and serious cases who cannot be turned at all there are two methods of changing the drawsheet. One is to lift the patient, while a third nurse inserts the drawsheet. If a third person is not available the patient may be rolled very slightly while the drawsheet is inserted.

To change the bottom sheet (when the patient cannot be rolled). Make two-thirds of the length of the clean sheet into a roll. One nurse lifts up the patient's feet, whilst the soiled sheet is rolled up lightly under the patient's thighs as far as possible. The roll of clean sheet is put beside it and the remainder (just sufficient) is tucked in under the bottom end of the mattress. The patient is lifted over the rolled sheets and is supported by

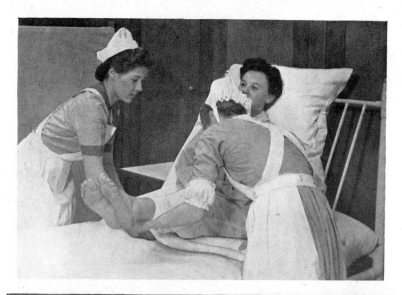

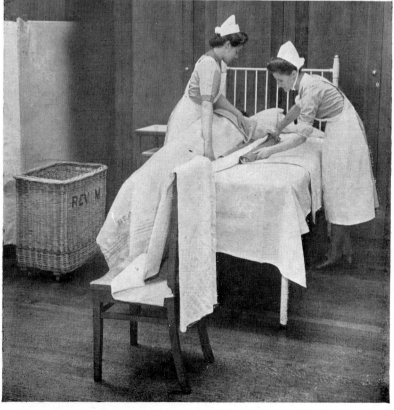

Plates 5 and 6. Changing bottom sheet. See page 45

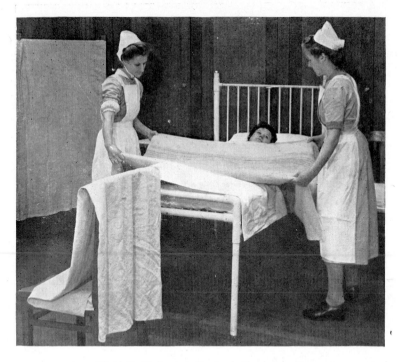

Plate 7. Stripping the bed. See page 44

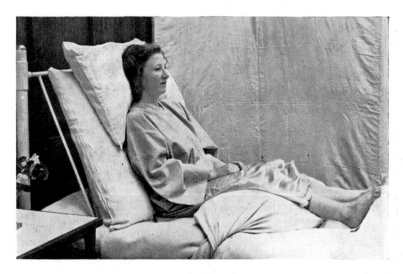

Plate 8. Fowler position. See page 46

one nurse whilst her partner places the under blanket and sheet in position at the top of the bed, removing the soiled sheet altogether (see plate 5).

Notes. (1) Whenever possible lift the patient on to an adjacent bed or stretcher for the changing of the bottom sheet and then the mattress can be thoroughly brushed and turned and the bed made up fresh and clean. This, of course, is not always practical.

(2) Find out how much the patient can be moved. Do all you can to avoid unnecessary handling and lifting.

(3) Most cases are rolled from side to side for bedmaking; among those that are lifted are:

a. Heart and lung cases with dyspnœa or orthopnœa.
b. Cases of peritonitis with drainage.
c. All leg cases, amputations, fractures, thrombosis, etc.
d. Fractured pelvis.

SPECIAL BEDS

Air and Water Beds. These are kept in store in hospitals, and in private practice may be borrowed from certain surgical supply depots or District Nursing Associations. Fracture boards are put in position to support the springs and a mackintosh is put over the mattress, then an old blanket. The air or water bed is then put in position and filled until there is a sufficiency of air or water to prevent the two sides from touching when the nurse presses her body weight upon it with her elbows. In the case of a water bed the spout should be at the bottom corner, a funnel is fitted into it and water, at a temperature of 98° F., poured into it by a jug. One pint of carbolic lotion 1—20 should be added to each gallon of water. When the bed is filled, the bedclothes are arranged in the usual way, remembering that rubber surfaces should never be in contact with each other. If a patient gets up for any leng h of time off a water bed, hot bottles must be put in to keep it warm. It should be emptied, washed and refilled at intervals if it is being used for a long time. When the bed is finished with it must be emptied, thoroughly scrubbed with soap and water and dried carefully. Great care must be taken that no grease gets on to the rubber and that the bed is not damaged by safety pins. Sorbo or Dunlopillo mattresses are used nowadays in preference to air and water beds.

The Lawson Tait Beds for postural drainage—are useful for maintaining patients in the prone position with the head lowered in cases of bronchiectasis and acute dilatation of the stomach.

Operation Beds. As soon as the patient has gone to the theatre make the bed in readiness for her return. Strip it, dust the bed frame, brush the mattress and turn it. Make it up with a clean bottom sheet, if the one already in the bed is soiled. Put the pillows on the chair by the side of the bed. Put two hot water bottles in the middle of the bed. Place the top

BEDMAKING

clothes over the bed in order. Do not tuck them in. Fold them sides to middle, making a long packet. Arrange this over the bottles so that all the clothes are warm when the patient returns. Put on the radiator a clean gown and blanket. Prepare on the locker a vomit bowl and cloth, mouth gag, tongue forceps and sponge holders, marine sponges or wool swabs and a bowl of cold water in case the sponges or swabs are needed. Close the windows nearby and have screens at the sides of the bed ready to place round the patient. Extra equipment should be at hand as required: bed, blocks, electric cradle, sandbag, tourniquet, extra pillows, pulse chart, carbon-dioxide mixture and oxygen (see plate 9).

When the patient returns, the packet of clothes and bottles are removed the patient is lifted on to the bed. The stretcher sheet is rolled out and the packet unfolded over the patient and the clothes tucked in. A hot blanket off the radiator is put next to the patient and the gown changed if necessary.

Fracture Beds. Fracture boards are placed under the springs to keep the bed rigid. Before treatment has been decided upon, patients are arranged in bed as follows:

1. *Fractured tibia and fibula.* Two fracture boards at the lower half of the bed, one head pillow, leg on back splint raised on a wedge pillow, steadied by sandbags, protected by bed cradle.

2. *Fractured femur.* At least three fracture boards required, one small head pillow, patient kept flat. Leg immobilized from the hip with sandbags. The patient is probably on a temporary splint, Thomas's or long Liston's. Cradle to take the weight of bedclothes.

3. *Fractured spine.* Four or five fracture boards, low head pillow, sandbags on either side of the trunk kept in position with towels. A sandbag to support the feet. Large bed cradle over trunk and legs, a long mackintosh next to the mattress. A thin pillow under the small of the back. Fracture-dislocations of the dorsal or lumbar spine are placed in the prone position with small pillows under chest, pelvis and ankles, and bed cradle over trunk and legs (see plates 11 and 12).

4. *Fractured pelvis.* Arrangement as for fractured spine nursed on the back, except that the sandbags and towels should be placed on either side of the pelvis.

5. *Fractured skull.* (a) The patient flat, no head pillow, mackintosh and drawsheet under the head. Long mackintosh next to the mattress. Light shaded. Pulse chart.

(b) Sitting-up position (according to surgeon's instructions).

N.B. In all accident cases a vomit bowl and cloth should be put on the locker.

Amputation beds. Patient has one head pillow at first. The stump is raised on a *small* protected pillow for not more than 24 hours and is kept in position by towel and sandbags. It is covered by a cradle, a blanket is

48

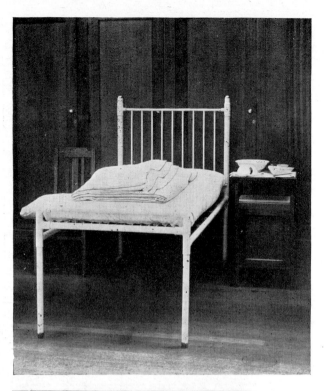

Plate 9 (above).
Operation bed. See
page 47

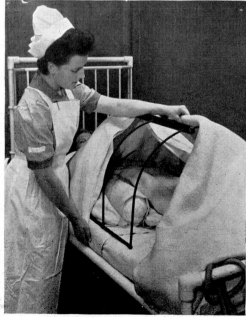

Plate 10.
Amputation bed. See
page 48

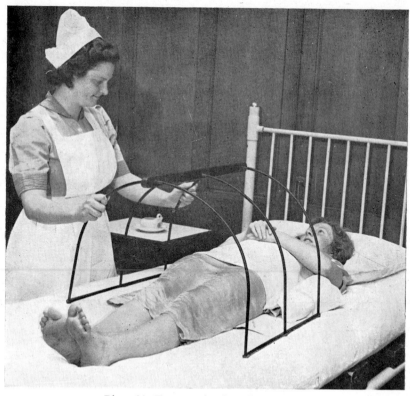

Plate 11. Fractured spine. See page 48

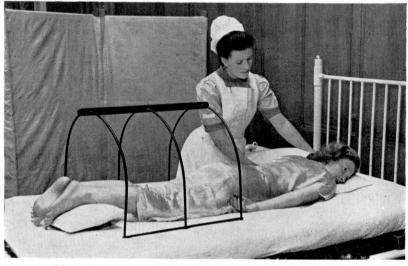

Plate 12. Fractured spine in prone position. See page 48

put next to the patient and the good leg is kept wrapped in it. The top bedclothes are arranged in two halves, the division being at a convenient place so that the stump can be observed without any disturbance to the patient. A tourniquet and wool is kept at hand but out of the patient's sight. Bed blocks may be required (see plate 10).

Plaster beds. When plaster of Paris has been applied, cover the part with a cradle. Arrange the bedclothes so that air can circulate around the plaster in order that it may dry. Hot bottles or an electric cradle are seldom used as they dry the plaster too quickly and they are liable to crack. A small pillow may be put under the knee to maintain 15° of flexion.

Rheumatism bed. Put a long mackintosh next to the mattress, then a sheet and an old blanket. A narrow drawsheet and mackintosh are placed under the buttocks. A blanket is put over the patient and a woollen gown is worn. One pillow only is allowed. A bed cradle may be required (see plate 14).

Renal cases. The bed is made as for acute rheumatism except that the patient may have two or three head pillows.

Cardiac cases. If possible these are nursed in an ordinary bed, flat, with one pillow. This is the best position. If, however, the patient's breathing is distressed, she must sit up in the most comfortable position, with three or four pillows and an air cushion and a small soft pillow under the knees to prevent her from slipping down. A stone hot water bottle filled with warm water may be put at the feet to keep her in position. A bed table is required, also a bedjacket and a chest blanket (see plate 13).

For Examination of a Patient

1. *Abdominal.* If the surgeon wishes to examine the abdomen of a patient, remove all pillows except one (if possible) and arrange the patient in the dorsal position. Remove the bedspread and arrange the bed as a half-bed, having one blanket folded down to the groins and the other covering the legs. Roll the night-gown up and tuck it under the axillæ. In the case of a female patient the surgeon will usually examine the breasts as well. The patient may flex the knees. The bed is well screened and the nurse explains to the patient exactly what the doctor is going to do, and encourages her to lie in a relaxed position (see plate 15).

2. *Rectal.* The bedspread is removed and the bed arranged as a half-bed as above. Place the patient in the left lateral position, buttocks well to the edge of bed. When the surgeon is ready, turn the corner of the bottom blanket back, just exposing the buttocks.

3. *Vaginal.* Arrange the patient exactly as for a rectal examination, but instead of the left lateral position, Simm's position may be required. Draw the patient on to the extreme edge of the bed and tell her to lie in a semi-prone position with her right arm above her head, the left arm behind her, and the right knee flexed (see plate 16).

CARE OF BEDDING AND BEDSTEADS

Bedsteads. Enamel bedsteads should be cleaned with turpentine at intervals. Wooden bedsteads are cleaned with furniture polish. All bed frames should be dusted each time the bed is made. Springs should be tightened as required so that the mattress does not sag.

Sacking or Platforms. These are made to cover the springs and protect the mattress. They must be washed frequently and the tapes must be sewn on again if they are torn off or loose. Loose mattress covers, if supplied, are easily changed and washed.

Mattresses and Pillows. These should be kept in good condition and sent to be remade when necessary. Mattresses should not be allowed to become thin and lumpy. They need brushing and turning every day whenever possible. Pillows and mattresses must be sent to be fumigated after they have been used for an infectious case, or after a patient has died.

Blankets. Blankets which have been used next to a patient are always sent to the laundry when the patient is discharged. If a blanket is stained or soiled the nurse should at once take it away and wash the soiled part, otherwise the blanket may be ruined if neglected at this stage. Blankets, other than the one used next to the patient or for the blanket bath, are used on the beds again and washed as often as the supply allows. They are sent to be disinfected after infectious cases and deaths. When they are returned they are sent to the laundry.

Linen. Sheets, pillow cases, and towels are sent to the laundry when necessary. Linen soiled by fæcal matter, including babies' napkins, are kept in special linen bins. They are listed and sent to the laundry separately for special treatment there.

The alternative method for dealing with soiled articles is to soak them in a bucket of water containing disinfectant turning them about with a stick. The water is changed several times until the articles are clean enough to be dried and mixed with the other linen which is to be sent to the laundry. This method is most undesirable in a hospital and special arrangements ought to be made for grossly soiled articles to be dealt with at the laundry.

The linen is prepared for 'change' each month. All worn-out articles are put on one side when the clean laundry is put away and once a month they are counted and listed. One bundle is for repair, a second bundle if condemned by the superintendent of the linen room is replaced by new articles. A third bundle of articles is sent for remarking as it is important for the name of the ward or department to be legible if the articles are not to be lost. Nurses should not put linen on the beds if it is in need of repair. Small repairs are often done by the nurses, and the convalescent patients in the women's wards are pleased to do a little mending. The

50

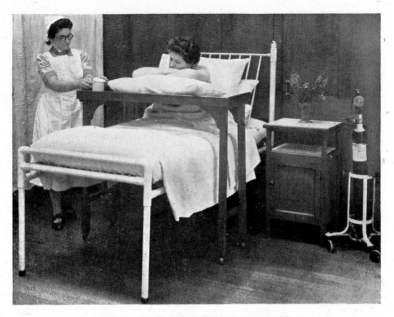

Plate 13. Cardiac bed. See page 49

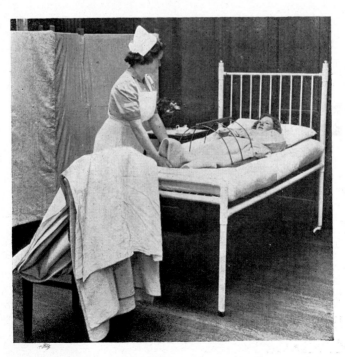

Plate 14. Rheumatism bed. See page 49

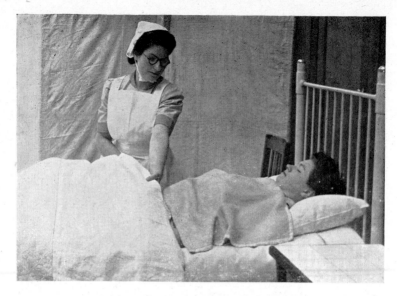

Plate 15. Preparation of patient for examination of abdomen.
See page 49

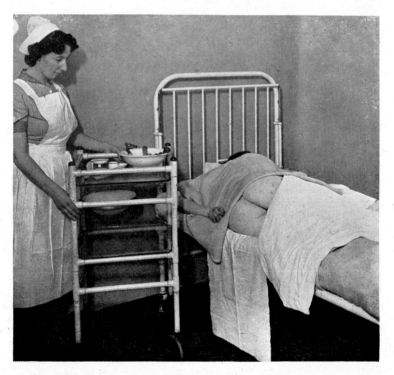

Plate 16. Sims' position for vaginal examination. See page 49

larger patches and renovations are done by the linen room staff. Gowns may be the responsibility of the night nurses who look them over and sew on buttons and tapes.

The care of the linen in a ward is a collective responsibility and the linen can be kept in very good order if every nurse does her share. In this connection every new probationer in the Preliminary Training School, before she goes to the wards, should understand how linen is cared for, then she will realize that she must never tear up, or use for cleaning purposes, any article, however old it may be. Unless it is shown intact with the name of the ward, a new one cannot be obtained in its place.

The above details regarding the care of linen hold good if the system is *decentralized*, i.e. if each ward is issued with a certain quota of linen. Inventories are taken at regular intervals, and the ward sister is responsible for the upkeep and good condition of the stock. In some institutions (perhaps the majority), a *centralized* system is organized, i.e. all linen is kept in a central store; the storekeeper issues a certain amount of clean linen to each ward and department daily. All clean linen is returned from the laundry direct to the store, where it is sorted, repaired, etc. Thus the ward sister has less work, and less responsibility. On the other hand, she has not the same pride and interest in her linen, and the nurses do not get the valuable practical experience in its care.

Chapter Five

OBSERVATION OF EXCRETA

An important part of a nurse's work is the observation and examination of excretions. In the altered metabolism of diseased conditions many abnormalities occur. The nurse learns to know what to look for and the physician is very dependent upon her accuracy of report.

URINE

Normal urine is light yellow in colour, clear and has a characteristic but not unpleasant odour. The average amount passed is 50 oz. per day, and about 10 oz. are voided at a time. Specimens for examination should be obtained in clean vessels which have been previously rinsed with water.
Note:

1. Colour

a. *Pale:* specific gravity is usually low and the urine pale when large amounts are being passed, except when sugar is present.

b. *Darker colour:* shows concentrated urine and has a high specific gravity when small amounts are being passed. This is particularly so in cases when the patient is dehydrated due to diarrhœa and vomiting, or excessive sweating.

c. *Blood:* urine may be bright red, if the blood is fresh and present in large quantities. Clots may be seen. If only a little blood is present, the urine may be smoky or darkish brown.

d. *Bile:* the urine is dark brown. Bubbles of gas are seen on the surface.

2. Naked-Eye deposits

1. *Urates*—brownish pink or brick-red deposits seen when the urine is cold.

2. *Uric acid*—small red grains resembling cayenne pepper.

3. *Phosphates*—white deposit.

4. *Blood*—clots or brown deposit.

5. *Pus*—thick yellow deposit.

3. Smell

a. If the urine smells strongly of ammonia: this is a decomposition product of protein and is found in cases of cystitis and when the urine has been standing for some time.

b. If a fishy odour is detected: This may indicate infection of the bladder by bacillus coli.

c. There may be a peculiar sweet smell of acetone, as found in diabetes mellitus. This is unmistakable once it is recognized.

4. Reaction

This varies according to the diet and other factors. On a mixed diet the reaction of normal urine is slightly acid, i.e. it turns blue litmus red. If it turns red litmus blue, it is alkaline. If no change occurs in the colour of the litmus paper, it is neutral.

5. Specific Gravity (or relative density)

This depends upon the amount of solid constituents in solution or in suspension in the urine. The specific gravity is compared with that of distilled water which is taken as 1,000. It is estimated by means of a urinometer, which is floated in a specimen glass containing urine.

N.B. Make sure:

1. That the urinometer is floating and not touching the bottom of the glass.

2. That the glass is standing on a steady surface.

3. That the reading is taken at eye level. The nurse should bend down to the table to read the figure.

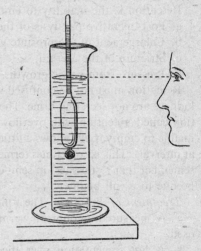

Fig. 15. Taking the specific gravity

Normal specific gravity: 1,010—1,025.

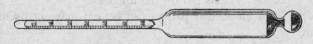

Fig. 16. Urinometer

6. Amount

This must be accurately measured in diseases of kidney and bladder, also in high fevers and severe heart conditions. The urine is all saved for twenty-four hours in a Winchester bottle and is measured. The patient should be discouraged from opening the bowels into the same bedpan into which the urine is passed. If this should happen, the nurse should estimate and note as far as she can the amount of urine excreted before the bedpan is emptied.

Polyuria

The passing of abnormal quantities of urine, as in diabetes mellitus and insipidus, and also when the patient is taking large quantities of fluid.

Oliguria

The passing of small quantities of urine during the twenty-four hours in cases of nephritis, cystitis and other urinary conditions.

Anuria

Suppression of urine, in which the kidney function is very gravely disordered, as in uræmia, and renal disorders of pregnancy.

Retention

Retention is the inability to empty the bladder, owing to:

a. Post-operative paralysis of the bladder.

b. Enlargement of the prostate gland.

c. Stricture of the urethra.

d. Pressure from pelvic growths or the pregnant uterus.

Retention must not be confused with suppression; in the latter case the kidneys are not secreting urine. The nurse must not be misled by a condition called 'retention with overflow', in which the full bladder, although unable to empty itself, allows a little urine to escape through the sphincter at intervals. This is sometimes termed 'false incontinence'. She should also remember that restlessness in semi-conscious or unconscious patients may be due to a full bladder.

Treatment of Retention. The following measures may be tried:

a. A measured amount of warm water put in the bedpan before it is used.

b. A hot fomentation over the pubic area and changed every few minutes.

c. Lemon water and imperial drink may be given.

d. A few boracic crystals put on the tongue.

e. A tap turned on so that patient can hear it may act by means of suggestion.

f. Irrigation of the vulva with a measured amount of warm water from a jug.

g. Change the position of the patient, if possible. In some cases it may be possible for a male patient to sit on the edge of the bed or to stand up.

If these measures fail, a hypodermic injection of carbachol 1.c.c. may be ordered or catheterization may be necessary.

Incontinence

This means inability to control the sphincter of the bladder. It is due to:

1. Local condition, such as irritation of the bladder by stone or inflammation.

2. Injury to the nerve from: (a) lesion of the spinal cord, e.g. fractured spine injuring the cord, tabes dorsalis, or spinal tumour; (b) cerebral conditions. In the latter the patient is usually unconscious.

In cases of incontinence, e.g. in spinal injury, the bladder action becomes automatic. That is to say, the sphincter will relax and the bladder be emptied when a certain amount, perhaps 10 oz., has collected. The nurse, after a time, can sometimes avoid the bed becoming wet by anticipating this. A urinal can be kept in position in the case of a male patient. Unfortunately, a bladder which acts in this automatic way, never quite empties itself. The residual urine which is left becomes stagnant and infected and cystitis results. The greatest nursing care is required for incontinent patients. Bedding must be well protected, sheets changed as often as necessary and the back and thighs, and groins, washed and rubbed every four hours. If the urine is strongly acid or alkaline, an ointment may be rubbed into the skin, e.g. zinc and ol. ricini, to render it waterproof. Rubber bedpans are of use in this condition.

Stress Incontinence. A condition due to pressure on the bladder. A little urine is passed when the patient coughs, strains or sneezes, etc. The pressure may be from a uterine growth, a pregnant uterus or a prolapsed uterus.

Frequency

This does not necessarily coincide with the passage of large quantities of urine. The patient may ask for a bedpan very frequently, but the total excretion for the day may still be small. It is due to:

1. Irritation of the bladder by a stone, growth or inflammation.
2. Strongly alkaline or acid urine.
3. Pressure on the bladder from uterine growths, etc., as above.

Pain on Micturition

This is associated with acute retention, due to:

1. Enlargement of the prostate gland or stricture of the urethra.
2. Cystitis.
3. Stone or growth in the bladder.
4. Pyelitis.

Hot fomentations may be applied to relieve the pain in acute cases. The patient may be able to sit in a hot bath. The drug used to relax the sphincter is tincture of hyoscyamus, dose m. 15—40, usually made up into a mixture.

TESTING THE URINE

When examining a specimen of urine for abnormal constituents, note on a slip of paper the following points:

1. Colour.
2. Deposits seen by the naked eye, if any.
3. Smell.
4. Reaction.
5. Specific gravity.
6. Abnormalities.

After testing the urine, wash the hands thoroughly.

Abnormal Constituents of Urine (Chemical)

(For bacteriological examination a catheter specimen is required to be sent to the pathological laboratory.)

Albumen

Albuminuria is found in the following conditions: acute nephritis, chronic parenchymatous nephritis, fevers, pregnancy (abnormal) and after the taking of certain drugs, e.g. gold. Small quantities of albumen are found in the urine of children and adolescents of nervous temperament and poor physique, especially after vigorous exercise. In these cases it disappears with rest. Postural albuminuria is not uncommon in bedridden patients: it disappears when the patient gets up.

Tests for Albumen

1. *Hot test*. Fill two-thirds of a test tube with urine, add a few drops of acetic acid, unless the reaction is already acid, and boil the upper part. A cloud may form, due to the presence of phosphates or albumen. Add a few drops of acetic acid and if the cloud is caused by phosphates, it will disappear. If the cloud remains, albumen is present.

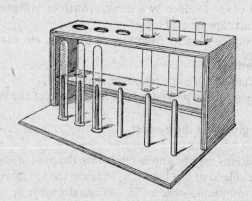

Fig. 17. Test-tube rack

2. *Heller's Test*. Pour half an inch of nitric acid into a test tube. With a pipette add about the same amount of urine, allowing it to trickle down

the side of the tube. If albumen is present, a white ring will appear at the junction of the fluids.

3. *Quantitative Test.* For estimating the amount of albumen present. Esbach's albuminometer is a thick glass tube, graded from 0 to 7 and marked with the letters U and R. The specific gravity of the urine is taken and if it is more than 1,010, it is diluted to bring it to a figure below 1,010. If cloudy, the urine must be filtered and if alkaline, one or two drops of acetic acid added. The tube is then filled with urine up to the letter U and Esbach's solution is added until it reaches the letter R. A rubber stopper is inserted into the neck of the tube which is inverted to allow the fluids to mix. It is kept upright in a stand for the next twenty-four hours at an even temperature. The level of the precipitate is read on the scale. The tube is graded to show parts per thousand, so that dividing by ten will give the percentage. If the urine has been diluted, the result must be multiplied by the degree of dilution. If, after the first trial, the precipitate level is above 4, the urine must be diluted and a fresh estimation made. e.g, (a) If the specific gravity of the specimen is 1,016, dilute with an equal quantity of water. Multiply the result by 2. (b) If the specific gravity is 1,024, dilute by adding twice the amount of water. Multiply the result by 3.

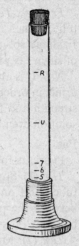

FIG. 18.
Esbach's
Albuminometer

Blood

The urine may be bright red or smoky in appearance. Hæmaturia is found in the following conditions: acute nephritis, renal calculi, tuberculous kidney, cystitis, growth and stones in the bladder, and after operations or accidents involving the renal tracts.

Guaiacum Test. Stir the specimen, take one inch of urine in a test tube and add two drops of tincture of guaiacum. Shake it gently and then float one inch of ozonic ether on the surface by pouring it gently down the side of the test tube, taking care not to shake it. If blood is present a blue colour appears at the junction of the liquids. If iodides are present, a blue colour may also result when the test is made, but it is distinguished from the colour due to blood by the fact that it appears more slowly throughout the fluid and not only at the junction of the fluids.

Sugar

The urine is copious in amount, pale yellow in colour and of high specific gravity. Glycosuria is found in diabetes mellitus and in small amounts in some persons after excitement and in association with exophthalmic goitre and pituitary tumours.

Benedict's Test. Five c.c. of Benedict's solution (about one inch) are put in a test tube. With a pipette, 8 drops of urine are added. This is boiled for five minutes and left to cool. If a small quantity of sugar is present, the reagent turns green, a larger quantity gives a yellow or copper-red deposit. The urine should be filtered before it is tested.

Fehling's Test. Into a test tube put an inch of urine and into a second tube an inch of Fehling's solution. Both are boiled. Add the urine to the Fehling's solution and reboil it. The reagent changes colour in the presence of sugar, as with the Benedict's test.

N.B. It is always necessary to boil the Fehling's alone before adding the urine, in order that it is clearly shown that the Fehling's solution is at full strength and fresh. A colour change denotes reduction of the copper in solution even before the addition of urine.

Pus

Pyuria is found in cystitis and pyelitis.

Test (1). Stir the urine and pour an inch (containing sediment) into a test tube. Add an inch of liquor potassæ. Rotate the test tube vigorously between the palms of the hands. If much pus is present, the mixture will be 'ropy'. If small quantities only are present, a flocculent deposit is seen.

Test (2). Mix and shake together in a test tube one inch of urine and one inch of ozonic ether. Effervescence shows the presence of pus. In many cases pus can only be detected by microscopical examination, and the above tests are only useful if pus is present in large amounts.

Bile

Choluria is found in jaundice. The urine is a dark porter colour and frothy.

Gmelin's Test. With a pipette put a few drops of urine and a few drops of fuming nitric acid separately on a white receiver. The two fluids are then allowed to run together. The presence of bile will be denoted by a play of colours, one of which is green.

Acetone, and diacetic acid (Ketone bodies)

Acetonuria found in cases of diabetes mellitus, chloroform poisoning and acidosis (ketosis).

Rothera's Test. Add to one inch of urine in a test tube an inch of ammonium sulphate crystals and shake thoroughly. Add 5 drops of freshly prepared 5 per cent solution of sodium nitro-prusside, followed by one inch of concentrated liquid ammonia. Mix well together. A purple colour denotes the presence of acetone. Some minutes may elapse before the colour fully develops.

Indican

Indicanuria is the result of putrefactive processes within the intestines. It is also found in some skin conditions.

Test. To a quarter of a test tube of urine add an equal amount of strong hydrochloric acid. Then slowly drop in a freshly prepared solution of bleaching powder (1—20), shaking the mixture all the time. Add half an inch of chloroform and shake thoroughly. A blue or pink colour indicates the presence of indican.

Chlorides

Add a few drops of silver nitrate solution (3%) to a little urine in a test tube. If chlorides are present there will be a cloudy deposit. If chlorides are absent, the need is indicated for giving more. It is a useful test for deciding whether it is necessary to give saline intravenously, etc., in cases of dehydration, when chlorides are lost in appreciable amounts.

FÆCES

Normal fæces are light brown in colour and formed. They have an inoffensive odour and should float in water. The bowels should be opened once or twice a day.

Composition of fæces

Water, undigested food, some bacteria, products of bacterial decomposition, fats, soaps, salts and pigments derived from the bile.

Constipation

Constipation is undue delay in the passage of contents through the intestines. The quickest time in which the residue of a meal is normally passed is nine hours, i.e. it stays about 3—4 hours in the stomach and about five hours in the intestines. After the absorption of water in the large intestine, the residue may accumulate in the pelvic colon for another twenty-four hours before being evacuated. Normally the bowels are opened in the morning after breakfast, as the entrance of fluid or food into the stomach sets up the gastro-colic reflex, which cause muscular contractions propelling the fæces from the pelvic colon into the rectum.

Scybalæ. This is a term used to describe hard, detached masses of fæces which have accumulated near the anal orifice. An enema may fail to remove them, in which case a nurse must put on a rubber glove, well lubricated with vaseline, and evacuate the fæces with her finger. She should then wash the glove thoroughly with cold soapy water and boil it. The hands should be thoroughly scrubbed. It is a good plan to put vaseline under the finger nails before doing a rectal examination for any purpose.

Causes of constipation

1. Unsuitable diet and insufficient roughage.
2. Lack of fluid.
3. Lack of exercise, as in bedridden patients.

4. Probably the most important—due to neglect of the habit of regular defæcation. The term given to this type of constipation is 'dyschezia'.

Treatment of constipation. Aperients should be quite unnecessary for normally healthy individuals. Patients in bed, however, are given drugs with discretion. The fundamental rules for the correction of constipation in an otherwise healthy adult are:

1. Insist upon the establishment of a habit. The patient should make an attempt to open the bowels at the same time every day (usually after breakfast) even if unsuccessful.

2. Reorganize the diet, giving plenty of residue-forming foods, e.g. wholemeal bread, prunes, figs, fresh fruit, vegetables, etc.

3. Encourage the patient to drink a full glass of water on waking in the morning and to omit the early morning cup of tea, also to take plenty of fluids throughout the day.

4. To lead as active a life as possible; walking, riding, cycling and games are most helpful.

5. Abdominal exercises.

In very obstinate cases at the onset of treatment a small enema may be required for several days and such bulk producers as petroleum agar and lubricants such as liquid paraffin are permissible until the new regime accomplishes defæcation without their aid.

Diarrhœa

This means abnormal rapidity in the passage of the contents through the alimentary canal. The stools are loose, offensive and often green in colour, owing to imperfect digestion and absorption; decomposition takes place. They are often passed with violent peristaltic waves, causing spasms of pain called colic.

Causes. (1) Unsuitable and bad food, such as unripe or over-ripe fruit, meat and other foods which are not fresh.

(2) Infections; in the case of children.

(3) Colitis, dysentery and cholera.

(4) The typhoid group of diseases.

Treatment of diarrhœa. (1) Rest in bed.

(2) Warm blankets and hot water bottles.

(3) Withhold all food and fluids by mouth.

(4) If the cause is definitely bad or unsuitable food, an aperient may be prescribed, e.g. magnesium sulphate 2 drachms. This may help to clear away the poisonous materials. Kaolin is often prescribed.

(5) Record the temperature and pulse.

If diarrhœa persists, medical aid should be sought before the patient is exhausted and dehydrated. In milder cases, when the condition begins to clear up, suitable foods to give are: arrowroot, Benger's food. Half an ounce of neat brandy can be given at the onset of the attack if the patient seems cold, shivery, and collapsed.

Tenesmus. A term used to describe ineffectual straining to defæcate. The patient expresses an urgent desire for a bedpan, but there is no result. It often occurs in colitis and is distressing for the patient.

Abnormalities of the Stools

1. Black—after iron medicines.
2. Green—in food poisoning and after arsenical medicines.
3. Clay coloured—as in jaundice.
4. Bright orange and constipated—found in pyloric stenosis.
5. Grey, glistening, fatty, large stools—as in cœliac disease.
6. Blood and mucus—resembling red currant jelly—found in intussusception.
7. Bright red blood—as in cases of carcinoma recti and internal piles.
8. Melaena—dark, tarry stool, due to the presence of digested blood—as in duodenal ulcer, typhoid fever, or if blood has been swallowed after mouth operations.
9. Pea soup stools—in typhoid.
10. Rice water stools—found in cholera.
11. Sloughs resembling pieces of washleather—are found in typhoid stools.
12. Mucus—as in colitis. (Mucus appearing after constipation for several days suggests fæcal impaction).
13. Pipe stem stools—i.e. flattened stools denoting a growth in the pelvis.

Worms

1. **Thread worms.** They appear as small fragments of white thread. They inhabit the rectum and are fairly common in children. The symptoms are: capricious appetite, grinding of the teeth during sleep and itching around the anus.

Treatment. Saline enema ($\frac{1}{2}$ oz. of sodium chloride to 10 oz. of water), followed by quassia infusion 6 oz. Prepare the quassia in the following way. One ounce of quassia chips and $1\frac{1}{2}$ pints of water are boiled down to 1 pint, and 6 oz. of this solution is given. Repeat the treatment three times per week. For children over ten years butolan 1—3 tabs. per day up to twenty doses may be given. The anus should be smeared with a mercurial ointment. Knickers should be worn in bed at night. Finger nails must be kept short and the hands washed regularly, especially before meals. If necessary the elbows should be splinted, so that the child cannot scratch the anus. Larvæ collect under the nails and re-infection may occur if the child sucks the fingers.

Sources. Infected hands, drinking water, vegetables.

2. **Round worms.** These resemble garden worms, but are pale pinkish white and the ends are more tapering. They vary from eight to twelve inches in length and inhabit the small intestine. They are usually in pairs and occasionally they enter the stomach and are vomited.

Source. Contaminated water or food, or vegetables, etc., grown on contaminated land.

Symptoms are irregular appetite, grinding the teeth, emaciation and loss of weight.

Treatment. The drug used is santonin. The patient is given an aperient two days before the treatment and then is kept in bed for twenty-four hours on a starvation diet. Santonin gr. v is then given, followed two hours later by a dose of Epsom salts and an enema if necessary. The patient must be kept in bed and starved until the bowels have been well opened and examined.

3. **Tape worms.** These may be six feet in length. The worm has a small head armed with hooklets with which it clings to the mucous membrane of the duodenum. The body is segmented throughout its length, and each segment contains male and female elements which can continue to reproduce themselves. Hence it is essential that the head be evacuated before a patient can be pronounced cured.

Source. Uncooked pork and beef. Very prevalent in Northern Europe.

Treatment. Liquid diet is given for two days. On the afternoon of the second day an aperient is given. On the morning of the third day black coffee (if liked) is given, followed by extract of filix mas. This is usually in capsule form, each containing m. xxx. Three are given at half-hourly intervals. Vomiting is likely. After two hours a saline aperient is given. The stools must be carefully examined and passed into a vessel filled with water, to avoid breaking the worm, and then strained through black muslin to make it easier to recognize the head. After three weeks the stools must be examined for ova; if present the treatment must be repeated.

VOMIT

Emesis is the emptying of the stomach contents. Four types of vomiting may be recognized:

1. *Reflex.* If some unsuitable food or poison irritates the stomach, the muscles will contract by reflex action and eject the contents. Anæsthetic vomiting is reflex.

2. *Toxic vomiting.* The patient suffering from severe illnesses, e.g. scarlet fever, pneumonia or measles, often vomits on account of the toxins circulating in the blood stream.

3. *Cerebral vomiting.* This is unexpected and forcible emptying of the stomach and is in no way related to food, nor is it accompanied by nausea.

4. *Emotional.* Some people are sick at unpleasant sights or smells.

SPUTUM

Observations with regard to Vomit

1. The time in relation to food.
2. Whether effortless, projectile or accompanied by nausea or pain.
3. The amount.
4. Contents or type of vomit,

    a. Food, i.e. the contents of the stomach.

    b. Bile-stained, i.e. contents of duodenum.

    c. Fæculent, i.e. smelling of fæcal matter. This is seen in advanced cases of intestinal obstruction.

    d. Blood (hæmatemesis): (i) bright red, if fresh and in large quantities; (ii) coffee ground, i.e. partly digested blood, stale and dark brown after delay in the stomach. The cause of blood in the vomit is usually a gastric ulcer.

    e. In cases of suspected poisoning all vomit is saved and the reaction is tested.

SPUTUM

The amount of sputum should be measured and charted. If a specimen is required it should be collected in the early morning. The expectoration from the bronchial tubes is characteristic in certain conditions. The cough accompanying the sputum may also be typical. The following list describes the outstanding types, which the nurse may easily differentiate:

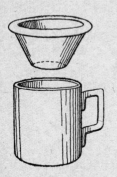

1. *Bronchitis.* In the first stage the cough is dry, hard, and painful and in the second stage, loose. The sputum is scanty at first. Later it becomes copious, muco-purulent and frothy.

2. *Broncho-pneumonia.* The patient has a loose cough with copious muco-purulent sputum.

3. *Lobar pneumonia.* There is a hard, dry, painful cough; unproductive at first. Later there is scanty sputum containing a little altered blood. It is described as 'prune juice' or 'rusty' sputum.

4. *Congestive Heart Failure.* The patient has an irritating unproductive cough. If there is any sputum it is scanty and may be streaked with blood.

FIG. 19. Sputum Cup

5. *Phthisis.* There is a severe 'hacking' cough. The sputum may be copious and nummular (i.e. coin-shaped). It consists of dead lung tissue which floats in water. It is often bloodstained (hæmoptysis) and is very infectious.

6. *Bronchiectasis.* Severe and exhausting attacks of coughing occur at intervals. The sputum is copious, purulent and greenish-yellow in colour, and very offensive.

7. *Whooping cough.* A series of coughs on expiration followed by a long

inspiration, 'the whoop'. This may be followed by vomiting. The sputum is white, ropy, sticky and frothy.

8. *Asthma*. The patient suffers attacks of exhausting, ineffectual coughing, accompanied by severe dyspnœa. The sputum consists of scanty, small pellets.

9. *Aneurysm of the Aorta*. The cough is hard, with a metallic ringing sound due to pressure on the recurrent laryngeal nerve. There is no sputum.

Chapter Six

FEEDING THE PATIENT

A very important part of a nurse's work is preparing and serving meals to her patients; not only does she need to understand the principles of dietetics as applied to special diseases, but she should be able to supply good nutritious food which the patient will enjoy. The better the general health of the 'soil' (that is, the tissues) the more resistant are the tissues to disease. It is an excellent thing for the nurse to have had a preliminary course of dietetics and cookery. She must be able to cook simple dishes and serve meals daintily, and she should understand how to arrange a balanced menu. Whether she is in hospital or later engaged in private or district nursing, at any time the domestic arrangements may make it necessary for her to fill the gap and take a lead in preparing food for her patient.

CLASSES OF FOOD

A balanced diet contains the following types of food:

1. *Protein.* Examples: meat, fish, cheese, legumes (peas, beans, and lentils). These foods are required to build up the cells and to replace tissue wear and tear. During the process of digestion they are broken down into their simple forms—amino acids—of which there are many types, some more valuable than others. Thus we speak of first and second class protein. Most animal protein is first class and vegetable protein second class.

2. *Carbohydrates.* These comprise the starches and sugars. Cane sugar, milk sugar, cereals, potatoes and all starchy foods are included in this class. They are broken down into their simple form, glucose, before they are absorbed into the blood. Glucose is required in the tissues to provide heat and energy.

3. *Fats and oils.* These include animal fats, as found in milk, butter, cheese, meat, etc., and vegetable oils such as nut oil and olive oil extensively used in cooking. Fats are the 'fuel' foods producing heat in the body.

4. *Salts.* These are contained in many foods, and a sufficient quantity of iron, calcium, potassium, and magnesium are required in the metabolism of the body.

5. *Vitamins.* Vitamins are accessory food factors, and are important constituents of food, in the deficiency of which certain diseases declare themselves.

6. *Water.* All the chemical changes of digestion take place through the

E   65

medium of water, and water is required in all the body tissues; at leas
three pints should be taken daily.

Calorific requirements. A Calorie is the unit of heat. It is the amount o.
heat required to raise one litre of water one degree centigrade. Food value
are estimated according to the amount of heat which they yield for the
body's use.

1 gramme (1/30 of an ounce) of protein yields 4·1 Calories.

1 gramme of carbohydrate yields 4·1 Calories.

1 gramme of fat yields 9·3 Calories.

THE SERVING OF MEALS

The Midday Dinner. In hospital this is the most important meal of the
day, and it needs careful organization if the twenty to forty patients in the
ward are to receive the meal well served and really hot.

1. First, the patients should be prepared. Any medicines which are due
are given twenty minutes beforehand. Make sure that the patients are
comfortable and not likely to require bedpans during the meal. If a patient
has just had a bedpan sponge the hands with a flannel and moisten with
- a little eau-de-Cologne, if available. Sit the patient up comfortably, adjust
the pillows and draw the locker or bed table conveniently near. See that
the locker is clear of all unnecessary articles and that, as far as is possible,
all signs of dressings and treatment are removed from the vicinity of the
patients. See that each one has a knife, fork, spoon, glass of water and
a serviette. In some hospitals each patient has a tray on which these may
be placed. If there is no tray, the knife, fork and spoon should be put on
the locker on the serviette. See that the ward is well ventilated and smells
fresh. The head nurse should go round the ward just before the meal is
served to make sure that the patients are ready.

2. The kitchen should be prepared. First tidy up generally; clear
away any dirty dishes, etc., from the sink, and clear the dresser and table.
Put a cloth on the table with a sufficient number of sharp carving knives,
forks and spoons. Prepare a plate of cut bread. Make out a list of diets—
full, light full, farinaceous, milk, special diets, etc.—with the names of
patients (classified) under each heading. In a medical ward where the diets
are very important and varied, it is a good plan to mark the plates with
the names of the patients in ink so that there can be no mistakes. See that
a sufficient number of plates have been put to heat, at least half an hour
before the meal is due to be served. Keep the oven hot while the meal is
in progress, in case a patient's dinner has to be left in it. Meals are often
served from a heated trolley in the ward, instead of from the ward kitchen.

3. All nurses should be ready when the food arrives. They should have
washed their hands, and their aprons and cuffs should be clean.

4. The actual service is arranged somewhat as follows: One nurse prepares special feeds and fluids which are distributed just before the main
diets are served. A second nurse is detailed to feed helpless patients. The
sister serves these first, and their foods are put into the oven until the nurse
is ready to feed the patient. The rest of the available staff, and this should
be arranged so that two or three nurses are helping, take round the dinners
as they are served to the other patients. The sister usually carves and one
nurse helps with vegetables, gravy, and condiments, and puts a piece of
bread on each plate. She should have a clean towel at hand to wipe round
the edge of the plates so that they are clean and free from splashes of
gravy, etc. The potatoes and greens should be arranged in neat little piles.
A corner of bread may be stuck into the potato so that the whole plate
looks attractive, and as appetizing as possible. A little fresh parsley for
garnishing should be used as required. The nurse taking round meals must
be very careful that the patients get the correct plates. They must be taken
round quickly so that each patient gets the meal really hot. The fish
and chicken diets may be served first and followed by the full diets. Each
dish is kept in the oven until it is ready to be served.

When the first course is finished the dirty plates, etc., are collected and
the pudding distributed. As soon as she has served the meal the sister or
the staff nurse goes round the ward to see if the patients have eaten their
meal, noticing what has been left, and hearing if the meal has been enjoyed.
By this means, and by the careful observation and report of every one of
the nurses, a very good idea of the likes and dislikes of each patient should
be obtained. These should be remembered and as far as possible catered
for. Thus the patient feels she is being considered as an individual and it
makes a great difference to her enjoyment of food and her satisfaction and
happiness in the ward. It is a good plan not to serve the meal in the same
sequence each day or certain patients at one end of the ward may begin
to feel that they are always last on the list. Sometimes it may be found that
some patient has not been able to eat her dinner. She may not be feeling
well enough, and in this case the sister or nurse should ask her what she
fancies. Perhaps a glass of milk or a cup of bovril may be acceptable, or
it may be that the sister has something special in reserve for a particularly
difficult or ill patient. On the other hand, in hospital it is not possible to
allow the convalescent patients to indulge too much in fancies, otherwise
meals become unmanageable. It should be the most ill patients who receive
special consideration, and no amount of trouble should be spared to
encourage them to take sufficient nourishment. Some special thought
should be given to the diet of patients who have been in hospital for a long
time and who naturally get very tired of the same type of food. Any little
variation in the menu or in the method of serving it is appreciated.

Hospital diets as provided are generous in quantity and usually of good quality. The food is bought by contract and good buyers know that it i never economy to buy food of poor quality. It is in the cooking an serving of food that the failure is more likely to lie, and the sister an nurses of the ward can help considerably with this. Complaints of reall bad cooking, for example, meat, potatoes and vegetables under- or over cooked, puddings undersweetened or the reverse, should be reported t the proper quarter, but the nurses can improve on the food that is ser up in many ways. For instance, she can sometimes beat up the potatoe with butter and milk, or make white sauce to serve with fish; thin toas can be made for the ill patients if it is desired. She can also chop and drai the cabbage if necessary. It is usual for the nurses to make jellies, junkets and egg custards, or other little delicacies in the ward kitchen. Som hospitals do not encourage this, but there is no doubt that where it is don the nurses are really interested in improving the regular diets and it als gives them scope and an outlet for their initiative. It is a most useful par of their training for their future career, wherever they may be nursin patients.

It is sometimes possible to serve a cup of tea after the midday meal, an it is always much appreciated.

Washing up after meals is done by a ward maid or ward orderly, but i is most important that the nurse should scrutinize the cutlery and silve and glasses before giving them to the patient. Nothing is more distastefu than a spoon or fork which is not perfectly clean, and the nurse should giv them and the glasses a final polish if necessary. The final responsibilit for all these details rests with the nurse whether she is in hospital or privat nursing. If the food is served on trays they should be scrupulously clean Cloths and mats should be in a good condition, and the private nurse i often able to put a small vase of flowers on the tray to add to its attraction bright and attractive china should also be chosen. In children's hospital it is often possible to obtain very attractive mugs and plates for the gener wards.

Breakfasts. These are served at different times in different hospitals What most patients appreciate more than anything is a good cup of tea This should be served first. The night nurses usually prepare breakfasts as far as possible during the night and again it varies in different hospital as to how much cooking is done by the nurses, and how much of the mea comes prepared from the central kitchen. In some cases the nurses cook porridge, bacon, tomatoes, fish, boiled, scrambled and fried eggs, according to each patient's diet, and according to what is provided. There is usually a good deal of variety. To have all this properly cooked and ready to serve needs good management, and a capable nurse enjoys doing it, and giving the patients as far as possible what they like. Bread and butter is prepared during the night and is kept moist by being covered with damp loths. It is a good plan for the sister or head nurse to have a cup of tea out of the pot or urn to see that it is really well made. The patients should be prepared and the meal organized in the same manner as for the midday meal.

Mid-morning Lunch. This is served between 9 and 10 a.m. in hospitals where the patients have early breakfast. It usually consists of milk, cocoa or coffee and bread and butter. Very often the convalescent patients enjoy biscuits, cake, etc., brought to them by their friends, in addition to food provided.

Tea. This usually consists of tea and bread and butter, with watercress, lettuce, jam, paste, cake or whatever is served on successive days. Once again it rests with the nurse to see that the very best use is made of the food provided, the bread and butter cut thinly, the watercress, etc., well washed. The trolley on which the tea is served should be arranged in an orderly and attractive manner. China, spoons, etc., should be clean and well polished.

Supper. This is served between 6 and 7 p.m. and is usually a light meal consisting of milk or cocoa and bread and butter. Jellies, junket, fruit and custard may be given to the ill patients, and sometimes the remains of the midday meal are made up into soup, rissoles or cottage pie and the vegetables fried. Convalescent patients appreciate such things if served occasionally, but it is not the custom in most hospitals to serve a hot meal every night. On the other hand soup and special supper dishes are in some hospitals sent up from the central kitchen for this meal.

Feeding the Helpless Patient. The meal should be kept very hot and the patient put in as comfortable a position as possible. She should not be hurried, and if she is lying down drinks are given from a feeder. If it is a feeder with a spout it should be tilted as high as possible. There is no danger of the patient taking too much with this type of feeder, and she can usually control it herself with her tongue. It is difficult to drink out of a feeder and the nurse should herself try one so that she knows how unsatisfying it is to get little sips when a long drink is what is really needed.

FIG. 20. Types of feeding cup

It is most important that the nurse's hands and cuffs should be very clean. The patient notices these at close quarters, and nothing is more distasteful than to see food being handled by nurses whose hands are not scrupulously clean.

Some patients can feed themselves if the food is cut up. It should be remembered, however, that the food becomes cold whilst being prepared Unless specially heated plates are provided, the food should be reheated before being taken to the patient.

Feeding a Semi-Conscious Patient. There are many patients who though they appear very drowsy or semi-conscious are nevertheless able to swallow and do not need feeding artificially. The nurse should test the swallowing reflex by putting the spout of the feeder—containing a little water—to the patient's lips to see if she can swallow. It is important with this type of patient not to give a second mouthful until she has swallowed the first one. In some cases the patient can be asked to say 'more' before continuing the feed.

DIET IN DISEASE

After Operation. Most patients after operation may have a light diet and anything they fancy as soon as vomiting has ceased. While they are still vomiting sips of water only should be given.

Operations on the stomach. These patients are often allowed nothing by mouth for twenty-four hours. Salines may be given rectally or intravenously. On the second day one ounce of boiled water may be given hourly by mouth, gradually increasing to two-hourly feeds of milky fluids. Many surgeons, however, now advocate a more normal diet from the first day, the patient being allowed a cup of tea twelve hours after the operation and drinks of milky fluids at hourly intervals. The surgeon will give instructions in these cases.

Other abdominal operations. These patients may be given 'surgical fluids' until the bowels have been opened, which is usually on the third day. 'Surgical fluids' are fluids which leave little or no residue, such as tea (with little milk), coffee, fruit drinks, bovril, etc. Jellies may be given with this diet. Again the surgeon's instructions vary with regard to the feeding of these patients. The old rule of 'surgical fluids' for three days and then a dose of castor oil is practically obsolete. It is more usual to give liquid paraffin morning and evening on the second day, and there is no objection to the patient having a little bread and butter or toast, or some very light food which he may fancy, before the bowels are opened. Again the surgeon's instructions must be followed.

Operations on the mouth. (Example: Compound fracture of the jaw, excision of tongue, cleft palate.) The feeds should be sterile for the first four days and should be preceded and followed by long drinks of boiled water. Water can be given freely between meals. The feeds should not be given too hot. In cases of fractures of the jaw which are fixed in position by internal splints or bandage, feeds should be given from a feeder with sterile rubber tubing attached. The tubing is inserted at the side of the mouth in a gap between the teeth, if there is one. In some difficult cases

70

tooth is extracted so that the patient can be fed in this way. These patients' mouths are carefully syringed after meals.

Pneumonia. In this exhausting illness the patient needs a good nourishing diet to enable him to fight the infection. Two-hourly feeds, of five ounces, should be given. The feeds should be planned well ahead and given somewhat as follows.: Coffee, Horlick's, tea, Benger's food, soup, etc., and in addition to these nourishing feeds plenty of fruit juice with glucose, and water should be given. A minimum amount of five pints of fluid should be given daily in these cases. Fresh pineapple cut into little pieces is also very refreshing and cleansing. Boiled sweets such as acid drops help to keep the mouth clean if the patient likes them. Stimulants such as brandy, sherry, or champagne are given in small quantities with advantage during the critical stage of the disease. If the patient does not take sufficient nourishment with two-hourly feeds, smaller quantities must be given hourly. It is of vital importance that the patient should take sufficient nourishment and stimulant. There is no objection to his having a little solid food, such as fish, egg, or thin bread and butter, if he can take them. 'Brand's Essence' of meat juice and calves' foot jelly and such delicacies are also helpful in these cases. If sulphonamide drugs are prescribed, sulphur-containing foods, e.g. eggs, onions, may be omitted from the diet.

Phthisis and other Tuberculous Disease. A full and generous diet is demanded for these patients, as the aim of treatment is to enable the body tissues to resist the infection. Nursing the patient out of doors helps to stimulate the appetite, and the patient will eat better. The diet is not usually reduced, even when the temperature is raised, except that at these times the patient is not inclined to eat so well. Every effort must be made to provide appetizing food. Articles of particular value in the diet are milk, cream, eggs, fresh meat, fish, cheese, in fact everything in a well-balanced diet of the highest quality. Vitamin D, as found in animal fats, has a beneficial effect on patients with this disease, also vitamin A.

Nephritis. The diets prescribed for the different forms of inflammation of the kidneys, acute and chronic, are problems for the physician. The nurse should understand the principles underlying the dietetic treatment. There are four points to be considered :

1. *The amount of fluid.* In acute nephritis this is usually restricted to thirty ounces a day, consisting of fruit juice only, for the first three days. The amount given is increased as the amount of urine passed increases, and as the œdema lessens.

2. *Milk.* This used to be the standard diet prescribed by most physicians for acute nephritis. Some, however, consider it contains more protein than a damaged kidney can cope with, and therefore practically no milk is given in the first stages. Others give a pint of milk a day, saying that it is important to give the patient food to keep up the general condition, and

that the amount of protein contained in milk makes little difference to the condition of the diseased kidney.

3. *Salt.* It is a fairly general rule that salt should be omitted from the diet of patients with œdema, as it tends to retain fluid in the tissues to keep it in solution. Most physicians, however, allow food to be cooked with salt, but discourage extra salt being taken with it.

4. *High protein diet.* Patients whose urine contains albumen in a large quantity are losing protein constituents from the blood. This alters the osmotic pressure, and fluids tend to leak into the tissues. This is considered to be the chief cause of œdema in these patients. The giving of a high protein diet seems logical to replace the albumen lost. Before a high protein diet is given, however, a urea concentration test is done to ensure that the kidney can excrete urea, the waste product of protein metabolism, in sufficient quantity.

The diet which the nurse will have to give her patient will be based on one or other of these theories. Two special diets are in fairly common use—Epstein's diet and Blum's diet.

Epstein's high protein diet. Protein (lean meat, fish, white of egg, ham), 120—240 grammes. Carbohydrates (cereals), 150—300 grammes. Fat, 20—40 grammes. Fluid (milk, tea, coffee, fruit juices, etc.), 1½—2 pints.

Salt and protein-free diet for cases of uræmia (Blum's diet). *Morning.* Sweetened drinks, lemonade, tea without milk, raw fruit, coffee with cream.

Ten a.m. Boiled rice with butter and sugar, flavoured with cinnamon.

Midday. 500 grammes potatoes boiled or baked (without salt), butter, salad, fruit cooked or raw.

Three p.m. Sweetened fruit drinks, tea or coffee.

Five p.m. Tea or coffee with cream, fruit.

Evening. Cereals with fruit juice, sugar and cream. Rice croquettes with jam or honey, fruit drinks.

In cases where neither of these special diets is prescribed, perhaps an average diet in a case of acute nephritis would be arranged in the following stages:

1. Limited fluids, fruit juice and barley water, thirty ounces per day.

2. Fruit juices, thirty ounces, with milk, one pint.

3. Farinaceous diet; that is, bread and butter, cereals, milk pudding, with increasing milk and fruit juices.

4. One egg a day added to stage three.

5. A light diet with chicken, fish, vegetables, etc. Progress would be according to:

   i. The increase in the amount of urine passed.

   ii. Decrease in the œdema.

   iii. The disappearance of albumen from the urine.

Chronic parenchymatous nephritis. An average diet would contain fluids limited to thirty ounces per day, protein such as chicken and fish—and ordinary light diet with salt only used in cooking.

Chronic interstitial nephritis. All stimulants and most of the protein must be omitted from this diet, as high blood pressure is part of the condition, and the development of uræmia is probable.

Jaundice. These patients do not tolerate fat in the diet, and are usually nauseated at the sight of any food. The nurse should not, in the early stages, present food which she knows the patient cannot take, but at the same time she should encourage him to eat or drink what he will. She might try these feeds in the following sequence: Soda water, dry biscuits (water biscuits, cream crackers), tea without milk with a slice of lemon, China tea without milk, good black coffee, dry toast, lemonade, barley water, honey, jam, salads, bovril, cold chicken, potato, etc. Glucose should be put in drinks if the patient can take it.

High Calcium Diet. In cases of bone conditions, such as fractures, the diet should include an abundance of milk, cheese, eggs, and green vegetables.

Addison's Anæmia. Liver is the specific treatment for this disease, and in the past it was supplied by giving the patient half a pound of fresh calves' liver every day. This should preferably be given raw or very lightly fried, the outside just brown. It was almost impossible to persuade the patient to take a sufficiency, and moreover, it had to be taken for the rest of the patient's life. Now the liver is given by injection, and in addition the patients should have a generous diet with the addition of plenty of salads and vegetables.

Gastric and Duodenal Ulcers. The best-known medical treatment of these conditions is by the Hurst-Ryle diet, with the addition of certain drugs. The Sippy diet is similar. Most doctors prescribe one of these diets in modified form; an example is as follows:

Stage 1. Milky fluids, Horlick's, Ovaltine, milk jellies, junkets; five ounces two-hourly.

Stage 2. Two-hourly milky feeds with the addition of farinaceous foods, bread and butter, puddings, potatoes and cereals.

Stage 3. A light diet with a little chicken and fish, but mainly farinaceous with milky feeds between meals.

The progress depends upon the absence of blood from the stools as evidenced by chemical examination of the fæces, and the absence of pain. Medicines given with this diet include:

1. An alkaline powder to neutralize the acid, e.g. magnesium tricilicate; magnesium hydroxide.
2. Olive oil to inhibit the acid secretions of the glands.
3. Bismuth also to inhibit the gastric secretions.
4. Liquid paraffin to regulate the bowels.

5. Atropine or belladonna mixture to inhibit secretion, and to relieve the muscular spasm of the stomach wall which is partly responsible for the pain.

An experiment in the dietetic treatment of gastric and duodenal ulcers has been introduced by Meulengracht, a Danish physician, and has been used in a modified form in this country. It is a more generous and varied diet including purées and sieved foods. Eggs and white fish are given, bread and butter, and other carefully chosen cereals. Drug treatment is also modified.

After-Treatment of Gastric and Duodenal Ulcers. The following instructions are given to patients on discharge:

Articles to be strictly avoided. Alcohol in every form and all effervescing drinks, and strong coffee and tea.

All pips, skins, nuts, unripe fruits: for instance, oranges may be sucked but not eaten. Currants, raisins and figs are especially undesirable. All raw vegetables.

Green vegetables are best taken finely chopped or sieved, and mixed with butter.

Porridge may only be taken if prepared from the finest oatmeal.

Avoid vinegar, sour fruit, mustard, pepper, curry, pickles and chutney.

Avoid tough meat, twice cooked meat, cheese—except cream cheese—and new bread. Boiled fish is always preferable to meat. Avoid hot soups. Be very sparing with salt. After the first month, if all is well, a little cold boiled fatty bacon may be taken at breakfast, provided that it is not too salt. The most desirable foods are milk puddings, gruel, custards, Force, corn flakes, eggs, butter, cream, biscuits, cocoa, Horlick's, Benger's, well-mashed potatoes, etc.

Take a small feed between breakfast and midday, and at bedtime, and if awake in the night.

Eat very slowly and chew very thoroughly.

Smoke in strict moderation, if at all, and only after meals.

If there is the slightest indigestion, rest, avoid all meat and fish, take alkalies and seek medical advice. Do not wait for symptoms to become severe.

Indigestion. (For irritable conditions of the stomach and intestines, gastritis, and colitis, including ulcerative colitis.)

Instructions to patients. Avoid all pips and skins of fruit (whether raw, cooked, or in jam, and currants, raisins and lemon peel in cakes), nuts and all unripe fruit. For example, an orange may be sucked, but not eaten. Currants, raisins and figs are particularly undesirable, and all fruit is better stewed than raw. Red currant, apple and other fruit jellies allowed, but no ordinary jams or marmalade.

Avoid all raw vegetables, whether taken alone (celery, watercress), or in pickles and salad; green vegetables must be passed through a sieve and mixed with butter in the form of a purée. Porridge is only allowed if made with the finest oatmeal.

Avoid alcohol, vinegar, pepper, mustard, curry, chutney, new bread and tough meat.

Eat slowly and chew very thoroughly. Do not smoke excessively. No smoking at all if any indigestion is present.

Have the teeth attended to by the dentist regularly every six months.

Intestinal carbohydrate dyspepsia

No potatoes. No carrots, onions, beetroot, artichokes, parsnips, green peas or lentils. *No rice.*

No bread, toast or biscuits with lunch or dinner.

Puddings containing starch not more than once a day.

Anti-fat Diet for Obesity (for maintenance)

Instructions to patient. Avoid sugar (saccharine may be used as a substitute), potatoes, turnips, beetroot, parsnips, peas, onions, salmon, turbot, herrings, mackerel, sardines, pork and ham, cream, beer, bread with lunch and dinner.

Take no second helpings.

Take no food apart from breakfast, lunch, tea and dinner or supper.

Take plenty of green vegetables, salads (without oil), and clear soup.

Diabetes Mellitus. In this condition, insulin, the secretion of the Islets of Langerhans in the pancreas, is deficient in quantity, and therefore the carbohydrates in the body are not assimilated. This is not the only trouble, for where the metabolism of carbohydrates is deficient the burning up of fats does not take place properly, and poisons called ketones are formed. They accumulate in the blood and may precipitate the patient into a diabetic coma. Hence the importance of finding a balanced diet with a sufficient dose of insulin given hypodermically, which will enable the body to function adequately with a correct metabolism.

An average diabetic diet consists of 400 grammes of carbohydrate, 100 grammes of fat, and 100 grammes of protein. Careful menu building is required while the diet is being stabilized. It may be adjusted day by day according to the results obtained from the injection of a certain dose of insulin. Careful tests for sugar and acetone in the urine and sugar in the blood are carried out. These investigations are done many times and the diet and dose of insulin adjusted until a diet has been found which:

1. Keeps the urine sugar-free.

2. Keeps the blood-sugar normal.

3. Is sufficient to keep the patient satisfied, well nourished and able to do his work.

While in hospital, the patient must be taught:

1. To understand his diet.

2. The importance of keeping to it.
3. To give himself the insulin.
4. To test his urine.

In diabetic clinics this teaching is done, and members of the patient's household are taught to co-operate in his careful feeding. A useful scheme of diet which some doctors follow is the Lawrence Line Ration Diet, of which a sample is given on page 82.

Typhoid. The diet is of the utmost importance in this disease. The Peyer's patches in the ileum are ulcerated and during the third week the sloughs come away from the ulcers. The two main principles in feeding these patients are:

1. That the food should contain nothing which can irritate the ulcers and cause bleeding or perforation.

2. That the diet should be adequate to maintain the patient's strength during a long and emaciating illness. In the past it was the custom to give a milk diet only for several weeks, but this treatment is now practically obsolete. The patient disliked it so much and it was difficult to keep the mouth clean. There seems to be no particular advantage in giving such a limited diet. Nowadays the foods which are included are: citrated milk (one grain of sodium citrate to one ounce of milk), milk diluted with barley water or flavoured with a little tea or coffee, fruit drinks, chocolate, barley sugar, thin bread and butter, lightly boiled eggs, pounded fish with butter, carefully prepared potatoes, stewed apples sieved and beaten up with sugar and cream, etc. *N.B.* Glucose and sugar should be given as freely as possible as it needs no digestion and is very sustaining and nutritious. The patient may chew rusks, and fresh pineapple, ejecting the remains from the mouth. The chewing stimulates the flow of saliva, thus keeping the mouth clean and fresh. Stimulants are not given in the acute stage, if there is any risk of hæmorrhage. The diet is ordered by the physician.

Ketogenic Diet. This diet is seldom ordered nowadays, but in the past it has been prescribed for pyelitis and epilepsy. It consists of a high fat content and practically no carbohydrate. Such foods as milk, butter, cream, eggs, tomatoes, salads, dry biscuits are given in as large a quantity as possible. The idea was to make the blood less alkaline by the production of ketones or fatty acids which result from the combustion of fatty foods. The diet was never a success, as the patient could not take it in sufficient quantity without being sick. Fortunately, for pyelitis an alternative treatment was discovered, that is, the giving of mandelic acid by mouth. Sulphonamides also are prescribed.

Albuminuria of Pregnancy. The principles of the diet in this condition are those outlined in the dietetic treatment of nephritis. It consists usually of fruit drinks, very little milk and foods of low protein content. It is ordered in stages by the obstetrician, who does so after examination of the urine and blood pressure.

PRACTICAL HINTS FOR THE PREPARATION OF PATIENTS' FOOD

To make tea

    a. Rinse the kettle and fill it with fresh cold water.

    b. Heat the teapot.

    c. Infuse the required amount of tea with water which has just, and only just, boiled.

Tea made in any other way tastes stale, and is not refreshing. Milk which has been boiled should not be used.

    d. Study the amount of milk the patient likes in tea.

To make coffee

There are many ways of making coffee; a good way of making it in large quantities for a number of patients is as follows:

    a. Place the required amount of coffee (five heaped tablespoonfuls for twenty patients) in a saucepan with cold water. Add as much milk as can be spared and a good pinch of salt.

    b. Bring to the boil very gently.

    c. Turn off the heat and allow the coffee grounds to settle for a minute. Then strain through a heated strainer into a hot jug.

Cocoa

    a. Mix the cocoa powder with cold water to a smooth paste.

    b. Add to it equal parts of cold water and milk if sufficient milk is available; if not less milk and more water can be used.

    c. Bring the mixture to the boil, stirring carefully the whole time.

Lemonade

    a. Wash and wipe the lemon with a clean cloth.

    b. Peel the rind very thinly and put into a jug.

    c. Peel off the white pith and throw it away.

    d. Cut the lemon across in slices and put into the jug, throwing away the pips. Add one tablespoonful of sugar and a pint of boiling water.

Orangeade

Cut the orange across and squeeze into a glass. The orange juice can be drunk pure, or with sugar and water added.

Whey

Heat a pint of milk to 98° F. Put it in a dish and add one teaspoonful of essence of rennet: stir and let it stand until it is set. Break it up with a fork, and pour it into a muslin bag. The whey is drained into a basin and the curds are left behind. It can be flavoured with sugar or salt or lemon if required. It contains water, salts, sugar and a little fat. The protein of the milk is in the curd.

Albumen water

a. Break up an egg and separate the yolk from the white.

b. Beat the white to a froth and then stir it into five ounces of water. If it is to be given to an ill baby the water should be previously boiled, and the fork and receptacle should be sterile. A little lemon and sugar may be added if allowed.

Egg flip

This is a very nutritious drink for an ill patient.

a. Break an egg and separate the yolk from the white. Put the yolk in a glass and beat it up with a tablespoonful of sugar.

b. Add the juice of half a lemon and a small tablespoonful of brandy.

c. Add two ounces of milk.

d. Beat up the white of the egg with castor sugar and stir it into the mixture.

Barley water

a. Take two tablespoonfuls of pearl barley and add to it a pint of cold water. Bring it to the boil, strain and throw the water away.

b. Add another pint and a half of water and bring it slowly to the boil.

c. Let it simmer until it is reduced to about a pint. It will then be slightly pink in colour and thickened.

d. Lemon may be added as a flavouring, also a little sugar if desired.

Arrowroot

a. Take one tablespoonful of arrowroot and mix with a little cold milk to a smooth paste.

b. The remainder of half a pint of milk is stirred into it and the mixture is then brought to the boil and kept simmering until it is the consistency of thick cream.

To boil an egg

The water should be boiling. The egg is put in and removed after it has been boiling exactly three and a half or four minutes, according to whether the patient likes it just set or a little harder. Boiled eggs are completely spoiled unless they are done to a turn.

When boiling a number of eggs, say twelve or twenty together, some device must be used so that all the eggs are put in at the same moment. They may be put in a muslin bag which should be large enough to allow the water to circulate around every one, or a wire basket, such as is used for frying fish would serve. Eggs which are boiled in large quantities should be cooked for four minutes, as the immersion of the cold eggs brings down the temperature of the water. Crack the top of each egg as soon as it is removed from the water.

To make toast

The bread should be a quarter of an inch thick, though in some cases thinner toast is preferred. The toaster should be red hot. The bread is put an inch away from it and should brown quickly. The crusty edges should be cut away thinly to avoid waste and the toast should at once be stood in a rack. Toast which is put flat on a plate becomes hard and leathery, and loses its crispness. The crusts can be eaten by the children in the ward or they can be made into bread crumbs for cooking purposes.

If the toast is to be served already buttered the butter should be put on when the toast is made. It can be kept hot and moist by being placed in the oven with a hot basin covering it.

Butter

If served on a tray the butter is made into small butter balls, each garnished with a small leaf of parsley. The balls can be made in quantity once a day and kept in the refrigerator.

The heating of milk

The saucepan must be scrupulously clean and if possible kept for milk only. If an enamel saucepan is used the enamel must not be chipped, otherwise the milk will burn. Rinse the saucepan with cold water, before putting in the milk; then bring the milk to the boil.

When preparing milky drinks during the night it is customary to put the milk in a jug and stand it in a saucepan of water to heat it. This method ensures that the milk will not burn or boil over, and the nurse does not need to watch it. It should not, however, stand in the hot water indefinitely, otherwise the flavour of the milk is altered.

The nurse should keep the pantry or kitchen where the patients' feeds are prepared scrupulously clean; slabs and tables should be scrubbed; dishcloths and towels should be clean and free from grease. Cupboards and refrigerators should be turned out daily, so that scraps of stale food do not accumulate. Buckets for scraps of waste should be inspected by the sister at frequent intervals, so that the nurses are trained not to be careless and wasteful with food.

Sample Daily Diet of a Patient in Hospital in Peacetime
1. Full Diet.

Food	Amount in ounces
Bread	9
Oatmeal	1

FEEDING THE PATIENT

Food	Amount in ounces
Potatoes	6
Sugar	3
Milk pudding (made with rice or other cereal)	6
Uncooked milk (in addition to that in the pudding)	20
Butter	1
Cheese	1
Cooked meat	4
Dried fruit or fresh fruit	1 or 8
Second vegetable, greens or root vegetables or bulbous vegetables	4

2. Light Full Diet.

Bread	9
Oatmeal	1
Potatoes	6
Custard	5
Uncooked milk in addition to that in custard	30
Chicken, fish or rabbit or brains or tripe	4
Butter	1
Cheese	1
Jelly or fresh fruit or dried fruit	4 or 8 or 1
Second vegetables (greens, roots or tubers)	4

3. Fluid Diet.

Milk	60
Sugar	4
Fruit juice	3

CALORIE REQUIREMENTS

Average man	requires	3,000	*Calories per day*
Pregnant woman	,,	3,000	,, ,,
Boy 14 to 18 years	,,	3,500/4,000	,, ,,
Nursing mother	,,	3,500/4,000	,, ,,
Adult woman	,,	2,500	,, ,,
Child 12 to 14 years	,,	3,000	,, ,,
Baby	,,	45/50	*Calories per lb. of body weight per day.*
Patient in bed	,,	1,800/2,000	*Calories per day*

(These figures vary with sex, health, climate and occupation of the individual.)

80

VITAMINS

VITAMINS

Vitamin A present in:
  Cod Liver Oil
  Calves' Liver (raw)
  Ox Liver
  Rose Hips
  Turnip Tops
  Dried Apricots
  Cream Cheese
  Butter
  Egg Yolk
  Carrots

Vitamin B present in:
  Yeast
  Marmite
  Bemax
  White Grain Cereals
  Dried Pulses
  Egg Yolk
  Green Vegetables
  Nuts
  Wholemeal Bread

Vitamin C present in:
  Ascorbic Acid
  Parsley
  Black Currants
  Brussels Sprouts
  Oranges
  Lemons
  Watercress
  Cauliflower
  Turnips and Swedes
  Grape Fruit
  Red Currants
  Gooseberries, Loganberries,
    Raspberries
  Tomatoes
  Cabbage
  Leeks
  New Potatoes

Vitamin D present in:
  Halibut Liver Oil
  Cod Liver Oil
  Body Oils of Sardines, Salmon,
    Turbot, Herring
  Butter
  Cream
  Milk

Foods Rich In:

Protein
  Meat
  Fish
  Milk
  Eggs
  Poultry
  Cheese
  Legumes
  Soya Beans

Carbohydrates
  Sugar
  Cereals
  Potatoes
  Bread
  Flour
  Oatmeal
  Dried Pulses
  Treacle

F

81

FEEDING THE PATIENT

Foods rich in:

Protein
  Nuts

Fats
  Butter
  Cream
  Cheese
  Eggs
  Nuts
  Chocolate
  Oatmeal
  Oily Fish
  Fat Meat and Bacon
  Bone Marrow

Phosphorus
  Cheese
  Egg Yolk
  Beef, lean
  Chocolates, Almonds
  Dried Peas, Beans, Whole Wheat
  Lentils, Liver
  Walnuts
  Mackerel
  Eggs
  Salmon, Poultry
  Halibut, Cod

Carbohydrates
  Jams
  Honey
  Dried Fruits (apricots, figs, raisins, dates)

Calcium
  Cheese
  Turnip Tops
  Black Treacle
  Almonds
  Watercress
  Egg Yolk
  Milk
  Dried Beans
  Lentils
  Spinach
  Dried Peas
  Carrots
  Whole Wheat
  Cabbage

Iron
  Lentils, Egg Yolk
  Liver
  Dried Beans
  Black Treacle
  Oatmeal
  Dried Peas
  Whole Wheat
  Dried Currants, Almonds, Lean Beef
  Turnip Tops, Spinach, Dates
  Eggs, Dried Figs and Prunes
  Green Peas, Asparagus

THE 'LINE RATION' DIET SCHEME FOR DIABETES

(Based, by permission, upon the Line Ration Card, by Dr. R. D. Lawrence, published by H. K. Lewis & Co., Ltd.)

One Black Portion added to one Red Portion = One Line Ration
Carbohydrate Foods (containing sugar and starch)
Black Portions (10 gm. Carbohydrate)   *ounces*

Flour, rice, sago, tapioca (raw) $\frac{1}{6}$

82

THE 'LINE RATION' DIET SCHEME FOR DIABETES

ounces

Biscuit, toast or breakfast cereals, oatmeal, macaroni (all dry)	½
Bread (all kinds)	⅔
Potatoes, peas or beans (dried or tinned), banana or grapes; dried apricots (stewed)	2
Parsnips; ripe greengages; prunes (stewed)	3
Raw apple, pear, cherries, gooseberries, plums, damsons, orange (skinned); young peas or beetroot	4
Peach or apricot (ripe); greengages (stewed); broad beans	5
Strawberries, stewed pears, damsons or plums	6
Milk; raspberries or melon (ripe)	7
*Apples or cherries (stewed); carrots or leeks	8
*Jerusalem artichokes; loganberries, blackberries (stewed)	10
*Grapefruit (in skin), tomatoes, red or black currants (stewed)	12
*Onions, turnips or radishes	14

Negligible starch content in average helpings of:

Asparagus, green artichokes, french beans, brussels sprouts, cabbage, cauliflower, celery, cranberries, cress, horse-radish, lemons, lettuce, macaroni, marrow, mushrooms, radishes, rhubarb, salsify, scarlet runners, seakale, spinach.

Extras of no food value:

Tea, coffee, soda water, Bovril, Oxo, etc., ordinary condiments and flavourings.

*—Half portions of these are usually enough.

Red Portion (protein and fat) 7½ gm. protein and 9 gm. fat

One egg.
Bacon or ham (both lean) 1 oz.
Kidney 1¼ oz. and fat ¼ oz.
Liver 1 oz. and fat ¼ oz.
Tongue (tinned or fresh) 1 oz.
Tripe or sweetbreads 1¼ oz. and fat ¼ oz.
Lean beef or veal 1 oz. and fat ¼ oz.
Lean lamb or mutton 1 oz. and fat ¼ oz.
Lean pork 1 oz.
Chicken or pigeon 1 oz. and fat 1 oz.
Duck 1 oz.
Pheasant, grouse or partridge ¾ oz. and fat ¼ oz.
Rabbit or hare ¾ oz. and fat ¼ oz.
Crab or lobster 1¼ oz. and fat ¼ oz.
Herring 1 oz. and fat ¼ oz.
Kipper 1 oz. and fat ¼ oz.

Salmon 1 oz. and fat ¼ oz.

Sardines 1 oz.

White fish (all kinds) 1¼ oz. and fat ¼ oz.

Cheese ¾ oz.

Fats are meat fats, suet, dripping, butter, margarine, olive oil, thick cream in twice the amount stated for other fats.

Notes

1. A certain number of rations are ordered per day.

2. One ration is one complete line (i.e. one black and one red portion). Any *black* portion may be combined with any *red* portion to make one ration.

3. Each line has a calorific value of 210 calories.

4. All foods are to be weighed cooked, except fats like butter and the articles marked 'raw'.

5. No flour or sugar must be used in cooking. Saccharine can be used for sweetening.

6. Insulin is given according to the doctor's instructions.

CALORIES AND COMPOSITION IN GRAMMES OF 1 LB. OF COMMON FOODSTUFFS

Foodstuffs	Calories	Protein A*	P* Fat	Carbo-hydrate
		g.	g. g.	g.
Meat				
Beef steak	715	100	— 31	—
Lean of beef	618	100	— 23	—
Lean of veal	493	93	— 11	—
Lean of mutton	688	95	— 31	—
Lean of lamb	630	93	— 29	—
Lean of pork	612	85	— 29	—
Lean of meat, average	608	93	— 24	—
Liver, sheep's	573	95	— 13	11
Liver, calves'	504	66	— 4	47
Sweetbread, calves' pancreas	684	100	— 29	—
Tongue, ox, canned	1340	88	— 105	—
Tripe, ox	382	72	— 9	—
Bacon, streaky	2478	46	— 246	—
Brawn	840	71	— 51	14
'Breakfast' sausage	1420	51	— 99	71
Corned beef	1280	128	— 82	—
Ham, slices	2206	57	— 173	—
Pork pie	1670	34	11 113	142
Sausages	1238	51	— 80	69

CALORIES AND COMPOSITION

Foodstuffs	Calories	Protein A*	P*	Fat g.	Carbo-hydrate
Poultry, Game, Eggs		g.	g.	g.	g.
Chicken, turkey flesh	515	100	—	11	—
Rabbit, hare flesh	550	105	—	13	—
Hen's egg, with shell	659	50	—	46	6
Hen's egg, without shell	734	54	—	48	7
Hen's egg yolk	1730	71	—	150	8
Hen's egg white	229	77	—	—	6
Eggs, dried	2598	183	—	179	43
Fish					
Cod, flesh only	330	80	—	—	—
Herring, fresh, whole	662	69	—	49	—
Herring, fresh, flesh only	920	82	—	62	—
Kippered herring	978	85	—	68	—
Haddock, dry smoked	377	91	—	—	—
Salmon, fresh, Scotch	1012	85	—	74	—
Salmon, canned, Pacific	915	100	—	54	—
Sardines	1257	85	—	95	—
Lobster (flesh only)	415	89	—	1	9
Oyster flesh	370	40	—	4	39
Milk and Dairy Produce					
Milk, human	310	9	—	17	29
Milk, cow's (per pint)	378	19	—	20	27
Milk, cow's dried, full cream	2126	110	—	110	159
Milk, cow's condensed, unsweetened	976	37	—	54	65
Milk, human, condensed, sweetened	1712	45	—	62	236
Cheese, Stilton	2341	119	—	194	11
Cheese, Cheddar	1939	113	—	150	14
Fats					
Butter	3503	1	—	376	—
Clotted cream, Devonshire	2416	31	—	264	9
Dairy cream (average)	—	—	—	—	—
Dripping, lard, nut butter, olive oil	4218	—	—	454	—
Suet	3958	3	—	426	—
Margarine	3579	1	—	386	—
Bread, Cake, Cereals, etc.					
Bread, wheat, average	1014	—	31	1	215
Biscuits (average mixed)	2050	—	43	46	335
Biscuits, plain	1673	—	57	3	334
Cake, fruit	1566	—	17†	46	261
Cake, sponge	1536	—	32†	17	282

Foodstuffs	Calories	Protein A*	P*	Fat	Carbo-hydrate
Cereals, etc.		g.	g.	g.	g.
Macaroni (average)	1656	—	53	1	348
'Shredded Wheat'	1674	—	44	5	352
'Grape Nuts'	1687	—	43	2	363
Barley 'Kernels'	1655	—	36	6	353
Cornflour (maize)	1648	—	4	—	397
Oatmeal (average)	1866	—	54	38	315
Rolled oats (average)	1809	—	59	29	315
Rice (average)	1640	—	30	2	368
Sago, tapioca (mean)	1656	—	1	2	399
Sugar, Jams, etc.					
Sugar, white	1860	—	—	—	454
Sugar, brown	1823	—	—	—	444
Golden syrup	1427	—	—	—	347
Black treacle	1118	—	1	—	272
Honey	1335	—	2	—	324
Jam and marmalade (average)	1296	—	1	—	315
Chocolate (average)	2515	—	22	141	271
Cocoa	2215	—	82	121	183
Dried Pulses					
Beans, butter	1532	—	84	3	282
Beans, haricot	1552	—	81	2	293
Lentils, red split	1579	—	91	2	290
Lentils, whole	1595	—	97	3	286
Peas, green, whole	1467	—	92	3	259
Peas, yellow, split	1576	—	92	3	286
Peanuts or 'ground-nuts', kernels	2793	—	91	—	100
Nuts					
Almond, kernel	2900	—	92	246	70
Brazil, kernel	3366	—	60	319	37
Coconut, flesh	2267	—	19	220	35
Walnut, kernel	3314	—	62	301	63
Vegetables, fresh, raw per lb. as purchased allowing for waste in preparation					
Artichoke, Jerusalem	360	—	7	—	79
Beans, broad	177	—	11	—	31
Beans, green runner	93	—	5	—	16
Beetroot	142	—	5	—	28
Cabbage and other greens	88	—	3	—	18
Carrots	205	—	5	—	43

CALORIES AND COMPOSITION

Foodstuffs	Calories	Protein A,	P,	Fat	Carbo-hydrate
Vegetables, fresh, raw per lb. as purchased allowing for waste in preparation		g.	g.	g.	g.
Cauliflower	80	—	4	—	14
Celery	76	—	2	—	15
Cucumber	42	—	2	—	7
Leek	98	—	5	—	19
Lettuce	41	—	3	—	5
Marrow	48	—	2	—	10
Mushroom	119	—	19	1	8
Onion	219	—	6	—	47
Parsnip	385	—	7	2	83
Peas, green	172	—	10	1	29
Potatoes, new	410	—	7	—	92
Potatoes, old	373	—	9	—	82
Rhubarb	68	—	2	—	14
Spinach	59	—	5	—	8
Swede turnip	145	—	4	—	31
Turnip, white	95	—	5	—	18
Tomato	101	—	3	—	20
Watercress	60	—	3	—	10
Fruits, Dried, 1 lb. as purchased, allowing for waste, stones, etc.					
Apple rings	1134	—	4	3	266
Apricots	1037	—	25	1	225
Dates	1131	—	6	—	268
Figs	1109	—	9	2	256
Prunes	685	—	11	1	154
Raisins, currants, sultanas	1090	—	8	1	254
Fruits, Fresh, 1 lb. as purchased, allowing for waste of stone, peel, etc.					
Apples	196	—	1	1	44
Bananas	279	—	3	—	64
Blackberries	162	—	6	1	32
Cherries	227	—	3	—	51
Currants	146	—	5	—	29
Gooseberries	128	—	3	—	27
Grapes	261	—	3	—	60
Lemon	31	—	1	1	4
Orange	137	—	3	—	30
Pear, pineapple	146	—	1	—	34
Plum and damson	156	—	2	1	33

A=Animal.   P=Plant.   †Contains some animal protein.

87

Chapter Seven

TREATMENTS AND APPLICATIONS

ENEMATA

An enema is an injection into the rectum. It may be given for the following purposes:

1. Purgative or evacuant, to empty the rectum.
2. Anti-spasmodic or carminative, to relieve flatulence.
3. Sedative, to induce sleep or anæsthesia, or to inhibit peristalsis.
4. Nutrient, to feed the patient.
5. Anthelmintic, to expel worms.

Requirements

1. Warm mackintosh.
2. Receiver.
3. Piece of wool three inches square.
4. Rectal tube (Jacques pattern No. 12/14, or a smaller one if preferred), clip, funnel and rubber tubing, with glass connection.
5. Lubricant (e.g. vaseline) and lint square.
6. Bedpan and cover, wool, tow or toilet roll.
7. Solution to be injected in a suitable container.
8. Lotion thermometer.

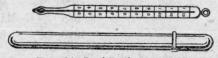

FIG. 21. Lotion thermometer

The use of a Higginson's syringe is a time-honoured method of giving an enema. The bone nozzle, however, is very rigid, and unless carefully used may damage the delicate mucous membrane of the rectum, nor is the interrupted flow with which the fluid is injected desirable. It is much better to use a rectal tube whenever available.

Method. Screens are arranged round the patient, the windows closed, and the bedspread turned back. The patient is put in the left lateral position, the buttocks well to the edge of the bed. The warm mackintosh is inserted and the piece of wool placed under the anus to absorb any fluid which may return. The bedclothes are arranged so that only the anus is exposed, the blanket being put over the trunk, and the rest of the bed-

othes folded over the legs. The tube is lubricated three to four inches
~~~d~~ the fluid at a temperature of 99° F., is run through the connected
~~~~pparatus in order to expel air from the tube, which is then clipped at its
~~~wer~~ end. The tube, now full, is inserted three inches into the rectu m, as
~~~e~~ clip is removed. X-ray evidence has shown that if the tube is intro duced
~~r~~ five or six inches into the rectum it doubles back on itself. The solution
~~~~run in fairly slowly.

After the bed-pan has been used (in cases where the enema is to be

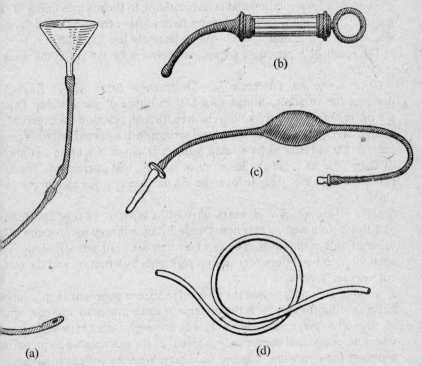

Fig. 22. (a) Rectal tube and funnel. (b) Glycerine enema and syringe.
　　　　　(c) Higginson's syringe.　　　(d) Flatus tube.

~~~~turned), the buttocks are dried, and powdered, and the mackintosh is
~~~~emoved. The bed is remade, the pillows turned, and the patient made
~~~~omfortable.

It is important to remember that the patient should be told what is going
~~o~~ be done before any treatment is started. What seems a simple procedure
~~o~~ the nurse is probably a new and alarming experience to the patient.

Remove the screens, open the windows, and remove all apparatus. Wash
~~~h~~e tube and boil it before putting away.

Soap enema (enema saponis). Four ounces of purified soap solution
one pint of water, or a solution made with a small piece of pure soap
large as a walnut shredded and beaten up until it is dissolved. Castile
white windsor soap are the best kinds to use if available; soft green soa
one tablespoon to a pint of water, may also be used. A strong soap ma
cause an enema rash on the buttocks and thighs. A pint is a reasonab
quantity for most adults, although ten to fifteen ounces of solution are ofte
found sufficient.

Some authorities consider that plain warm water is in many cases a
efficient as a soap solution and is less irritating to the mucous lining of th
rectum. In dealing with patients who have to have frequent enemata it
well worth trying, and if successful is definitely less harmful.

The result of a purgative enema must always be saved for the sister
inspection.

Glycerine enema. Glycerine ʒi—ʒii drachms for a child, ʒiii—ʒ
drachms for an adult, diluted with half an ounce of warm water. It is
purgative enema used for young children, though occasionally ordered fo
adults. The special vulcanite or metal syringe with a curved nozzle is used
but again it is better to fix a small catheter (Jacques No. 6) on to the en
of the nozzle to avoid the insertion of such a rigid instrument. The so
rubber tube is less likely to damage the delicate mucous membrane of
child.

Olive oil enema. ℥iv of warm olive oil is injected by tube and funne
and this is followed in two hours' time by an ordinary soap enema. Th
olive oil softens the fæces in cases where they are hard and scybalous. Th
soap solution two hours later sets up peristalsis by irritation and the recta
contents are evacuated.

Another method is to add the olive oil to sixteen ounces of soap solutio
and mix it thoroughly. It is the practice of some nurses to add one ounc
of olive oil to every soap enema. This is, however, rather extravagant, an
where an occasional enema only is given, as for example when preparin
a patient for operation, it is not necessary. Where a patient is having a
enema frequently it is a good plan to add olive oil to counteract th
irritating effect of the soap.

Turpentine enema (carminative and anti-spasmodic). Medicinal turpen
tine ℥i to Oi of soap solution. The turpentine must be thoroughly mixe
with a little of the solution before the rest is added, to make sure that no un
broken globules of turpentine float on the surface. This method is quit
safe though there are other methods of emulsifying the turpentine befor
mixing the solution. It may be mixed thoroughly with an ounce of oliv
oil, or beaten with the yolk of an egg before adding it to the soap solution
or it is sometimes given well mixed in half a pint of thin starch mucilage
It should be noticed whether flatus is passed when the bedpan is used.

Treacle enema. Five ounces of old-fashioned black treacle mixed with
n ounces of warm water. This enema is used in cases of distension. Some
rgeons prefer it as being less drastic and irritating than turpentine and
ually efficacious.

Oxbile enema. Liquid ox bile ℨii—iv in ℥x of warm water, or grs. xx
˙ powdered extract of ox bile (extr. fel bovis) in ℥vi of warm water
arminative).

Gruel enema. ℨi of fine oatmeal mixed to a smooth paste with cold
ater. To this add ℥xv of water and bring it slowly to the boil until it
ickens. Strain carefully through muslin. The gruel should be of a con-
stency of thin cream. This is a useful enema for patients who suffer from
ainful hæmorrhoids. It should be given through a fine rectal tube in order
˙ avoid unnecessary pain and discomfort.

Magnesium sulphate. ℨii of Epsom salts in ℥viii water (25 per cent solu-
on), or ℨii in ℥vi of water (33⅓ per cent solution). These strong saline
lutions are prescribed to relieve intracranial pressure in head injuries
nd other cerebral conditions. The solution is hygroscopic in its action,
nd results in a large watery stool.

Starch and opium enema (sedative). ℨii of thin starch mucilage and ♏xxx
ncture of opium. An ounce of the starch is given, then the opium fol-
wed by the rest of the starch. It should be given almost cold. It is pre-
cribed in cases of intractable diarrhœa, as in cases of typhoid and
ysentery.

Paraldehyde. ℨi of paraldehyde per stone of body weight, given in
iii of saline. In this proportion it is often given to children as a basal
næsthetic before tonsillectomy.

Avertin (bromethol). Dose: 0·1 gramme per kilogram (2⅕ lbs.) of body
eight. This is often used as a basal anæsthetic. The patient is weighed and
he solution is made up accordingly by the dispenser, who is also told the
ime of the operation. He sends up the freshly made bromethol which is
o be given half an hour before the patient goes to the theatre. The solution
hould stand in warm water until the nurse is ready to give it. The patient
s screened, wool may be put into his ears and a quiet atmosphere should
revail. He is turned on to the left side, the right arm on the pillow, above
he head. The nurse first pours a little of the solution into a test tube to-
;ether with a few drops of solution of Congo red. If the mixture does not
etain the red colour it should not be used, as it is not fresh and will have
lecomposed into hydrobromic acid. After testing, the bromethol is run
nto the rectum fairly quickly, taking two or three minutes. An evacuant
:nema will have been given previously to empty the rectum.

Bromethol has several advantages as an anæsthetic. The patient loses
:onsciousness until an hour or two after the operation is over and there
s no vomiting. It is quite safe in skilled hands, but it is a respiratory de-

pressant and the nurse must watch the patient carefully all the time whi
he is unconscious, the pulse and respiration being taken every fiftee
minutes and the colour noted. If the breathing becomes shallow and t
patient a bad colour she should:

1. Report to the sister.
2. Give inhalations of carbon dioxide and oxygen. This mixture
obtained in various proportions, one commonly used being 7 per ce
CO_2, 93 per cent O_2.
3. Give coramine (nicamide) 1 c.c. by injection. The giving of this drug
usually left to the discretion of the sister.

Ether. A prescribed amount of ether mixed with four ounces of oli
oil, warmed, was a basal anæsthetic used in the past, especially for cas
of thyroidectomy. It has been entirely superseded by bromethol ar
paraldehyde.

Sleeping draughts. Smaller doses of paraldehyde and bromide in salir
are sometimes given per rectum for their sedative effect. The dose is usuall
twice that given by mouth. They are given with a small catheter, so tha
they are better retained.

Suppositories. These are made of gelatine or cacao butter in which
incorporated some drug, usually a sedative, such as morphia or cocain
They are useful in preparation of the patient for examination of the rectu
when pain is present, and also before a sigmoidoscope is passed. A glyce
ine suppository, or soap suppository is used sometimes instead of a purga
tive enema, either for an adult or a small child.

The nurse should wear a glove on the right hand and lubricate the sup
pository before insertion. It should be placed one to two inches inside th
rectum. Afterwards the glove should be well washed with cold water an
soap and boiled. The hands should be scrubbed.

Flatus Tube. This is a rectal tube with the hole at the end. The patien
is put in the left lateral position and the tube lubricated and inserted thre
inches into the rectum. The other end is put in a bowl of disinfectant, fo
example, 1 in 20 carbolic. The tube stays in position for fifteen to twent
minutes, and the nurse should be able to report if the patient obtains relie
by the passing of flatus. It is a good plan to put a hot water bottle on th
patient's abdomen at the same time.

Rectal Examination. The patient is arranged as for a rectal injection i
the left lateral position.

Requirements. A tray containing:

1. Rubber glove or finger-stall.
2. Receiver.
3. Lubricant (vaseline).
4. Lint squares.
5. Powder.

6. Warm mackintosh.
7. Electric switch (if necessary).

LAVAGE

The cavities of the body and passages leading to the exterior are washed
t for the following reasons:
1. In preparation for treatment and operations.
2. To remove discharge, infection, or poisons.

Rectal Lavage may be ordered:
1. In cases of patients having regular rectal feeds.
A washout is often ordered daily to keep the mucous membrane clean
d fresh and to remove debris.
2. After a barium enema has been given.
3. Before a rectal operation.

Requirements
1. Warm mackintosh.
2. Receiver.
3. Rectal tube, funnel, and rubber tubing, clip and glass connection.
4. Lubricant and lint square. Piece of wool.
5. Lotion thermometer.
6. Four pints of tap water, or normal saline, or solution of soda bicarbonate, one drachm to a pint of water.
7. Pail.

Method. The patient is prepared as for an enema, well covered up and
ith the buttocks to the edge of the bed. The mackintosh and piece of wool
e placed in position under the buttocks. The fluid at a temperature of
° F. is run through the tube to expel air, and the tube is clipped at the
wer end. The lubricated end of the tube is inserted three inches as the
ip is removed. The lotion is run in four or five ounces at a time and re-
rned into the pail by lowering the funnel: each time before raising and
wering the funnel the tube must be clipped to prevent air entering. An
ternative method is to inject Oiss of solution as an enema and allow
e patient to return it into a bedpan after retaining it for one or two
inutes.

Colon Lavage is ordered in cases of chronic colitis.
Requirements. As for rectal lavage.
Method. (1) The patient is arranged in the left lateral position. The
ctal tube is inserted three inches and one and a half pints of tap water,
a temperature of 99° F., is run fairly quickly into the rectum. He is asked
retain it for a minute or two before being put on a bedpan, into which
e fluid is returned. This procedure may be repeated once.
With the patient well over in the left lateral position the fluid runs round
the cæcum and the colon is well washed out, with the minimum of

discomfort to the patient. A hot water bottle should be applied to t abdomen whilst the lavage is in progress.

Method. (2) The patient is arranged in the knee-elbow position, t elbows well supported on a soft pillow, and light blankets arranged ov the patient's back and legs. As much as four to six pints of solution 99° F. are run in, a few ounces at a time, and returned into the bucket the side of the bed. This treatment is a very exhausting and unpleasant o for the patient and the results do not justify it. Many authorities are i sistent that it should be discontinued. Some physicians, however, st prescribe it. A similar method may also be used with the patient in th left lateral position which is not so tiring for the patient as the knee-elbo position.

Other solutions for colonic lavage are: Soda bicarbonate ʒi to Oi wate normal saline, silver nitrate 1 in 15,000 followed by plain water.

Appendicostomy Lavage is occasionally done in cases of colitis. Tl appendix is brought to the surface of the abdomen and opened. A sma catheter is inserted. Rubber tubing, glass connection and funnel a attached to the catheter. The patient sits on a bedpan, the irrigating sol tion is run through the tube, thus washing out the cæcum and colon. Tl fluid escapes via the rectum.

Colostomy Lavage. It is sometimes necessary to wash out the bow after colostomy. A small rectal tube, attached to rubber tubing gla connection and funnel, is put into the colostomy wound and the war. irrigating solution is run into the bowel and siphoned back into the bucke until there is little residue.

The solutions used are soda bicarbonate (ʒi to Oi water) or norm saline. After the lavage, the colostomy dressing is done.

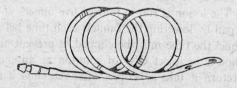

Fig. 23. Stomach tube

Gastric Lavage is prescribed in the following cases:
1. Before operations on the stomach.
2. In cases of poisoning.
3. In cases of gastritis, alcoholism, and persistent vomiting.
4. After a barium meal.
5. In cases of pyloric stenosis in infants and adults.

Requirements
1. Warm mackintosh.

2. Receiver.
3. Bucket.
4. Bowl marked 'residue'.
5. Stomach tube of suitable size, glass connection, rubber tubing and funnel.
6. Lubricant, e.g. liquid paraffin or glycerine.
7. Lint squares.
8. Three pints of solution (or more).
9. Lotion thermometer.

The tube should be boiled before and after use, but need not be sterile hen used.

Method. The patient is usually arranged in a sitting-up position; in me cases, however, the nurse is asked to give the treatment with the atient lying in the prone position with head over the side of the bed. he tube is lubricated and nine or ten inches of it are swallowed by the atient. Sometimes it is found that a fairly large tube is swallowed more asily than a finer one. The stomach contents are first returned into the owl marked 'residue'. Four or five ounces of fluid are run into the stomach nd returned into the bucket, and this is repeated until the fluid is clear.

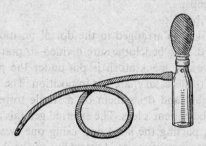

Fig. 24. Senoran's evacuator

An apparatus called Senoran's evacuator is sometimes used. The stomach ube is attached to the side of the bottle. The bulb is squeezed to expel the ir from the bottle through the hole in order to create a vacuum. The ole is kept closed by the finger, and the bulb is released. The con- nts of the stomach are thus emptied into the bottle by suction. The ulb is removed and the contents emptied into the bowl marked 'residue'; ur or five ounces of fluid are then poured into the bottle and allowed run into the stomach, which is emptied by suction as before. This rocess is repeated as often as necessary. It is claimed that the washout more thoroughly done by this method.

Lotions used. Water, soda bicarbonate solution $\mathfrak{Z}$i—Oi of water, normal aline, hydrogen peroxide $\mathfrak{Z}$i to the pint; in cases of poisoning the appro- riate antidote is used.

If continuous gastric lavage is required as in some cases of persisten vomiting, a Ryle's tube is left in the stomach. Small quantities of fluid ar injected every half an hour by means of a syringe—and are aspirated als by the syringe, thus keeping the stomach clean and empty.

Bladder Lavage is prescribed for the following conditions:

1. Cystitis.
2. Hæmorrhage.
3. After operations such as prostatectomy.
4. In cases where a catheter has been fixed in the bladder.

Requirements (for female).

1. Warm mackintosh and receiver.
2. Electric light (if necessary).
3. Measure bowl.
4. Two sterile catheters in a sterile bowl. Tubing, glass connection an funnel (all sterile).
5. Dry sterile wool swabs; swabs in warm boracic lotion.
6. Sterile towel.
7. Two pints of irrigating solution.
8. Lotion thermometer.
9. Lifting forceps.
10. Bucket or bowl.

Method. The patient is arranged in the dorsal position with the knee flexed and abducted. The bedclothes are divided so that the genitals onl are exposed. The warm mackintosh is put under the patient's buttock Receiver and light (if necessary) are put in position. The nurse then scrub her hands thoroughly and dries them on a sterile towel which she the arranges between the patient's legs. The external genitals are swabbed fro above downwards, parting the labia and using one swab only once, di carding it into the receiver after use. At least five swabs should be used. Th catheter is passed two inches into the bladder, and the urine runs into th measure bowl. The glass connection, tubing, and funnel are then attache to the catheter. Two or three ounces of irrigating fluid are run into th bladder, the funnel inverted over the bucket and the fluid returned. Th procedure is repeated until the two pints have been used. Each time befor raising and lowering the funnel the tube must be clipped near the funne to prevent the entrance of air.

Lotions used: Sterile saline; boracic lotion and boiled water, $\bar{a}\,\bar{a}$; silv nitrate solution 1 in 15,000; potassium permanganate, two crystals to on pint of water.

Temperature of solution (a) For cleansing purposes 99° F. (b) F hæmorrhage 118° F.

THE ADMINISTRATION OF FLUIDS

When patients are unable to take sufficient fluid by mouth, as in cases f extreme shock, hæmatemesis, oesophageal obstruction, and after opera-ions on the stomach, it may be introduced into the body in one of the ollowing ways:

Into the Rectum. The position of the patient and the requirements are he same as for giving an enema by the tube and funnel method. A small atheter (size 8 or 10, Jacques' pattern) is usually used, and the fluids given re normal saline, glucose 6% solution or equal quantities of each of hese. Experiment has shown that the mucous lining of the rectum absorbs hese fluids very satisfactorily.

Method. A pint of fluid is given at a temperature of 99° F. It is run in lowly, the time taken should be about twenty minutes, the flow being egulated by a clip. It is more satisfactory to put the solution into a Lane 3ag (see Fig. 25), douche can, or other similar container, and run it into he rectum, using a glass drip connection. If this method is used, the fluid hould be prepared at a temperature of 120° F., and the rate of flow should oe regulated to sixty drips per minute. Up to five pints of fluid can be absorbed per rectum before it shows sign of irritation.

Into the Subcutaneous Tissues. This is a sterile procedure. The fluid is absorbed more quickly by this method than by the rectum, and it has been, and still is, extensively used.

Requirements

1. Mackintosh.
2. Receiver.
3. Sterile towels.
4. Lifting forceps in sterile solution or disinfectant.
5. Skin cleaning materials (methylated ether, liquor iodi, 2 per cent).
6. Sterile sponges, large piece of sterile wool.
7. Two sterile gallipots.
8. Zinc oxide strapping.
9. Sterile container, such as rubber bag (Lane pattern), sterile rubber tubing, Y-shaped glass connection, two sharp hollow needles and three clips. *N.B.* If needles with taps are used one clip only is re-quired for the main tube.
10. Rubber hot water bottle with woollen cover if Lane Bag is used.
11. Flasks of hot and cold sterile normal saline.
12. Sterile measure jug and lotion thermometer.

Method. The saline is prepared sterile at a temperature of 120° F., poured into the bag or container and hung on a screen or infusion stand at a height above the patient's head, the tube leading from the bag being clipped off. The nurse who is to give the treatment scrubs her hands and

G

dries them on a sterile towel. She then assembles the rest of the apparatus Y connection, tubing, needles, and clips, attaching them to the bag; the second nurse assisting runs the fluid through the needles by releasing the clips, each one being tested separately to make sure it is patent. The first nurse cleanses the areas where the needles are to be inserted, usually the tissues of the axillæ, or the front of the thighs, using methylated ether and iodine 2 per cent. She gathers up the flesh with her left thumb and fore-finger and, while the fluid is running through, inserts the first needle below the skin in a slanting direction. Her assistant fixes the needle in position with a piece of strapping. The fluid is run through the second needle which is placed similarly in the opposite axilla or thigh, as the case may be. The large piece of wool is put over the chest if the axillæ are used, and is kept in position by the patient's gown. The rate of flow is

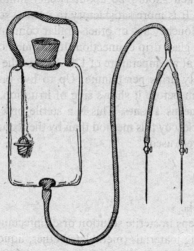

FIG. 25. Apparatus for subcutaneous infusion (Lane Bag)

regulated by the taps or clips. No drip connection is used, and the fluid is run in fairly quickly, twenty to thirty minutes being allowed for one pint. If the fluid is absorbed slowly the flow must be regulated until it disperses. The nurse should remember to feel round the patient's back to see that it is not accumulating there. A second or third pint of fluid may be given in this way, according to the amount the patient can absorb.

The subcutaneous method is a quick and efficacious way of relieving shock after operations, and it can be done by the nurse without any help from the surgeon.

Precautions. 1. Asepsis during the whole procedure is very important.

2. The fluid should reach the patient at 100° F., and the chest should be kept warm if the axillæ are used.

3. If the fluid is too hot, sloughing of the tissues will occur.

For babies a few ounces of saline can be given into the subcutaneous tissues by means of a 20 c.c. syringe; full aseptic precautions must be taken.

After the infusion is finished, the punctures are painted with iodine and sealed with strapping.

Into the Peritoneum. This is a reliable method of giving fluid, especially to babies suffering from diarrhœa and vomiting.

Requirements
1. Mackintosh and receiver.
2. Sterile towels and sponges; lifting forceps in disinfectant.
3. Skin cleaning materials.
4. Sterile bowl of saline, lotion thermometer and sterile jug.
5. Record syringe, 10 c.c. or 20 c.c. and two long sharp needles (sterile).
6. Strapping.
7. Sterile flasks of hot and cold normal saline.

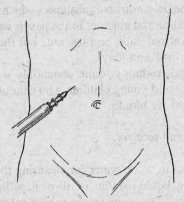

FIG. 26. Giving saline by the intraperitoneal route

Method. The saline is prepared in the jug at 105° F. The nurse scrubs her hands and dries them on a sterile towel. After the mackintosh and sterile towel have been arranged in position and the patient's skin prepared and cleansed she gathers up a fold of the abdominal wall to the side of the midline between the thumb and fingers of the left hand at about the level of the umbilicus. The needle is inserted in a slanting direction through the abdominal wall into the peritoneal cavity. She then draws up the prepared saline into the syringe which has previously been rinsed with saline, and attaches it to the needle, expels the air and injects the fluid into the peritoneum. Six to ten ounces of fluid may be given in this way, the syringe being disconnected and refilled as required. The needle is withdrawn and the puncture painted with iodine and sealed with strapping.

During an abdominal operation the surgeon sometimes pours a few ounces of sterile saline into the abdominal cavity before the peritoneum is sewn up, as absorption by this method is quick and has a restorative effect on the patient. The saline should be at a temperature of 105° F.

Into the Veins. This method is described in the next chapter as it is not a treatment done by the nursing staff.

ARTIFICIAL FEEDING

There are many conditions in which a patient is unable to take food by mouth, and an alternative route must be chosen. Conditions in which artificial feeding may be necessary are:

1. Diseases of the stomach, e.g. gastric ulcer with hæmatemesis.
2. Infants who cannot suck or swallow.
3. Unconscious patients.
4. After some operations on the mouth.
5. Œsophageal obstruction (e.g. carcinoma).

By the Rectum. This has already been described as a method of giving fluid to a patient. The only nutritive substances which are absorbed by the rectum are normal saline and glucose. In the past it was customary to give such fluids as pancreatized milk, beef tea, etc., but these are not absorbed and are never prescribed nowadays.

By the Nose. Nasal feeding is quite commonly used for unconscious patients or for babies and young children who cannot be induced to take sufficient nourishment by mouth.

Requirements

1. Mackintosh and receiver.
2. Diet cloth.
3. Wisps of wool in warm water for cleansing the nostrils.
4. Lubricant, e.g. liquid paraffin, or olive oil, gallipot and lint squares.
5. Nasal catheter, glass connection, rubber tubing and glass funnel, all boiled and placed in a clean bowl of cold water (not sterile).
6. Clip.
7. Two or three ounces of drinking water.
8. Feed prepared and strained; food thermometer.
9. Medicines, if prescribed.
10. Gag and tongue forceps.
11. Vomit bowl.
12. Swabs of dry wool.
13. Lanoline.

Method. If the patient is a child roll him in a blanket with the arms to the side, and arrange him in as comfortable a position as possible. Protect the bed with mackintosh and put the diet cloth over it. The nurse then washes her hands and dries them. The nostrils are cleansed with the wisps of wool. The tube is lubricated for eight to ten inches and directed along

100

the floor of the nose in a backward direction, being pushed down until it enters the stomach. There is very little danger of it entering the trachea, but if it should do so the patient will become distressed and cough violently, in which case the tube should be withdrawn. Usually there is a little cough and slight discomfort as the tube passes the back of the pharynx which is sensitive, but after this point it is usually swallowed quite easily. The tube should be a new and fairly rigid one otherwise it may pass through the naso-pharynx and curl up in the mouth. It is important to look carefully to see that this has not happened. When the tube is in the stomach a gurgling sound is heard through the funnel due to peristaltic action moving the contents of the stomach. When the nurse is satisfied that the tube is in the correct position, a little drinking water is run through it and then the feed (usually eight to ten ounces of some strained milky fluid) at a temperature of 100° F. When the feed is finished the remains of the drinking water are given and any medicines prescribed can conveniently be given while the catheter is in position. The tube is then withdrawn quickly by pulling in a downward direction. The nostrils are cleansed and dried very carefully with wool, and a little lanoline is smeared round the area to prevent irritation. Gag and tongue forceps should be at hand where the patient is restless, delirious or liable to have a fit. Feeds are given six-hourly.

By the Œsophagus. This method is very similar to the nasal one and is used in those cases where a catheter cannot be passed into the nose owing to obstruction. This method is preferred in cases of infants as it may not be possible to obtain a sufficiently small tube to pass through the nose.

Requirements. Requirements are the same as for a nasal feed except that

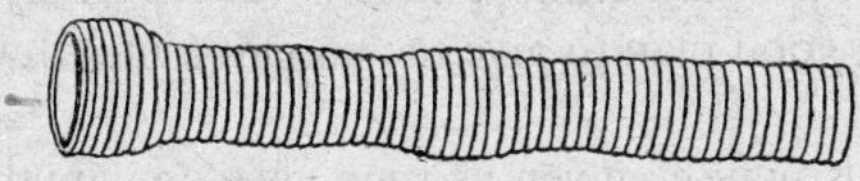

(a)

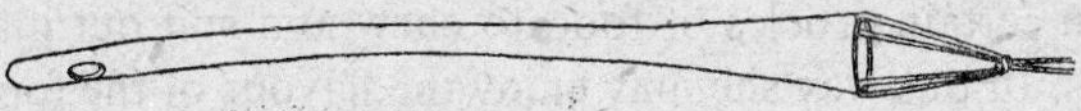

(b)

Fig. 27. Œsophageal tubes used in feeding patients with strictures of the œsophagus.

(a) Souttar's flexible gilt wire tube introduced into the œsophagus through an œsophagoscope and left in position indefinitely.
(b) Symond's silk web tube. This tube is put in position by a special introducer and the cords are secured to the side of the cheek.

a tube of a suitable size according to the age of the patient is chosen. The mouth must be cleansed beforehand and suitable materials and mouthwash are required.

Method. The method is also the same except that the tube is passed over the tongue into the pharynx and down the œsophagus. The same care must be taken to ensure that the tube is in the stomach before any food is passed.

By Gastrostomy Tube. In cases of œsophageal obstruction where neither fluid nor tube can be passed via the œsophagus, the surgeon makes an opening directly into the stomach through the abdominal wall. A catheter, about size 6, is passed obliquely through the walls of the stomach, and stitched in position. A sterile dressing is applied and the catheter either clipped or closed by a spigot. The feeds given through the tube must be sterile for the first five days, until healing has taken place. The first feed is often given by the surgeon in the theatre to make sure that the tube is in a satisfactory position.

Requirements

1. Mackintosh and receiver.
2. Glass funnel in clean water.
3. A few ounces of drinking water.
4. The feed strained through gauze.
5. Food thermometer and mouthwash.

Method. The nurse washes and dries her hands, releases the clip or spigot and attaches the funnel to the catheter. She runs a little water, then the feed at a temperature of 100° F. slowly followed by a little more water, into the stomach. Medicines are given as prescribed. When finished, the clip or spigot is fixed in position and the tube is tucked safely in the folds of the bandage. It is a good plan to give the patient a mouthwash at the time of the feed.

A variety of feeds may be given as time goes on; anything the patient fancies such as soup, tea, coffee, milky fluids, meat juice, in fact, any food which will pass down the tube without causing obstruction. The patient may be given certain articles of food to chew and spit out into a bowl if she so wishes. In this way she may enjoy the flavour of the food.

If gastrostomy is to be continued for any length of time the calorific value of the food should be estimated, to make sure that the patient is having sufficient (approximately 1,500—2,000 calories). Also she can learn to feed herself quite easily. The tube is taken out from time to time, and a fresh one inserted.

Inunction. The nutrition of a premature or jaundiced infant can be aided by rubbing oils into the skin. A warm bath should be given first, in a warm room, before a fire if possible. The warm water opens the pores. The nurse wears gloves and rubs olive oil, previously warmed, into the skin. The method of inunction is also used for treating congenital syphilis in infants. The prescribed amount (usually about the size of a pea) of a mercurial ointment (ung. hydrarg.) is rubbed into a different area of the skin each day, the axillæ, groins, and abdomen being the sites usually chosen. The nurse should wear gloves so that she does not absorb the mercury herself. The child's gums should be watched for signs of mercurial poisoning.

INHALATIONS

Inhalations of drugs are ordered for such conditions as colds, sinusitis, laryngitis, bronchitis and bronchiectasis. The drugs prescribed are usually antiseptics, e.g. friar's balsam (tinct. benzoin co.), camphor, eucalyptus, menthol; various combinations of these drugs are prescribed in the form of inhalants. The solution may be dripped on to a wool swab, wrapped in gauze and tied into a little ball by means of cotton. The patient is told to inhale frequently. Antiseptic powders or lotions such as orthoform and adrenalin may be introduced into the nasopharynx and back of the throat by

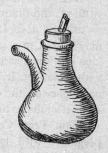

FIG. 28.
Nelson's inhaler.

means of an insufflator, similar to a scent spray. The medicament is put into the bottle; the nurse introduces the nozzle into the mouth or nose and usually gives six doses by squeezing the bulb half a dozen times.

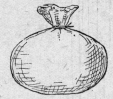

FIG. 29. Inhalant swab

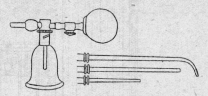

FIG. 30. Insufflator

Inhalations with steam. A Nelson's inhaler is commonly used. It is first warmed and the glass mouthpiece boiled. Half a pint of boiling water is put into the inhaler, then a teaspoonful of tinct. benzoin co., and another half a pint of water. This ensures thorough mixing and prevents the jug becoming coated with the drug. The mouthpiece is firmly fixed in and the inhaler covered with a flannel cover. If this is not available a towel should be pinned securely around it. The windows in the vicinity are closed, the patient made comfortable, usually sitting up, and the bed protected with a mackintosh. The inhaler is given to the patient in an enamel bowl, so that if an accident should occur both patient and bed are well protected. The patient puts the glass mouthpiece in her mouth and breathes through it. The spout for the escape of steam is directed away from her, her head

is covered with a blanket or shawl, and a face towel should be handy t
wipe the forehead and face as required. The treatment lasts for about te
minutes, after which the patient should be kept very warm for some time
The inhaler should be emptied at once down a drain, otherwise the sin
will become sticky and brown with the friar's balsam. The inhaler shoul
then be mopped out thoroughly with boiling water and the mouthpiec
boiled.

If a Nelson's inhaler is not available, a wide-mouthed jug may be sub
stituted, and the patient is instructed to breathe in the steam through th
mouth and nose. In cases of sinusitis, the boiling water and friar's balsar
may be put in a large bowl and the patient instructed to put the whol
face into the steam and breathe in and out. The head should be covere
with a blanket. By this method the steam thoroughly penetrates the nose
nasopharynx, throat, and sinuses and is found more effective than th
Nelson's inhaler in these cases.

Steam Tent. Certain cases are nursed in a steamy atmosphere im
pregnated with drugs. In these cases a tent is erected round the bed o

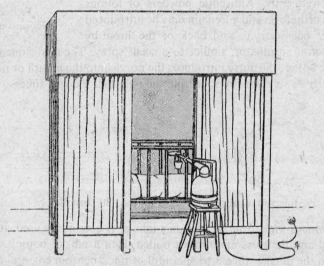

Fig. 31. Steam Tent

cot by means of screens and sheets. The treatment is most commonl
ordered for babies suffering from bronchitis or severe burns or scalds o
the throat. Also after tracheotomy the steam tent is a great help in nursing
as the air is warmed and moistened before entering the trachea. Ches
complications are avoided in this way.

Method. The tent is erected with an opening arranged at the side for nur
sing treatment. The special steam kettle, which has an elongated spout with
a fan-shaped end, is filled with boiling water and heated either by electri

current or methylated stove. If the latter is used a bowl of sand and a rug should be kept under the bed in case of accident. The water is kept boiling and the spout should face into the corner of the tent away from the patient, so that the steam circulates round the tent. A mackintosh should be placed on the bed under the spout of the kettle to catch the drips of moisture unless there is a special little bowl attached for this purpose. Drugs (friar's balsam, menthol, etc.) are put into the water as ordered. A thermometer should be placed over the head of the patient and the tent kept at an even temperature of 75° F. The patient should be kept sitting up, and if he is a restless child the nurse should be there all the time. When the treatment is discontinued, the screens are still left in position and the windows kept closed for some time so that the patient gradually becomes accustomed to the cooler atmosphere of the room or ward.

N.B. When the kettle needs to be refilled boiling water should be used to avoid a sudden fall in the temperature of the tent.

Administration of Oxygen

Inhalations of oxygen are prescribed in the following cases:
1. Pneumonia.
2. Certain cases of heart failure.
3. Shock.

It may be administered in the following ways:
1. By tube and funnel.
2. By nasal catheter.
3. By Tudor Edwards's spectacles.
4. By B.L.B. mask.
5. By oxygen tent.

Of these methods the tube and funnel method is obsolete. It is wasteful and ineffective. In certain cases of emergency, however, the rubber tube attached to the cylinder can be put to the back of the patient's mouth.

By Nasal Catheter

Requirements
1. Receiver.
2. Nasal catheter, glass connection and rubber tubing.
3. Cylinder and key.
4. Woolf's bottle, half full of hot water standing in a bowl of warm water.
6. Wisps of wool in warm water and dry wool swabs.
7. Lubricant, lint squares, strapping and lanoline; safety pin.

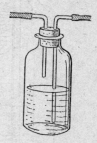

Fig. 32.
Woolf's Bottle

Method. The oxygen and nasal tubes are attached to the Woolf's bottle,

105

making sure that the glass tube to which the rubber tubing going to the patient is joined is well above the level of the water. The nostril is first cleaned. The oxygen is turned on and tested before it is brought to the patient. It should bubble through the water as fast as possible, short of blowing out the rubber bung of the bottle. The catheter is lubricated and inserted in a backwards direction for two inches and then strapped to the patient's temple and fixed by means of a safety pin to the pillow. This is a comfortable method of giving oxygen, and a concentration of 30 per cent oxygen reaches the patient.

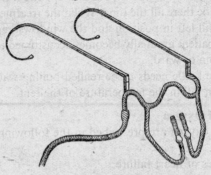

FIG. 33. Nasal Spectacles

Tudor Edwards's spectacles (see diagram). The same requirements are prepared as for giving oxygen by means of a nasal catheter, except that two small rubber tubes are attached to the spectacle frame, one for insertion in each nostril. A concentration of about 37 per cent is obtained by this method.

B.L.B. mask. This is the latest method of administering oxygen and by far the most efficient. The apparatus consists of a rubber bag, a face piece which can be modelled to the shape of the face to ensure a perfect fit; by means of a spring adjustment a tube is connected to the cylinder and there are four portholes to regulate the amount of air and oxygen received by the patient. The tubing from the bag to the cylinder is interrupted by a flow-meter containing warm water. This serves a double purpose of warming the oxygen and regulating the amount given. In the central metal column are holes marked 2, 4, 6, and 8. If oxygen bubbles through the holes marked up to 4 it is flowing at the rate of four litres per minute; up to the hole 6—6 litres per minute, etc.

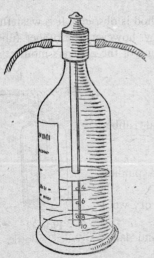

FIG. 34. Flow meter

106

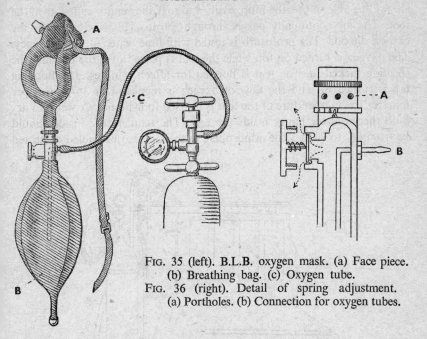

FIG. 35 (left). B.L.B. oxygen mask. (a) Face piece. (b) Breathing bag. (c) Oxygen tube.
FIG. 36 (right). Detail of spring adjustment. (a) Portholes. (b) Connection for oxygen tubes.

The facepiece is strapped to the patient and he is asked to breathe steadily through it. When he becomes accustomed to the apparatus and if all the portholes are closed and the oxygen flowing at 6 litres per minute a concentration of 90 per cent oxygen can easily be maintained. This is a most valuable piece of apparatus widely used in cases of severe shock after air raids and war injuries. It was invented by members of the American Air Force, Messrs. Boothby, Lovelace, and Bulbullian.

After use, the facepiece and breathing bag are detached from the metal part. All three pieces are washed and boiled for five minutes. They are then drained, dried and reassembled.

Oxygen Tent.

For a continuous high concentration of oxygen the oxygen tent is excellent and is specially useful for children who do not tolerate the B.L.B. mask. It follows the principle of the steam tent. The patient is not irritated by wearing a mask and the surrounding air is moist and contains the high percentage of oxygen required (50—60 per cent). No oxygen is lost because there is a long rubber mackintosh underneath the mattress and the rubber sheeting of the tent is tucked well in between this and the mattress so forming an almost air-tight join.

Before assembling the tent, ice is placed in the container at the side. A pail is placed underneath to catch the water. The patient is reassured that she will be able to breathe more easily and that she cannot suffocate in the tent. The air continually passes through 'protosorb' which absorbs the carbon dioxide. The protosorb is tested with lime water for its efficiency. The oxygen is turned on full while the tent is placed over the bed and the sheeting tucked in. The tent is flooded for fifteen minutes. The flooding tap is turned off and the flow of oxygen is regulated at 3—4 litres per minute. The temperature of the tent is charted four-hourly. A wet and dry bulb thermometer hangs inside the tent. The temperature inside should be from 64° to 70° F. The atmosphere in the tent can be cooled or heated

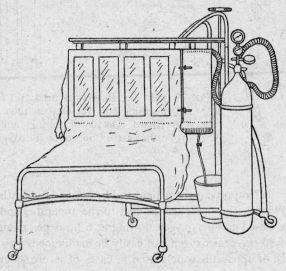

FIG. 37. Oxygen Tent

by ice or hot water bottles as required. Oxygen pressure is generally charted four-hourly at the same time as the temperature of the tent is recorded. The patient is attended to through special apertures in the tent which are tightly tied when not required. The oxygen tent has been the means of saving hundreds of lives from pneumonia, after chest injuries, and after extensive operations when the surgeon has removed a large portion of the lung.

Precautions to be taken in the use of oxygen.

1. Lighted matches and cigarettes, etc., are forbidden. Electric lights, pads and bells must not be used in the tent. Notices should be put up to this effect. Substances which burn in air burn vigorously in oxygen.

2. Alcohol must not be applied to the patient's skin.

3. The joints and fittings of cylinders must not be lubricated with vaseline or oil of any kind, or an explosion may occur.

APPLICATIONS OF HEAT

4. Cylinders, before they are changed, should always be tested away from the bed to avoid alarming the patient. Spare cylinders should always be at hand and the used ones should be clearly marked 'Empty'.

APPLICATIONS OF HEAT

Heat is a physical agent used in the treatment of both surgical and medical cases. It dilates the blood vessels, induces a hyperæmia, helps the healing process, and by relieving tension in the tissues, relieves pain.

Hot Water Bottles. A hot water bottle applied to any painful area is very comforting but is dangerous where the patient is a child or unconscious or paralysed. Its use is forbidden in such cases.

A funnel is used for filling the bottle. Water, not quite boiling, is poured through the funnel until the bottle is half full. Before the stopper is replaced air and steam are expelled. The bottle is inverted to make quite sure that the stopper is firm and not leaking. A woollen cover of sufficient thickness is then tied round it.

The greatest care must be exercised in the use of hot water bottles given to patients. There is no excuse whatever for carelessness on the part of a nurse. They must be so arranged that folds of blanket protect the patient from being burnt.

For warming a bed where rubber hot water bottles are not available, bricks or bags of sand heated in an oven serve the purpose very well.

FOMENTATIONS OR STUPES

Medical fomentations are used for relieving pain. They consist of a double piece of lint or flannel wrung out in boiling water in a piece of cloth called a wringer. They should be well wrung out and shaken before applying. They are put on very hot, covered with gutta percha tissue and a piece of wool larger than the fomentation, and bandaged in position. They should be renewed as often as necessary, every ten minutes if required.

Hot flannels applied frequently in this way over the bladder are often valuable in cases of acute retention.

The following drugs may be added to the boiling water:

1. Turpentine, ℥i to Oi of water for abdominal flatulence.
2. Brandy, ℥i to Oi for a 'tight chest' in bronchitis.
3. Tincture of opium, ℥i to Oi for painful joints.

Surgical fomentations are applied with the technique described under 'surgical dressings', as they are used for cleansing open wounds. Surgical lint is used.

109

POULTICES

Linseed

Requirements

1. Kettle of boiling water.
2. Poultice board and enamel bowl.
3. Spatula standing in jug of hot water.
4. Two enamel plates.
5. Linseed meal.
6. Linen cut to required size, wool, bandage, and safety pin.
7. Olive oil, lint squares, and gallipot.

Notes. (1) The patient should be prepared beforehand; she should be arranged suitably, the bed-gown removed, if necessary, and in the case of a poultice being applied to the abdomen, a many-tailed binder should be rolled in position.

(2) Everything used in the making and application of the poultice should be very hot, e.g. the bowl, wool, plates, etc.

(3) The skin may be treated with olive oil if it is tender.

Method. Pour a little boiling water into the enamel bowl, take the spatula in the right hand and with the left sprinkle in the linseed. Stir quickly until the mixture is smooth and thick. Spread it on the linen, dipping the spatula into the jug of hot water now and again before smoothing the surface. Quickly fold over the edges, put between the two plates and take to the patient's bed. Test it with the elbow and apply it to the patient with care so that it is really hot but does not burn. Cover it with the wool and bandage comfortably. If the linseed is of the right consistency it will come away from the skin without sticking; it should not be lumpy or hard, nor too heavy (about a quarter of an inch thick). Linseed poultices are very comfortable, retain the heat well and are cheap. Linseed contains valuable oils. Poultices should be renewed every four hours; when the old one is removed, the wool is left in position until the new one is applied.

Mustard Poultice. This is made in exactly the same way as the linseed poultice. The mustard is well mixed with the linseed, in a proportion of one part mustard to five parts of linseed, before mixing with the boiling water. Great care should be taken not to burn the skin and the poultice should be removed if any sign of redness appears. Olive oil may be smeared on the skin before the poultice is applied.

Charcoal Poultice. Powdered charcoal is mixed with linseed meal in a proportion of one part of charcoal to two parts of linseed. The poultice is made with boiling carbolic lotion, 1 in 60, and the bowl, spatula, etc., used for its preparation must be sterilized. Charcoal poultices are useful in cases of sloughing bedsores. They are very cleansing.

Antiphlogistine Poultice. The required amount of antiphlogistine (kaolin with glycerine) is heated in a gallipot in boiling water. It is spread about ⅛ of an inch thick on lint or old linen and covered with a piece of gauze. It is a very favourite application of heat for almost any type of pain.

Antiphlogistine is expensive, and nurses in hospital should remember that it is not always obtainable in private or district practice. Linseed poultices are generally as efficacious and much cheaper. One advantage that antiphlogistine possesses, however, is that it holds the heat exceptionally well, and need only be changed every twelve hours. It can also be used as a poultice for small open wounds. The glycerine in it is hygroscopic and helps to keep the wound open, drawing infected fluid to the surface.

N.B. The antiphlogistine should not be spread on the lint or linen cold and the poultice then heated on a radiator or in front of a fire. This has the effect of drying the antiphlogistine by evaporating the glycerine. The result is a hard, dry, less effective poultice. It is also much more difficult to spread when cold.

Other Useful Methods of Applying Heat

Bread poultice. Breadcrumbs boiled in a little water, thoroughly squeezed and spread quickly on linen make a good poultice that holds the heat very well. It is an aseptic form of poultice, very useful in home nursing for boils, septic fingers, whitlows, etc.

Fig poultice. For toothache, or an abscess at the root of a tooth, a cooking fig can be boiled. It is then slit open and packed between the cheek and gum. It is a very efficient application of heat which brings the abscess to a head.

Onion poultice. A small Spanish onion or shallot can be boiled and the end where the stem is cut off is inserted into the auditory canal, after the onion has been well squeezed. This is a homely method of obtaining relief in cases of earache and meatal boils. It is best to wrap the onion in a piece of gauze before applying it.

Nurses in hospital are apt to forget these simple remedies and how commonly they are used in private and district practice.

Electric pads and coils. They are useful for applying heat to eye and ear cases. The pad is heated by means of an electric battery or is plugged in to the main current. The heat must be carefully regulated before the pad is bandaged to the patient. There is usually an indicator marked 'hot', 'medium', and 'cool' which is easily adjusted by the nurse or the patient herself. They can be usefully applied to almost any part of the body.

APPLICATIONS OF COLD

Cold applications constrict blood vessels and are used:
1. To relieve cerebral irritation and headache.
2. To prevent swelling in cases of sprains.

3. To control hæmorrhage.
4. To reduce inflammation.
5. To reduce temperature (ice cradle).
6. To reduce hernia.

1. **Ice Compress.** A double piece of linen or lint is wrung out in ice cold water and applied to a painful area, e.g. forehead for headache. Vinegar or eau-de-Cologne or methylated spirit added to the water makes the compress more refreshing. It is used very frequently after certain eye treatments, e.g. after the granulations under the eyelids in trachoma have been expressed.

2. **Cold Water.** Cold water is used as a mouthwash to control bleeding from a tooth socket.

A cold water sponge squeezed over the face helps to control nose bleeding.

A bleeding finger is controlled by being held under a running cold water tap.

3. **Ice-Bag.** This is suspended from the head of the bed to relieve headache, e.g. in meningitis.

It may be applied to the epigastrium in cases of bleeding from an

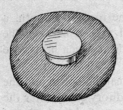

FIG. 38. Ice bag

ulcer, or over the abdomen in cases of bleeding in typhoid fever. The ice is broken into small pieces about the size of a walnut The bag is filled half full and to the ice a third of the quantity of salt is added. The air is expelled from the bag which is then securely stoppered and enclosed in a flannel bag. This prevents the extreme cold from freezing the skin, and absorbs the water on condensation. The bag is refilled as often as required. When finished with, it must be carefully dried and a layer of lint or wool put in the bag before it is put away.

4. **Ice-Poultice.** This is a convenient method of applying cold, e.g. to the nose-bridge in the case of bleeding after operations, or to the face for a bleeding tooth socket.

Requirements

1. Poultice board.
2. Gutta percha tissue.
3. Non-absorbent wool.
4. Ice.
5. Icepick.

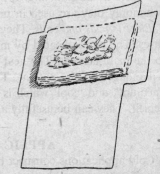

FIG. 39. Ice poultice

6. Salt.
7. Chloroform.
8. Gallipot.
9. Camel-hair brush.
10. Lint.
11. Dish.

Method. The gutta percha tissue is cut twice the size required to make a packet. A layer of wool, half-inch thick, and nearly half the size of the gutta percha tissue, is prepared. Pieces of ice are laid on the wool and sprinkled with salt; another layer of wool is laid on the top, then the poultice is enclosed in the gutta percha tissue; the air is pressed out and the three sides are sealed with chloroform. The salt is added to the ice to lower the melting point. The poultice is bandaged into position with a piece of lint next to the skin.

5. **Evaporating Lotion.** These lotions contain spirit (e.g. lotio plumbi, lotio spiritus, lotio plumbi cum opio). The evaporation takes heat from the surface of the skin thus cooling it and causing the vessels to contract. These applications are used for headaches and inflamed or sprained joints.

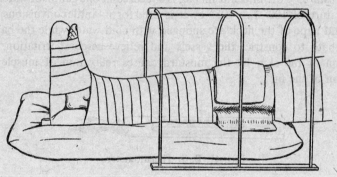

FIG. 40. Evaporating lotion applied to knee

Method. If the lotion is to be applied to a joint, e.g. the knee, the limb should be elevated on a pillow and if possible put on a back splint, covered with a piece of protective material. A double piece of lint soaked in the lotion is applied to the joint and lightly secured by one or two turns of a muslin bandage. The compress is renewed as soon as it is dry. Lotion can be poured over it at intervals. A bed cradle is put in the bed to allow circulation of air around the compress. The bed should be opened at the bottom from time to time to ensure this.

6. **Ice Cradle.** An ordinary bed-cradle is put in the bed and to it are suspended several ice-bags. This is a method of reducing temperature. A special ice-cradle is obtainable; this is an iron cradle under which a tray

is fixed. The ice is put on the perforated cover of the tray and as it melts the water drains into the receptacle underneath.

BATHS AND PACKS

Baths

1. *Hot* 100° F.—105° F. Used for cleansing purposes and to induce sleep.

2. *Warm* 90° F.—100° F. These have a sedative effect and help to soothe restless and excitable patients especially if the temperature is raised. A prolonged warm bath is sometimes ordered in cases of exophthalmic goitre. It is also a good method of inducing sleep in babies suffering from nervous unrest.

3. *Cold* 50° F.—55° F. This method of treatment is used in tropical climates to control the temperature in heat stroke and sunstroke. The condition may be critical and the treatment is a dangerous one. Every precaution must be taken against collapse.

Medicated Baths

a. Mustard. ½ oz. in a muslin bag is squeezed in one gallon of water at a temperature of 100° F.—105° F. It is used for infantile convulsions. The head and nape of the neck are sponged with cold water while the baby is in the bath to constrict the vessels and relieve cerebral irritation. The irritation of the skin by the mustard causes relaxation of muscle and cessation of the fit.

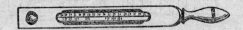

FIG. 41. Bath Thermometer

b. Alkaline. ½ lb. of sodium carbonate to thirty gallons of water. This is sometimes used to remove the scales from the skin before an ointment is applied in cases of psoriasis.

c. Antiseptic. Lysol 1 in 500 is used as an antiseptic bath when a patient has recovered from an infectious disease.

d. Sulphur. 4 oz. of sulphurated potash in an ordinary bath full of water—thirty gallons. Used for scabies and other verminous conditions. Sulphur is a parasiticide.

e. Emollient. Bran or oatmeal are used. 2 lb. to thirty gallons of water. The oatmeal or bran in a muslin bag is hung on to the tap and squeezed into the water, until the water feels soft to the touch. These baths are very soothing for irritating skin conditions, such as serum rashes, or the irritation sometimes met with in cases of jaundice.

One pound of pure starch made into a thin mucilage and stirred into the bath full of water has the same effect.

f. Normal saline. Baths at body temperature are useful for cleansing babies with infantile eczema. In these cases soap or even plain water is irritating, but saline, the same strength as that in the body tissues, is soothing, cleansing, and non-irritating. One ounce of common salt to a gallon of water is approximately the right strength. Baths of sterile saline are also used extensively for the treatment of burns.

Foam Bath used to produce sweating in fibrositis and chronic rheumatism. An ordinary bath is used and into it is put one and a half ounces of a special vegetable foam preparation and about ten inches of water at a temperature of 115° F. A perforated wooden rack, known as a foam distributor, is put into the water and attached to an electric motor which generates pressure. The patient is put into the bath and soon the foam fills it. A cold compress or ice poultice is applied to the head, and hot drinks are given. The treatment lasts 10—20 minutes. The patient is then taken out and the reaction of the skin observed. She is wrapped in warm blankets and left to rest and perspire for twenty minutes, after which a cold shower may be given to close the pores and superficial capillaries thus preventing the patient from getting cold. The treatment is followed by vigorous massage and exercises.

Wax Baths. Used to produce sweating and heat in fibrositis and joint affections. Paraffin wax is heated in a large deep container and the part— arm or leg—is immersed in it at a temperature from 100° F.—110° F., or as hot as the patient can bear. (The sensitivity of the skin varies in different patients.) The limb is dipped five or six times until it is enclosed in an unbroken casing of hot wax about a quarter of an inch thick. It is then quickly covered with mackintoshes for 10—15 minutes. The wax is peeled off and the treatment is concluded by vigorous massage and movements.

Vapour Baths. This treatment is occasionally prescribed to induce sweat-

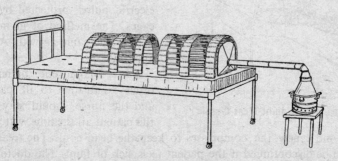

Fig. 42. Allen's Apparatus

ing in cases of chronic Bright's disease and uræmia. An Allen's apparatus (see diagram) with a steam kettle is used. A wicker cradle covers the patient from shoulder to feet. The gown is removed and a long bed mackintosh and blanket are put under the patient and another mackintosh over the cradles. Blankets are arranged over the bed well tucked in around the neck and sides. A thermometer is put inside the cradle. The temperature is raised to 115° F.—120° F. Cold compresses are applied to the head and careful watch kept on the pulse. Hot drinks such as lemon or weak tea are given by a feeder and the nurse should have a face towel at hand to dry the face when sweating commences. After twenty or thirty minutes the patient usually breaks out into a profuse sweat. The apparatus is removed, and the patient dried with hot towels. A warm flannel gown and hot blankets should be in readiness.

Hot Air Baths. Prescribed in cases of chronic Bright's disease and uræmia to make the patient sweat. Allen's apparatus is used without the steam kettle. The methylated spirit lamp heats the air which circulates through the perforations around the bottom of the apparatus. The hot air rises and enters the bed through a large funnel. The patient is arranged as for a vapour bath. A little ventilation is allowed for by opening the bedclothes at the bottom of the bed or the air in the bed would become saturated. Hot drinks are given to encourage diaphoresis and a cold compress and a face towel are required as before. The temperature of the bath is raised to 120° F., for 20 minutes after which the heating apparatus is removed. The patient is covered with a hot blanket and left to perspire for another thirty minutes. At the end of this time she is dried with hot towels, the under blanket and mackintosh are removed and the patient is left comfortable with a warm dry gown and blanket. If perspiration continues these may need to be changed again.

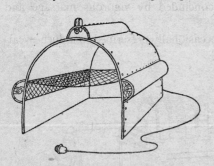

A radiant heat cradle is often used instead of Allen's apparatus. This consists of an aluminium cradle under which are fitted 6—8 electric bulbs, protected by wire cages. The method of giving the bath is the same as with Allen's apparatus.

Note. Diaphoretic baths are often exhausting to ill patients and the nurse should stay with the patient all the time, watch the

FIG. 43. Radiant Heat Cradle

pulse and renew the compresses to keep the head cool. The treatment should be discontinued if the patient feels sick or faint. The doctor will inquire as to success of the treatment and the nurse should be able to report accurately as to whether the perspiration was scanty or profuse, how long the bath lasted and the degree of heat the thermometer registered. Baths may be ordered to be given on alternate days or possibly every day, if the patient can stand them.

Hot Dry Pack. When an Allen's apparatus or electric cradle is not available, a hot dry pack is a useful method of making the patient perspire. It is used in district and private nursing particularly for patients with nephritis and uræmia.

Requirements

1. Three or more hot blankets.
2. Four hot water bottles.
3. A cold compress and face towel.
4. Hot drinks.
5. Hot bath towel, gown and blanket in readiness.
6. Hypodermic outfit and an injection of pilocarpine nitrate.

Method. The patient's gown is removed and the three hot blankets are rolled under her. She is wrapped in each one separately, tucking them in round the neck and folding loosely over the feet. All folding should be loose so that layers of air are enclosed between the blankets. The hot water bottles are put between the second and third blankets at the sides and feet of the patient. An injection of pilocarpine gr. $\frac{1}{10}$ is often prescribed to produce diaphoresis. The head is kept cool by the cold compress and the patient is given hot drinks such as weak tea or hot lemon. As no artificial means of heat is used, the pack may need to be continued for 1 to 1½ hours. The face is wiped with the towel when the patient begins to sweat. When the treatment is finished she is taken out of the blankets, rubbed down with a hot towel and made comfortable in a warm gown and blanket.

As in the case of the hot air bath described above, the nurse must be able to report in exact terms to the doctor the reaction of the patient to the treatment.

Hot Wet Packs. This treatment is more drastic in its results than the hot dry pack, and is ordered to produce sweating in patients for whom other treatments have failed. It is prescribed for patients with severe nephritis or uræmia.

Requirements

1. Two long mackintoshes.
2. Three or four blankets.
3. Three hot water bottles.
4. One old blanket, folded in a drawsheet as a fomentation is folded in a wringer.
5. Bath, jugs of hot water.
6. Hot drinks.
7. Cold compress and face towel.

8. Hypodermic outfit and an injection of pilocarpine nitrate.
9. Stimulants, e.g. brandy, medicine glass.
10. Hot blanket, gown and bath towel.

Method. Teamwork is essential if treatment is to be successful; at least three people are required. The patient's gown is removed and she is covered with a blanket. A long mackintosh and blanket are rolled under her. The old blanket in the wringer is put into the bath and hot water is poured over it. Four people may be required to wring it out, or sticks may be twisted round the ends of the drawsheet to ensure more thorough wringing. The blanket is then taken out and shaken and the patient is quickly wrapped in it. A second mackintosh is then put over the patient and two more hot blankets. The hot water bottles are put at the sides and feet. Pilocarpine, gr. $\frac{1}{10}$ is usually ordered to be given with the pack. The steam from the hot blanket penetrates the pores of the skin better than dry heat and the results are usually good. Within ten minutes the patient will probably be in a profuse sweat. She is taken out of the pack after fifteen to twenty minutes, rubbed down with the hot towel and made comfortable with the fresh gown and blanket. Drinks are given throughout the treatment and a cold compress is applied to the head. The pack must be discontinued if the patient shivers and looks blue, or if the pulse fails. Brandy and other methods of restoring the patient may be required. Pilocarpine is contra-indicated in cases of bronchitis because it increases the bronchial secretions to a dangerous degree (see plate 17).

Cold Pack. This is seldom used in temperate climates, but in the tropics it is prescribed in cases of heat stroke in order to reduce pyrexia and hyperpyrexia.

Requirements
1. Clinical thermometer.
2. Long bed mackintosh.
3. Twelve huckaback towels or three sheets.
4. A bath of cold water, ice and cold compress for the forehead.
5. Bath thermometer. Stimulants and hot water bottles.
7. Cold drinks.
8. Clean gown and bed linen, and a dry towel.
9. Bed cradle.
10. Bucket.

Method. The patient's temperature is taken and recorded and the bed is screened. The mackintosh and a sheet are put underneath the patient, the bed-gown is removed and she is covered with another sheet. A cold compress of lint wrung out in ice water is placed on the forehead. The towels are wrung out in the bath of cold water at a temperature of 55° F. They are applied in turn to the body, one round each arm, one or two to each leg, one over the front and one over the back of the trunk. The nurse

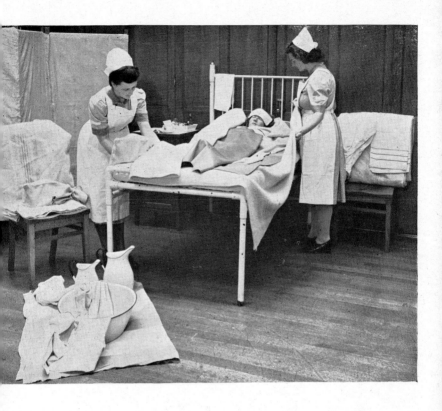

Plate 17. Hot wet pack. See page 117

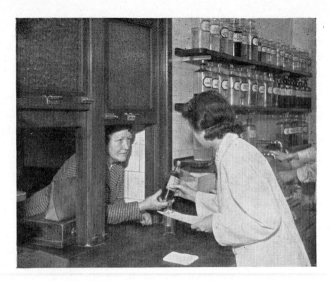

Plate 18. A corner of a hospital dispensary

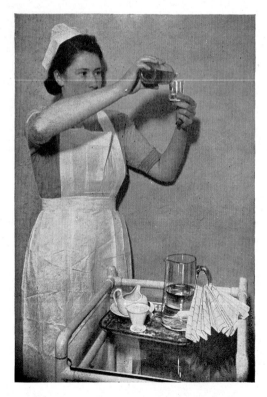

Plate 19. Administration of medicines.
See page 150

rubs the patient down over the towels with a lump of ice, and ice is packed in the axillæ and groins. The bath water is kept cold by adding ice to it. The towels are changed in rotation beginning with those on the arms. As a towel is removed it is put in the bucket so that the temperature of the bath water should not be raised.

If towels are not available, the patient is put between two wet sheets and the third is kept for changing. The temperature of the patient is taken after ten minutes of the treatment and if it is not falling too quickly and the patient is comfortable, the treatment can be continued for twenty to thirty minutes or even longer in the tropics. The temperature should not be allowed to fall below 101° F.

If the patient feels chilly or faint, or if the pulse fails, the treatment must be discontinued and restoratives and warmth applied. With an observant nurse, however, this should not happen.

When the pack is finished the bed is remade with clean, cool linen, and a bed cradle is put over the patient. Fresh air should be kept circulating round the bed, although draughts must be avoided. Treatment may be repeated as often as ordered.

Tepid Sponging. This treatment is frequently prescribed in this country to reduce hyperpyrexia or pyrexia. If well given it is very effective and is a much safer method of reducing temperature than by means of drugs. As well as its antipyretic effect, sponging often helps the patient to obtain soothing and refreshing sleep.

Requirements
1. Clinical and bath thermometers.
2. Long bed mackintosh.
3. Two bath blankets or sheets.
4. Jugs of hot and cold water and one large washing bowl.
5. Two marine sponges.
6. Cold compress.
7. Bowl of ice.
8. Cold drinks.
9. Stimulant, e.g. brandy.
10. Clean linen and bed-gown, face towel.
11. Hot blanket and hot water bottles in case of necessity.
12. An extra bowl.

Method. The patient's temperature is taken and recorded. A bed mackintosh and bath blanket are rolled under the patient, the gown is removed and he is covered with a second bath blanket. (*N.B.* In hot weather sheets may be substituted for blankets.)

The water is prepared in the washing bowl at a temperature of 90° F. The face, neck, and behind the ears are sponged, the hair being smoothed away from the forehead and nape of the neck. The skin is dried with a smooth face towel, using patting movements only to absorb excess water The compress, wrung out in iced water, is then applied to the forehead. The sponge is wrung out in the second bowl, and a piece of ice or more cold water is added to the bowl containing the sponging water. An arm is next treated, from the shoulder to the hand, using long, slow, sweeping strokes, allowing the water to evaporate from the skin surface. Each time, the sponge is squeezed into the second bowl, to avoid making the sponging water warmer. If several large marine sponges are available, the extra ones can be wrung out in the tepid water and placed in the axillæ and groins as these parts are treated. When the arm has been sponged, the excess water is dried by dabbing movements, no friction being allowed in this treatment. The idea is to allow the moisture to evaporate, thus losing latent heat from the skin surface. The second arm is sponged in the same way, the temperature of the water being reduced to 70° F. by the addition of ice. The legs are treated in turn, and then the chest and abdomen, using long slow sweeping strokes. The patient is turned on his side and the back is sponged last of all. A complete sponging should take about ten minutes, after which the temperature of the patient should again be recorded. If desired he can be sponged all over again a second time. Treatment should be finished in twenty minutes, and the temperature usually falls about two degrees. It should not be allowed to fall below 101° F.

This treatment should be done in a leisurely fashion and is very restful and soothing. If the patient begins to shiver or feel faint, sponging is discontinued; half an ounce of brandy should be given, and warm blankets and hot water bottles applied. Otherwise, after the treatment is finished the mackintosh and bath blankets are removed, and the bed is remade with a cool clean drawsheet and pillow case. The patient is given a clean cotton gown and is covered with a cradle, sheet and one blanket. The amount of bedding put over the patient must be left to the discretion of the nurse, as it depends on the weather and the temperature of the room or ward. The whole treatment is spoilt if the patient is clad too warmly afterwards. On the other hand, in this treacherous climate she should not be allowed to get cold. The fall in temperature after antipyretic treatments is recorded in red ink on the chart.

COUNTER IRRITANTS

Counter irritants are agents which irritate the surface tissues in order to relieve pain or inflammation in a deepseated part. They alter the distribution of the blood, thus relieving inflammation. Methods of counter irritation include the use of turpentine, mustard, leeches, blistering agents and cupping glasses.

1. **Turpentine.** Turpentine ʒi to boiling water Ol. A flannel is wrung out in the mixture, and is applied over the painful area as a medical fomenta-

ion or stupe, covered with gutta percha tissue and wool. It is removed when the skin becomes red and is only applied once unless otherwise ordered. It gives relief in cases of flatulence or abdominal pain.

2. **Mustard.** The making of a mustard poultice has been described elsewhere; it must always be removed when the skin becomes red.

A *mustard plaster* can be made by mixing mustard with flour, in the proportion of one to four, making a paste which is spread on brown paper. This is called a mustard leaf, or sinapism, and it can be bought ready made from the chemist. Mustard applications are used a good deal in private practice or district nursing to relieve a 'tight chest' in bronchitis, or to relieve intractable vomiting by applying the plaster to the epigastrium. The mustard leaf is soaked in tepid water, the skin is well washed and the leaf applied. It is removed when the skin is red. The area is dusted with talcum powder and a piece of warm wool is applied. Medicated wools such as thermogene and capsicum wool have largely taken the place of these homely remedies.

3. **Application of Leeches.** This is an old-fashioned remedy which in the past has been ordered for pericarditis, congestion of the liver, pleurisy and other conditions. To-day almost the only cases for which leeches are applied are eye cases, such as iritis and glaucoma. The leech is applied to the temple. It sucks the blood from the surrounding tissue, relieving pain and tension in the eyeball.

Requirements

1. Mackintosh and receiver.
2. Lifting forceps.
3. Soap, water, and towel.
4. Solution of sugar and water, or a little milk.
5. A leech in a test tube with wool stopper.
6. A piece of lint in which a small hole has been cut in the centre.
7. Dressing forceps, liquor iodi 2 per cent, gallipot, sterile sponges and bandage.
8. Bowl of water containing salt and a bowl of carbolic lotion 1 in 20.
9. Pressure pad.

Method. The area is washed with soap and water: the soap should be of a mild and unscented type, such as castile or white Windsor. It should be thoroughly washed off, so that neither smell nor taste is left behind. The area is swabbed with sugar solution or milk. The lint is then placed with the hole exactly over the part to which the leech is to be applied. The wool is removed from the mouth of the test tube, which is inverted over the hole so that the leech falls with its mouth on the spot where it is required to suck. Its position can be adjusted by holding it with the dressing forceps.

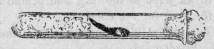

Fig. 44.
Leech ready for application

The nurse must stay with the patient all the time the leech is on the ski until it relaxes and falls off. It is put into saline solution in which it wi vomit the blood, and some idea is gained as to how much it has taken. Th bowl should be kept covered so that the leech does not escape. The bite then painted with liquor iodi and a sterile dressing is applied and bandage in position, using a certain amount of pressure. Leech bites are incline

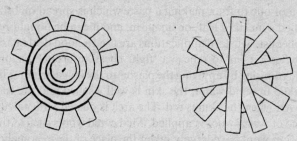

FIG. 45. A pressure pad for application to a leech-bite. Circular pieces of lint of increasing size are secured together by a thread. The pad is inverted over the bite, and fixed in place by pieces of strapping

to bleed owing to a secretion from the leech which lowers the clotting tim of the blood. This is a good thing up to a point, but if it becomes excessiv styptics such as methylated spirit, turpentine, adrenalin or ferric chlorid and a pressure pad may be applied. A leech takes a firm grip of the tissue and should not be pulled off until it is ready to relax its hold. If it i necessary to remove it, salt can be applied to cause it to relax its grip. A leech should never be applied over a superficial vein in case bleeding i difficult to control. Care must be taken that the leech bite does not becom septic. If the leech is not required again for the same patient it is kille by immersion in carbolic lotion. If it is likely to be used again, it is kep in a jar of clean cold water and is not fed. Leeching is an unpleasant treat ment for the patient, and the nurse should distract her attention while i is in progress.

4. **Blistering.** Blistering agents are fluids, plasters, and ointments con taining a substance known as cantharidin. This is a powerful irritan obtained from a species of Spanish fly. Blistering is seldom prescribe nowadays, but it may be occasionally ordered for cases of synovitis of the knee joint In the past it was used for sciatica in which case the blisters were raised along the course of the sciatic nerve. Blisters were also applie to the nape of the neck and behind the ear for headache, and on the forehead for eye conditions.

To apply a Blister for Synovitis of the Knee Joint
Requirements
  1. Knee pillow.

2. Mackintosh and receiver.
3. Lifting forceps.
4. Washing materials.
5. Vaseline and lint squares.
6. Blistering fluid and gallipot.
7. Camel-hair brush.
8. Dressing forceps and sterile dressings; sharp-pointed scissors (sterile).
9. Zinc oxide strapping; boracic and savin ointment.
10. Bed cradle.

Method. The leg is raised comfortably on the pillow. The mackintosh is placed underneath and the painful knee carefully washed with soap and water. The blistering agent is applied in the shape of a horseshoe round the patella, with the ends of the horseshoe directed downwards. Blistering agents should be applied over soft tissues and not over bone. The area is outlined by smearing vaseline around it to limit the fluid to the required area. The horseshoe is then painted with blistering fluid which is allowed to dry. Two or three applications are made. The part is covered with sterile gauze or lint square strapped at the corners or is loosely bandaged in position. Some hours elapse before the blister rises. The doctor usually asks the nurse to remove the raised epidermis by cutting it carefully away with the sharp sterile scissors. The fluid from the blister should be caught on a sterile swab. A soothing ointment dressing is applied or, if the irritation is to be continued, a horseshoe shaped dressing spread with savin ointment may be put on. This contains the blistering agent, cantharidin. The bed cradle is placed in the bed to keep the bedclothes away from the painful knee.

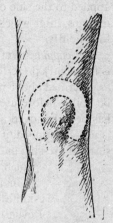

FIG. 46. Area of application of blister for synovitis of the knee

A blistering plaster (emplastrum cantharides) may be used instead of the blistering fluid. The plaster is cut horseshoe shaped and applied after the part has been washed. It is removed after the blister has risen, and the area is treated as described above.

5. **Cupping.** Cupping is an old-fashioned remedy for all types of deep-seated pain and congestion. It has been applied over the kidneys for nephritis, over the chest in bronchitis and pleurisy and is still used in certain continental countries.

Requirements for dry cupping
1. Mackintosh and receiver.
2. Cupping glasses, size and number as required.

3. Methylated spirit and pieces of blotting paper the size of postage stamps, matches.

4. Vaseline and lint squares.

Method. The patient is arranged in position with the part of the body exposed to which the cups are to be applied. The inside rim of the cup is smeared with vaseline; a square of blotting paper soaked in methylated spirit, is put at the bottom of the glass, or the cup itself may be smeared with a little spirit; the spirit is set alight with a match, and the cup quickly inverted over the part. The flame causes a vacuum in the cup which causes the tissues to be sucked up. The part will become blue and congested as the blood is brought to the surface. The cup is left in position for a few minutes, when it is removed by inserting the finger underneath it to allow air to enter. In continental countries as many as a dozen cups may be applied to the side of the chest in pleurisy, and are left in position for ten minutes, after which a linseed poultice is applied. The treatment is done four-hourly.

Wet cupping. Wet cupping for boils or carbuncles is a treatment which is frequently prescribed. After the boil has been incised the cup is applied as described above in order to draw out the pus. In this case the cup must be boiled before use and sterile sponges and vaseline used. After the cup has been removed a hot boracic fomentation or antiphlogistine poultice is usually applied. The cupping in this case, therefore, becomes part of a surgical dressing and is a very useful form of treatment, as the tissues are not bruised as they are if the boil is squeezed.

In the past, inflamed areas were 'scarified' by a sharp knife called a 'scarifier' and several small cuts were made even if pus was not present. The cups were then applied to draw blood from the tissues and congestion was said to be relieved in this way. This treatment is now obsolete.

Bier's Cup. A Bier's cup is commonly used for the treatment of boils and carbuncles. The vacuum is produced by squeezing the bulb.

FIG. 47.
Bier's Cup

OTHER TREATMENTS

1. **Belladonna Plaster.** This is commonly applied to inhibit the flow of milk in the breasts when, for some reason, the baby is not breastfed. It is a debatable point as to whether the belladonna does inhibit the secretion at all, but, at any rate, the application of the plaster and the support afforded by it and by the firm bandaging give relief to the patient. A hole is cut in the middle of the plaster and the edges are snipped to make it fit. It is then warmed. The breast is washed and the plaster is applied fixing it underneath first and fitting the nipple through the hole. The breast is then lifted up and the plaster fixed in position above; a large piece

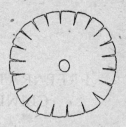

wool is applied and the breast is bandaged
rmly. Belladonna plasters are left on for twenty-
our to forty-eight hours.

2. **Unna's Paste.** This is a favourite applica-
on for the treatment of varicose ulcers of the
g. The paste consists of zinc oxide, glycerine
nd gelatine. It is heated until it is of a fluid con-
stency. The leg is cleaned with spirit and the
aste is spread thickly over the limb with a flat
aintbrush. A two and a half or three-inch ban-
age is applied firmly from below upwards. A

FIG. 48. Belladonna plaster prepared for application to the breast

econd coat of paste is painted on and then another bandage. If necessary
third coat may be applied. The paste is an astringent healing substance
nd as the dressing hardens the leg is kept splinted. It is renewed every
eek, or in some cases it may be left longer.

Scott's Dressing. This is a useful dressing which also acts as a splint.
is commonly used for synovitis and strains of the knee joint. It promotes
e absorption of fluid and splints the knee sufficiently to enable the
atient to walk.

Strips of soap strapping $1\frac{1}{2}$ inches wide are cut long
nough to encircle the limb and overlap two inches
t each end. Lint or linen is spread with mercurial
intment (ung. hydrarg. co.) and cut into strips, the
ime width and length as the strapping. The patient's
g is put on a flat surface with the knee almost straight.
Flexion should not be more than 15°.) The skin is
ashed and dried. A strip of the spread lint is put
ound the back of the upper part of the calf, the ends
re brought forward in an upward direction, crossing
ach other at the front. The other strips are applied
the same manner, each one overlapping the other
y half an inch. When the knee is covered the strips
f soap plaster, which have been previously warmed,
re put on in the same way over the lint. The dressing
then completed by the application of a firm calico
andage, put on in figure of eight fashion. The dress-
g is left in position for a fortnight.

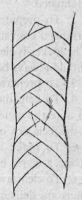

FIG. 49. Scott's dressing to knee, showing strips of plaster applied

Chapter Eight

PREPARATION FOR TREATMENT AND CLINICAL INVESTIGATIONS

Many investigations and treatments are done by the doctor in order to confirm diagnosis or to give the patient relief. The nurse is usually told at what time these are to take place and the following are her duties:

1. To explain to the patient what is going to be done. A treatment which is trivial to a nurse, who is accustomed to it, assumes alarming proportions to a patient who is ill and apprehensive and completely ignorant of medical and surgical practice. Simple and reassuring explanations are a great help to the doctor and prevent the patient from being frightened.

2. To prepare the patient. The bedspread is removed, the bedclothes arranged conveniently and the pillows adjusted to the required position. The locker is cleared, the windows closed and the bed screened. A bedpan should always be offered to the patient before the doctor arrives.

3. To prepare the apparatus required.

4. To help the doctor to do the treatment and while it is being done to note the condition of the patient, reassuring her and attending to her if she feels sick or faint.

5. To make the patient comfortable after the treatment is finished giving a warm blanket and stimulant or drink, as required.

6. To clear away, clean and sterilize all apparatus and to see that specimens are delivered to the appropriate laboratory without any delay and with all the necessary forms, correctly filled in and in order. If the collecting tubes are sterile test tubes, plugged with sterile wool, the nurse flames the wool before replacing it at the neck of the tube, after the specimen has been obtained.

1. **To Take Blood for Microscopical Examination, Cell Counts, etc.**
Requirements
1. Methylated ether, lint squares.
2. Receiver.
3. Glass slides.
4. One or two sharp sterile needles.
5. Sterile tubes.

126

Method. 1. *Dry.* The surgeon makes a puncture either on the thumb, und the nail bed, or on the lobe of the ear. The blood is smeared on the ide and the result is allowed to dry quickly and is examined by the ctor.

2. *Wet.* Very occasionally used for reticulocyte counts. A special slide used covered with brilliant cresyl blue. The smear is covered with a ver slip, the edges sealed with vaseline (to prevent evaporation), and en sent for examination.

2. **To take Blood for Certain other Tests, Sedimentation Rate, Urea, ugar, Wassermann, etc.**

Requirements

1. Pillow to support arm.
2. Mackintosh.
3. Sterile towel and dressings.
4. Receiver.
5. Light.
6. Tourniquet or rubber tubing.
7. Dressing forceps.
8. Methylated ether.
9. A sharp hollow needle and tubing.
10. Sterile test tube.
11. Solution of sodium citrate 3·8 per cent.
12. Gallipot.
13. Zinc oxide strapping.
14. Bandage.

Method. The arm is put on a pillow protected by a mackintosh and sterile wel. It is arranged in a supinated position; the patient grips the bandage d the tourniquet is lightly applied to make the veins at the elbow stand t. The doctor washes his hands and cleans the area with methylated her. He chooses the vein which he thinks most easily accessible and rces it with the needle. The tourniquet is removed and the blood runs to the sterile tube. The doctor takes the required amount of blood (see t below). The needle is then removed, the area swabbed with methylated er, putting a little pressure on the puncture until it ceases to bleed. A uare of strapping may be applied for twenty-four hours.

Blood urea. 1 c.c. to 2 c.c. of blood should be drawn into the syringe and t into a sterile oxalated tube (oxalate does not dilute blood in the same y as sodium citrate).

Blood sugar. As for blood urea.

Wassermann reaction. Blood serum is required so clotting is essential. ve c.c. of blood are drawn into a plain sterile tube and allowed to t.

3. Vein Puncture.

Requirements

1. Pillow and mackintosh.
2. Receiver.
3. Sterile towel.
4. Tourniquet or light rubber tubing.
5. Bandage.
6. Methylated ether, and lint squares.
7. Gallipot.
8. Hollow needle.
9. Short piece of sterile tubing.
10. Glass measure.
11. Zinc oxide strapping.

Method. The method is exactly as described above except that from te
to twenty ounces of blood may be removed from patients who have a hig
blood pressure or congestive heart failure. If the veins are difficult t
penetrate and the puncture is not successful, it may be necessary to us
cutting down instruments as described in the open method of giving fluid
intravenously (see below). This is called venesection.

4. The Giving of Fluids Intravenously.

This is done to prevent and relieve shock before and after operation
and to treat cases of dehydration. The fluids of choice are:

(1) Normal saline 0·9 per cent. (2) Glucose 5 per cent. (3) Gum acacia
(4) Blood. (5) Plasma.

For cases of shock normal saline and glucose are often given. During th
war 1914–18, and subsequent years, a solution of gum acacia was popular
This is a more viscid fluid than saline and stays in the blood vessels
longer time, hence its effects are rather more lasting than those of salin
which diffuses more quickly. The modern practice, however, is to giv
saline and glucose except in the more serious cases in which whole bloo
or plasma is given.

One pint of normal saline is usually given. Larger quantities of glucos
(5 per cent) can be tolerated, but if too much saline is given the kidney
may not be able to excrete the excess salts. Tissue œdema may result, an
this may be a cause of waterlogging of the lungs (pulmonary œdema
Testing of the urine for the presence of chlorides is a useful test for de
ciding if more salt is required.

The Red Cross Blood Transfusion Service has made it comparativel
easy to obtain blood in the quantities required and methods of storin
blood in blood banks at a temperature of 4—5 degrees Centigrade hav
been so perfected that the blood remains fresh for three to four week
The giving of plasma is a recent improvement in the treatment by bloo

ransfusion. It is chosen for those cases of dehydration in which whole blood, with its cell constituents, has not been lost, e.g. in cases of shock, burns, vomiting, diarrhœa and severe dehydration due to loss of fluid by the alimentary tract and skin. In these cases, to give whole blood would make the blood in the vessels still more concentrated.

Administration of Intravenous Fluids by the Drip Method

Requirements

1. Mackintosh and receiver.
2. Lifting forceps.
3. Sterile towel and dressings.
4. Splint, wool and bandage.
5. Pillow.
6. Sphygmomanometer or tourniquet.
7. Skin-cleaning materials: Methylated ether, 2 per cent iodine, two sterile dishes, two gallipots, and lint squares.
8. Local anæsthetic, hypodermic syringe and needles.
9. Vacoliter packet containing: Intravenous needle, glass connections—drip and plain—rubber tubing and glass tubing to fit the vacoliter.
10. Vacoliter of sterile normal saline or glucose 5 per cent.
11. Clip.
12. Strapping.
13. Distilled water or sterile saline.

Method. The patient is given a bedpan if necessary and made comfortable. A table is brought to the side of the bed and the arm, resting on a pillow, is stretched on it. The nurse then applies a well-padded straight splint and bandages it firmly to the fore-arm and again above the elbow, leaving it unbandaged at the region of the elbow joint. The patient grasps the bandage, or opens and closes her fist, if she is in a fit condition to do so, and a light tourniquet is fixed to the upper arm, in order to make the veins on the flexor surface of the elbow stand out.

Veins which may be chosen for the infusion of fluid or blood are the median basilic on the flexor surface of the elbow joint, or one of the superficial veins of the fore-arm, or lower leg.

The process is sterile throughout. The surgeon scrubs his hands and he has a nurse to assist him who will have prepared the patient as described. The nurse hands to the surgeon a sterile towel which he puts under the arm. He then cleans the area with sterile swabs soaked with methylated ether. He chooses the vein into which he will insert the needle, which has two inches of rubber tubing and a plain glass connection attached. A glass connection may be fitted directly on to the needle if a connection of suitable size can be obtained. The surgeon knows he has penetrated the vein when

I

the blood flows back through the glass connection. He then fits on the rest of the apparatus through which the saline is already running so that no air is allowed to enter the vein. Some surgeons prefer to connect the whole apparatus before injecting the needle into the vein. They then lower the part of the tubing attached to the needle so that it can be seen through the glass connection if the blood is flowing. When satisfied on this point, the container is hung at a suitable height and the flow regulated through the drip by means of a gate clip. A sterile sponge is put over the needle which is strapped into position. The arm is kept still on the pillow which is on the bed at the side of the patient. The shoulders should be well covered with a blanket and the patient kept comfortable and warm.

As much as 5—6 pints of fluid can be given continuously by this method and care must be taken when fluid is running low in the container. It must be refilled before it is empty, or the flow will be stopped by an airlock. If this happens, it is entirely due to carelessness on the part of the nurse and it is serious as the whole apparatus may have to be taken down and the needle reinserted.

The vessel containing saline should be a sterile douche can, Lane rubber bag, or a thermos flask with tube attached to it. The *Baxter vacoliter*, patented in America, is now obtainable and adds a valuable measure of convenience and safety to the infusion. The saline or glucose solution is in a sterile airtight bottle of which the bung is sealed by a thin rubber cap. The neck of the bottle is gripped by a tightly fitting metal cap. This is removed and a special glass connection is fitted into a hole in the rubber stopper, or bung, which is exposed when the thin rubber cap is torn aside. Sterile needles and tubing are supplied with the apparatus and the vacoliter is fitted with a suspension wire by which it can be hung when inverted. Although this type of apparatus is so safe and simple to use, the nurse must thoroughly understand other types which she has to sterilize and prepare herself when vacoliters may not be obtainable.

Open Method of Infusion. Sometimes it is not possible for the surgeon to pierce the vein with a needle. If the veins are very collapsed, as in cases of shock, it is necessary to make an incision. In addition to the requirements listed above, the following must be prepared (all sterile):

1. Scalpel and scissors.
2. Two pairs of small artery forceps.
3. Two pairs of small dissecting forceps.
4. Aneurysm needle.
5. Cannula.
6. Catgut and salmon gut and small curved cutting needles.

Method. The arm is prepared as already described. An incision about an inch long is made through the skin over the vein. The tissues are separated with the dissecting forceps and the vein picked up with the aneurysm

eedle through which fine catgut is threaded. The catgut is cut so that two
strands lie under the vein about an inch apart from each other. The
distal one is tied. A small incision is then made and the cannula to which
s attached the rubber tubing, glass connection, etc., is inserted into the
vein directed towards the heart, with the saline flowing through it to avoid
ntry of air. The proximal ligature is then tied in a single knot in order to
old the cannula in position. The tourniquet is released and a sterile
dressing bandaged into position. When the infusion is finished, the dressing
s removed and the cannula withdrawn before the saline has quite stopped
unning. The proximal ligature is tied firmly and one or two salmon gut
utures close the incision in the skin. A sterile dressing is applied. The
utures are removed in three or four days' time.

BLOOD TRANSFUSION

The patient's blood group must be known. The following table explains
he four groups:

Moss Classification	International Classification
Group I	AB
„ II	A
„ III	B
„ IV	O

There are two important factors in the blood called *antigens A and B*.
The blood of persons in Group I contains both of these and can therefore
receive blood from any group (universal receiver). The blood of persons
in Group IV contains neither of them and can therefore safely be given
to persons in any group (universal donor). Persons in Group II can only
receive blood from their own group, which contains Antigen A, and from
Group IV. Persons in Group III can only receive blood from their own
group containing Antigen B and Group IV.

The first thing to do is to obtain blood of a compatible group from a
donor who has not suffered any recent illness or from malaria.

To Take Blood from a Donor
Requirements
1. Mackintosh and receiver.
2. Sandbag.
3. Lifting forceps.
4. Sterile towel.
5. Sterile dressings and strapping.
6. Skin cleaning materials: Methylated ether and iodine 2 per cent.
7. Two sterile bowls.
8. Two sterile gallipots.
9. Hypodermic needles and syringe.

10. Local anæsthetic.
11. Intravenous needle.
12. Sterile rubber tubing.
13. Sterile flask containing sodium citrate.
14. Light tourniquet.
15. Distilled water or sterile saline.

Method. The donor is made comfortable on a couch and the arm i
arranged on a pillow protected by a mackintosh and covered by a sterile
towel. A light tourniquet or sphygmomanometer is applied to the uppe
arm and the skin is cleaned as before. The vein is pierced by a sharp
hollow, wide-bore needle (French's pattern),
through which sodium citrate solution, 3·8
per cent has been run to prevent clotting. To
this is fitted sterile rubber tubing and another
sharp needle. When the needle has entered the
vein, the needle at the distal end is plunged

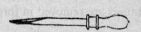

Fig. 50. Intravenous needle,
French's pattern

through the rubber cap of a collecting bottle. This collecting bottle has a
partial vacuum, containing only sodium citrate, 3·8 per cent. The amount of
citrate to be mixed with the blood is in the proportion of one to five. That
is to say, if fifteen ounces of blood are to be collected, three ounces of citrate
are required. The bottle should be gently shaken as the blood is collected.

After the blood has been taken, the vein is painted with iodine and a
piece of elastoplast or zinc oxide strapping applied. The nurse must be
quite sure that the bleeding has stopped before the donor goes home.

The blood may be stored in blood banks, labelled with the date when
it was taken and the group to which it belongs.

The Red Cross Transfusion Service does not permit the cutting-down
method to be used on donors.

Previously to being accepted as a donor, a preliminary blood test is
made for grouping. A few drops of blood are taken from the ear or finger
and put in a small quantity of sodium citrate, 3·8 per cent, and then grouped.

Nurses should remember that although the giving of blood is a simple,
painless procedure, in many cases donors feel nervous and apprehensive.
They should be allowed to rest for twenty minutes afterwards and should
be given a cup of tea before they leave the clinic. It may be wise to ensure
that they have had a meal fairly recently before blood is taken. A well
equipped blood transfusion centre should have a rest room furnished with
couches and easy chairs.

To give blood to a patient
Requirements
(1) Mackintosh and receiver.
(2) Lifting forceps.

(3) Sterile dressings.

(4) Sterile towel.

(5) Splint.

(6) Sandbag.

(7) Wool and Bandage.

(8) Skin-cleaning materials: Methylated ether; iodine 2 per cent; 2 gallipots; lint squares; two sterile dishes.

(9) Local anæsthetic and hypodermic syringe and needles, sterile water.

(10) Sphygmomanometer.

(11) Flask of blood, warmed to body temperature.

(12) 3·8 per cent sodium citrate.

(13) Packet containing: Sterile bung and filter; rubber tubing; drip connection, straight glass connection and intravenous needle.

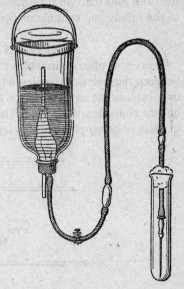

FIG. 51. Blood transfusion apparatus (closed method) showing intravenous needle and gas mantle filter

Cutting-down set (may be required):
2 pairs small dissecting forceps; aneurysm needle; catgut; 2 pairs small artery forceps; 1 pair scissors; scalpel; winged cannula; small curved cutting needles; salmon gut.

Method (closed). The technique is exactly the same as for giving an intravenous saline. Although the blood in the collecting bottle has been mixed with a solution of sodium citrate, it is wise for the nurse to have an extra supply of sodium citrate on the trolley, as some surgeons take the extra precaution of running this through the needle and

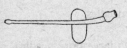

FIG. 52. Intravenous cannula (winged)

tubing before blood is allowed to enter the vein.

Some surgeons, too, filter the blood as it enters the tubing. Various kinds of filters are in use, the most common being the gas mantle filter.

The method of collecting and giving blood here described is by the use of special bottles, in which a vacuum has been created. If these are not available, of course, much simpler methods may be used.

One method is to run the blood from the donor into a glass measure, which has been boiled, together with a glass stirring rod, for twenty minutes. Into the measure, the required amount of citrate, 3·8 per cent, is put and the measure is stood in a bowl of hot water. As the blood is collected, it is stirred continuously with the glass rod. It is kept warm and then run into the vein through a sterilized glass funnel, which is attached to the tubing and cannula or needle.

EXPLORATION OF CHEST

In cases of pleurisy in which it is thought that fluid or pus is collecting between the layers of the pleura (pleural effusion or empyema), the doctor may explore the cavity, using a long needle and syringe, in order to find out the character of the fluid. This investigation often requires to be done in cases of developing phthisis and lobar pneumonia.

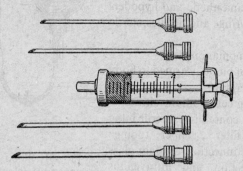

FIG. 53. Aspirating syringe with needles

Requirements
1. Mackintosh and receiver.
2. Lifting forceps.
3. Sterile towels and dressings.
4. Skin-cleaning materials; Methylated ether; iodine 2 per cent.
5. Two sterile bowls with two sterile gallipots.
6. Local anæsthetic, hypodermic syringe and needles.
7. Distilled water.
8. 10 c.c. or 20 c.c. aspirating syringe and two large bore needles.
9. Sterile specimen bottles with pathological laboratory form.
10. Adhesive strapping and collodion.
11. Brandy and cough mixture.
12. Medicine glass and sputum mug.

Method. The patient is arranged in a sitting-up position, leaning forward on a pillow, over a bed table. A warm mackintosh is arranged behind the patient to protect the bed and the patient's gown is rolled up round the neck, and tucked well out of the way, or, if more convenient, taken off. In the latter case, a woollen bed jacket or chest blanket must be put round the patient's shoulders. When the doctor has scrubbed his hands, a sterile towel is put over the mackintosh.

The fluid collects at the base of the lung. The skin over the area on the affected side is cleaned with sterile swabs and methylated ether. After he local anæsthetic has been given, the needle is inserted between the ower ribs into the pleural space. The syringe is attached, the piston withdrawn and the fluid evacuated. The syringe is detached from the needle and the fluid put into two sterile containers ready to be sent to the pathological department. The needle is removed, the puncture swabbed with methylated ether and a square of zinc oxide strapping applied. The patient s made warm and comfortable.

If the fluid withdrawn is clear, the diagnosis will probably be one of tuberculous effusion. In this case, the fluid is left in the pleural sac to splint the lung. This is nature's method of collapse therapy. If, however, the fluid is so excessive in amount as to cause the patient discomfort or dyspnœa, a little may be removed at intervals by aspiration with a two-way syringe.

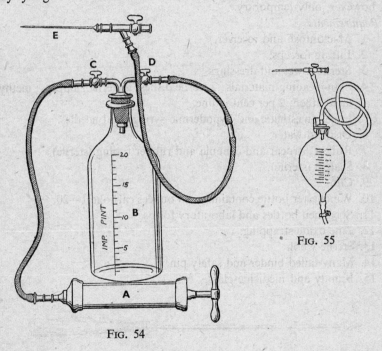

FIG. 54

FIG. 55

Fig. 54. Potain's Aspirator. Vacuum created in bottle (B) by pump (A), tap (C) being open and tap (D) closed. Tap (C) is then closed. Aspirating needle (E) inserted into pleural space; tap (D) is opened and fluid is aspirated into the bottle. Specimen of fluid may be obtained through needle before tap (D) is opened.

Fig. 55 Burrell's Aspirating Bottle with trocar for aspirating the pleural cavity. Suction is obtained by flow of water from the lower end of the reservoir.

If the fluid is purulent, the operation of rib resection and drainage of the empyema is performed. Potain's method of aspirating pus from the pleural cavity by means of a vacuum created in a Winchester bottle is seldom used nowadays, but the principle upon which it works is explained by the diagram on p. 135.

Paracentesis of the Abdomen. This is a method of removing fluid from the abdominal cavity by tapping. Sometimes several gallons of straw-coloured fluid collect in the abdominal cavity in cases of chronic heart failure, chronic Bright's disease, cirrhosis of the liver and inoperable malignant growths in the abdomen. The condition is called ascites. It causes the patient great discomfort, indigestion, and dyspnœa. It is relieved by the method of tapping explained below, or by giving injections of organic mercurial preparations, which aid the kidneys in excreting fluid. The relief is, however, only temporary.

Requirements

1. Mackintosh and receiver.
2. Lifting forceps.
3. Sterile towel and dressings.
4. Skin-cleaning materials: 2 sterile dishes; 2 sterile gallipots; methylated ether; 2 per cent iodine.
5. Local anæsthetic and hypodermic syringe and needles.
6. Distilled water.
7. Robert's trocar and cannula and rubber tubing (sterile).
8. Scalpel (sterile).
9. Clip.
10. Winchester bottle containing ten ounces carbolic 1—20.
11. Specimen bottles and laboratory forms.
12. Zinc oxide strapping.
13. Sterile wool.
14. Many-tailed binder and safety pin.
15. Brandy and medicine glass.

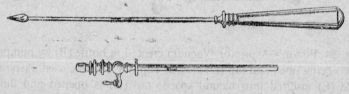

Fig. 56. Robert's trocar and cannula

Method. The bladder must be emptied before the instrument is inserted into the peritoneal cavity. The patient is arranged in the semi-recumbent position, with three pillows, and the bedclothes are turned down. The gown is rolled well out of the way and the chest and shoulders are covered with a blanket. The mackintosh (warmed) is arranged over the bedclothes and folded under, below the abdomen. The doctor scrubs his hands and arranges and covers the mackintosh with a sterile towel. The skin of the abdomen is cleansed with the sterile swabs and methylated ether. After the local anæsthetic has been injected, the trocar, with cannula, is inserted in the lower abdomen, usually below and lateral to the umbilicus. Sometimes a small skin incision is made with a scalpel. The trocar is withdrawn and specimens of fluid are collected into sterile bottles. The tap is then turned off while the connecting tubing is fixed in position. The cannula, with a sterile gauze swab packed round it, is fixed to the abdominal wall by a small piece of zinc oxide strapping. A large piece of sterile wool is put across the abdomen, and a many-tailed bandage is applied, with the cannula in position between two tails of the bandage. The distal end of the tubing should be below the surface of the antiseptic solution in the Winchester bottle. The tap is then turned on and the fluid allowed to escape gradually. Too rapid a removal of the fluid may cause unnecessary shock to the patient. The amount of drainage is measured and entered on the chart. The cannula is not removed until instructions are received from the doctor, and drainage may continue for twenty-four hours. The binder is tightened up from time to time, beginning from below and working upwards.

When the cannula is removed, the puncture is swabbed with methylated ether and sealed with a square of zinc oxide strapping.

If the abdominal wall is very thin, a much smaller cannula, perforated with small holes, is used. This is known as a Southey's tube. It is made of silver and four or six tubes with trocars and fine rubber tubing comprise a set. They are also used sometimes for tapping œdematous tissues.

Removal of Fluid from Œdematous Legs. Œdema is a collection of fluid in the subcutaneous tissues. The skin pits on pressure. The condition is most often found in chronic heart disease and chronic Bright's disease, as part of a general dropsy.

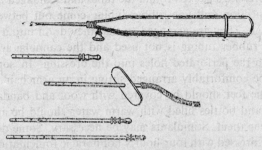

FIG. 57. Southey's drainage tubes

A modern method of removing the fluid is by stimulating the action of
the kidneys by the injection of mercurial drugs, but sometimes the fluid
is removed mechanically by means of Southey's drainage tubes, or by
puncturing the skin with six triangular spearheaded needles arranged with
their shanks in a cork (acupuncture). The legs are punctured in many
places and the fluid pours out from the cellular spaces. The important part
of this treatment is the preparation of the skin before the punctures are
made.

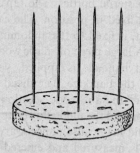

FIG. 58. Acupuncture needles

Method. The legs are shaved if they
are very hairy and are then thoroughly
washed with hot water and soap. The
skin is next cleaned with methylated
ether to remove grease and dirt from
the sweat ducts and hair follicles. The
legs are painted with methylated spirit
using forceps and sterile swabs. They
are wrapped in sterile towels which are
firmly bandaged in position. This skin
preparation should be repeated several
times as the circulation in the legs is extremely poor and sepsis would be
serious. An alternative method of cleansing the legs is by applying large
hot boracic fomentations four-hourly for twenty-four hours previous to
puncture. This method helps to soften the tissues and bring the fluids to the
surface. While the doctor scrubs his hands, the patient is arranged comfortably in a sitting position with high blocks at the head of the bed, to
assist gravitation. Mackintoshes are put under the legs and arranged so that
they drain into a pail or bucket at the foot of the bed. Before the legs are
punctured, they are again painted with methylated spirit, and surrounded
with sterile towels. If the acupuncture method is used, sterile gauze covered by sterile towels is loosely bandaged round the legs and an electric
cradle is put over them. Towels are changed as they become soaked in
fluid. If Southey's tubes are used for drainage, the legs are covered with
large sterile dressings packed round the tubes and bandaged in position so
that the connection and fine rubber tubing come out between the folds
of the bandage. They are arranged so that they drain into a bowl. Alternatively, the rubber tubing is not used and the cannulæ are allowed to
drain through the perforated holes into the dressing. In some cases the
patient can be comfortably arranged sitting in an armchair with the feet
in a bath. The feet should be covered with wool and bandaged to keep
them warm, and bottles filled with warm water should be arranged with
great care near them. Stimulants may be necessary. Some doctors prefer
the legs to be dressed with four-hourly hot boracic fomentations after they
are punctured. All aseptic precautions must be taken.

Lumbar Puncture. This is a treatment very frequently carried out for the purposes of investigation and for the relief of headache. Some of the diseases for which lumbar puncture is performed are: Encephalitis, and other conditions of the brain and spinal cord; for diagnostic purposes, e.g. syphilis.

Normal cerebro-spinal fluid is clear like water. In some cases of infection it becomes turbid and contains pus cells. The fact that the fluid appears normal, however, does not preclude the possibility of disease. The chemical composition varies in health and disease particularly in the protein content. In tubercular meningitis the fluid is usually clear.

Requirements
1. Mackintosh and receiver.
2. Lifting forceps.
3. Sterile towel and dressings.
4. Skin-cleaning materials: Methylated ether; 2 per cent iodine.
5. Two sterile dishes and gallipots.
6. Local anæsthetic and hypodermic syringe and needles.
7. Distilled water.
8. Two lumbar puncture needles.
9. Manometer attachment—in sterile towel on large dish.
10. Sterile specimen bottles and pathological form.
11. Zinc oxide strapping.

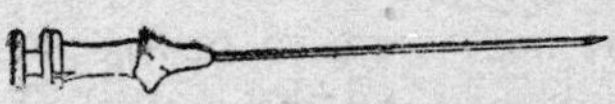

Fig. 59. Lumbar puncture needle

Method. The patient is arranged in the left lateral position with the knees bent up to the chin. The back should be arched as much as possible to open up the intervertebral spaces. It is easier for the doctor to do the puncture if the patient is on a theatre table, which is hard and rigid and of a more suitable height, but the treatment very often has to be done with the patient in bed. An alternative position is for the patient to sit up, bending the head forward between the knees. A mackintosh is put in position. When the doctor has washed his hands he arranges a sterile towel over the mackintosh. The area of the spine on a level with the crest of the ilium is cleaned with the sterile swab and methylated spirit and a local anæsthetic is given. As the needle is being inserted into the theca between the second and third lumbar vertebræ the nurse must help to keep the patient in a position of extreme flexion. Any sudden movement might cause the needle to break. The stilette is removed and two specimens of fluid are caught in the sterile

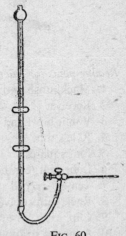

FIG. 60.
Lumbar puncture needle
with manometer

139

containers. Most modern patterns of lumbar puncture needles are pro
vided with a tap at the junction of a metal side arm. After the stilette i
withdrawn the tap is turned off while the manometer is attached to thi
little metal arm by a piece of sterile rubber tubing. The manometer i
held in the vertical position. The tap is turned on and the fluid is seen to
rise up in the marked glass tube. Thus the pressure of the fluid is estimated
The normal pressure is 80 m.m. If it registers higher than this it indicate
that the fluid around the brain is under pressure. The manometer is the
detached and specimens are collected. The needle is withdrawn, th
puncture is painted with methylated ether and a piece of zinc oxid
strapping is applied. The patient is made comfortable with one pillow
The bed is raised on six-inch blocks for twenty-four hours, to avoi
headache, and the patient should not sit up. The bed should be kep
screened for a time.

Test Meals. Investigations are carried out in cases of gastric disorde
to analyse the contents of the stomach at different stages of digestion
There are several varieties of test meal of which the fractional method i
in most common use. The preparation, giving, and withdrawal of a tes
meal is usually entrusted to a nurse. In teaching hospitals the student
often help.

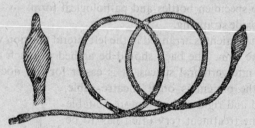

FIG. 61. Ryle's stomach tube

Requirements for fractional test meal
1. Mackintosh and towel.
2. Receiver.
3. Vomit bowl and cloth.
4. Ryle's tube.
5. Lint squares.
6. Lubricant (e.g. liquid paraffin) and gallipot.
7. Ten c.c. record syringe in bowl of water.
8. Rack with twelve specimen bottles and labels.
9. Clip.
10. Adhesive strapping.
11. One pint of gruel in jug (in bowl of hot water).
12. Cup and saucer and spoon.

140

13. Pathological form.
14. Mouthwash.

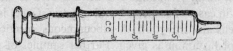

FIG. 62. Glass syringe for test meal

Method. The patient has nothing to eat after ten p.m. the previous evening. At nine a.m. the bed is screened and the patient is arranged comfortably, in a sitting position if possible. A mouthwash is given and a lubricated Ryle tube is passed over the tongue, through the pharnyx and œsophagus into the stomach. The second mark on the tube should be seen at the lips. The tube is secured to the cheek over the malar bone by a piece of strapping. There is seldom much difficulty in passing the tube. It helps the patient if he is told to take short breaths during the process of swallowing. The syringe is attached and the contents of the stomach are aspirated. They are put into the specimen bottle labelled 'gastric residue' and the time, 9 a.m., is written on the bottle. The patient then drinks the warm gruel—(two tablespoonfuls of fine oatmeal to two pints of water mixed smoothly and simmered down to one pint and then strained)—without the tube being disturbed. After this, at fifteen minute intervals, specimens of the gastric contents are taken. About 5 c.c. should be withdrawn each time and put into bottles labelled 9.15, 9.30, 9.45 a.m., etc., until eleven further specimens have been obtained. The tube is then withdrawn by pulling it quickly in a downward direction. The patient is given another mouthwash and may then have his midday meal. It is important that his mind should be kept occupied during the morning. He should have an interesting book to read, so that he does not think too much about the discomfort of having the tube in position. Nervous patients are inclined to retch and eject the tube at the slightest provocation, if their minds are not kept occupied. In some cases the patient may help the nurse by ringing a bell every fifteen minutes when the specimen is due to be taken. Many patients like to feel that they are co-operating in this way. Specimens are sent with the appropriate forms filled in to the chemical laboratory where the result is recorded as a graph which shows the amount and rate of secretion of hydrochloric acid (HCl) and any other abnormality of the digestive processes. The tube and syringe should be washed and boiled before being put away.

Excessive amount of hydrochloric acid (hyperchlorhydria) is found in cases of gastric and duodenal ulcers.

A deficiency (hypochlorhydria) is found in carcinoma of the stomach and Addison's anæmia.

Achlorhydria is complete absence of hydrochloric acid and is found in some cases of Addison's anæmia.

Histamine test meal. Histamine test meal is used to stimulate the production of acid in cases of suspected achlorhydria. Gruel is given and three or four specimens are drawn off. A subcutaneous injection of 1 mgm. of hydrochloride of histamine is given. Further samples of gastric juice are drawn off. In true achlorhydria no hydrochloric acid will be found. In others a flow of hydrochloric acid will be stimulated.

Alcohol test meal. 50 to 100 c.c. of a 7 per cent solution of alcohol in water is given, and the method of withdrawing is the same as for the gruel test meal. From the analyst's point of view the advantage of this method is that the gastric samples are cleaner and are more easily cleared. Some authorities, however, state that alcohol is not such a sure stimulus to gastric secretion as gruel.

Evacuation of Duodenal Contents. *Method.* A Ryle tube is passed in the same way as for a fractional test meal. The patient is then turned on to the right side, so that the end of the tube slips through the pylorus into the duodenum. The syringe is attached and the contents aspirated. They will appear green owing to the presence of bile. Sometimes a strong solution of magnesium sulphate, 25 per cent, is then passed into the tube, by means of a funnel attached. The magnesium sulphate stimulates the flow of bile. It is a treatment which has been tried in cases of gallstones and infections of the gall bladder. In the latter case the organisms which are commonly suspected are bacillus typhosus and bacillus coli.

Passing a Mercury Tube. The patient is arranged sitting up comfortably.
Requirements
1. Mackintosh and receiver.
2. Mouthwash.
3. Vomit bowl, and cloth.
4. Mercury tube.
5. Lubricant.

Method. The patient is given a mouthwash and the tube is lubricated. The tube is made of rubber with closed ends and contains mercury to increase its weight. A small-sized tube is first passed to dilate the spasm of the œsophagus which prevents the patient from swallowing (dysphagia). When a patient becomes accustomed to it he can pass the tube himself. It is passed before each meal and a tube of larger size is passed as the spasm is gradually overcome. In cases of carcinoma of the œsophagus, an X-ray picture taken while the tube is in position will show up the growth.

Gastroscopy. This is an examination of the stomach by means of an instrument called a gastroscope. This is a metal instrument fitted with a periscope and electric light, and is similar to a cystoscope. It is passed into the stomach via the œsophagus, and, by a system of lenses, the lining of the stomach wall may be examined. It is an investigation done in cases of gastric ulcer or growths.

Method. No food is given to the patient for six hours previous to the examination. The patient, sitting in a chair, is given an injection of morphia grs. $\frac{1}{4}$ and hyoscine grs. $\frac{1}{100}$. The throat is painted with 10 per cent solution cocaine. The stomach is then washed out with saline. The patient is put on a theatre table, and turned on to the right side with the head held well back and down whilst the instrument is passed. The nurse holds the head firmly during this part of the procedure. After the examination food is withheld for six hours in case there is a temporary paralysis of the throat muscles. Inhalations of steam and tincture of benzoin co. are given four-hourly while the throat is sore from the passing of the instrument.

Artificial Pneumothorax. This is a treatment performed in order to collapse the lung in cases of unilateral phthisis. Air is injected into the pleural cavity by means of a hollow needle and special apparatus, 500 c.c. being given at the first injection. This is followed at intervals of a day or two by smaller amounts until complete collapse is obtained. The patient has refills at intervals of two or three weeks for a period of two years. After the preliminary induction collapse therapy by artificial pneumothorax is done in the out-patient department if the patient's condition allows.

Requirements
1. Mackintosh and receiver.
2. Lifting forceps.
3. Sterile towel and dressings.
4. Skin-cleaning materials: Methylated ether; iodine 2 per cent; two sterile bowls and gallipots.
5. Local anæsthetic.
6. Sterile saline.
7. Artificial pneumothorax needles (sterile).
8. Apparatus.
9. Adhesive strapping.

Method. The patient is turned on to the unaffected side. The skin is cleaned, the local anæsthetic injected, and the pneumothorax needle, having been connected to the apparatus, is inserted into one of the inter-costal spaces. Part of the apparatus consists of a manometer which shows a free rise and fall as the patient breathes in and out. Filtered air is admitted into a glass reservoir which is controlled by a three-way tap. Water is pumped by a rubber bulb into the reservoir from below and displaces the air, which by adjustment of the tap is admitted in measured doses into the pleural cavity.

PREPARATION FOR TREATMENT

The Meaning of Special Tests

1. *Basal metabolism.* The metabolic rate is important in diseases of the thyroid gland. It is raised in hyperthyroidism and lowered in myxœdema and cretinism. The basal metabolic rate is the rate of metabolism when the body is at complete rest. The test is taken about nine a.m. The patient must have been in bed from the previous evening and is not allowed to have any breakfast nor is he allowed to get up for toilet purposes. Screens are placed round the bed so that other patients do not visit and talk to him. A special apparatus is used, part of which is a breathing bag which is fixed by a mask on to the patient's face. The patient breathes in and out for a few minutes, after which the contents of the bag are analysed. The estimation is made on the amount of oxygen breathed in. This is compared with the intake of a normal individual, taking into account age, sex, weight, and height. The calculation is made by means of tables and is expressed as a percentage above or below normal. Thus the standard being 100 a high metabolic rate would be 150. This would be expressed as plus 50.

Blood sedimentation rate. If citrated blood is allowed to stand the red corpuscles sink to the bottom of the containing vessel, leaving a clear fluid above. The rate of sedimentation is increased in the presence of infection, hence it is a useful test of the progress of the disease in such cases as phthisis and rheumatoid arthritis. If, for example, during the acute stages the sedimentation rate has been high the amount of exercise allowed to the patient may be increased as the figure falls.

Method (Westergren's). 0.4 c.c. of a 3.8 per cent solution of sodium citrate is drawn into a syringe. Blood from a vein is then drawn into the syringe until the total amount is 2 c.c. After thorough mixing the blood is sucked into a standard pipette to make a column 200 millimetres high. The pipette is fixed upright in a stand. After one hour the level of the sedimented corpuscles is measured. The reading is taken again two hours after. In normal health the clear fluid at the top measures 1—5 mm. In cases of active disease the red corpuscles may fall to 70 millimetres. This would be expressed as a blood sedimentation rate of 70. The pipette is often set up in the ward and the nurse is asked to take the readings.

Glucose tolerance test. The patient is allowed no food after supper the night preceding the test. A cup of tea is permitted at bedtime but this must contain no sugar.

1. A blood sugar test is done and a specimen of urine taken. The patient then drinks 50 grammes of glucose in a tumblerful of water.

2. Half an hour afterwards another blood sugar test is done.

3. Three more blood sugar tests are done and specimens of urine are taken at half-hourly intervals. The blood sugar curve should not rise above 180 mgs.

Galactose tolerance test. No food is allowed overnight or at breakfast.

The patient empties her bladder and then drinks 40 grammes of pure galactose in 500 c.c. of water. Urine specimens are then collected hourly for five hours. The six complete specimens are then sent to the laboratory. Normally 0—3 grammes of galactose are excreted.

Occult blood in the stool. Traces of blood from bleeding gastric or duodenal ulcers or growths may be detected in the fæces by chemical methods. For three days previous to the test, the patient has a diet free from red meat and green vegetables. The specimen is collected from a stool uncontaminated with urine. A sufficiently large specimen should be sent. If the patient suffers from bleeding gums or hæmorrhoids the result may be confused.

Urea concentration test. For this test the blood is flooded with urea and the power of the kidney to excrete it is estimated. Nothing is given to drink after 10 p.m. and the test is given the following morning. At 6.55 a.m. the bladder is emptied completely and the urine put into a container marked 'Specimen 1'. At 7 a.m., 15 grammes of urea are given in a glass of water.

At 8 a.m. a specimen of urine is collected and marked 'Specimen 2'.

At 9 a.m. a specimen of urine is collected and marked 'Specimen 3'.

At 10 a.m. a specimen of urine is collected and marked 'Specimen 4'.

Normally the figure rises to 3 per cent, but if it is below 2 per cent the functioning of the kidney is considered inefficient.

Urea clearance test is given to estimate the amount of healthy functioning tissue remaining in the kidney in the presence of disease. 70 to 80 per cent is a normal reading after calculations have been made based on the blood urea, the amount of urea in the urine, and the interval at which the urine is passed. Lower percentages indicate damage to the function of the kidneys. It may decrease to 10 per cent in which case the patient would be in a state of uræmia. The patient is given a normal breakfast, but without coffee or tea. Between breakfast and the midday meal:

1. The bladder is completely emptied and the contents thrown away.

2. The patient drinks a glass of water.

3. A specimen of blood for urea estimation is taken.

4. One hour after emptying the bladder, it must be emptied again (by catheter if necessary). Label this 'Specimen 1' and write the time when it is obtained.

5. One hour later take a specimen and label 'Specimen 2'.

6. Send the two specimens and the blood to the laboratory.

N.B. It is important that the bladder is completely emptied each time. The exact time of the withdrawal of the specimens must be recorded on the label, e.g. Specimen 1—One hour and four minutes; Specimen 2—Fifty-six minutes.

Guinea pig inoculation. Some urine is injected into a guinea pig which is killed a week or two later. If evidence of tuberculosis is found, it is

assumed that the urine specimen contained tubercle bacilli. This test i
also performed at monthly intervals in the case of patients who have had
a tuberculous kidney removed, in order to make sure that the condition
is clearing.

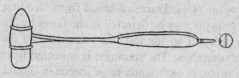

Fig. 63. Hurst's Percussor or tendon hammer with rubber
head for testing tendon reflex and guarded point for plantar
reflex

Normal Blood Count (Approx.)

Hæmoglobin (Hb.): 95 per cent to 105 per cent.
Red Cells: Males: 5,500,000 per cu. mm.
        Females: 5,000,000 per cu. mm.
Colour Index (C.I.) about 1.
Leucocytes: 6,000—8,000 per cu. mm.
Polymorphs. Neutrophil 60 per cent approx.
        Eosinophil 2—4 per cent approx.
        Basophil 0·5 per cent approx.
Lymphocytes: 20—30 per cent approx.
Large Monocytes: 4—6 per cent approx.

Blood calcium	9—11 mgms. per 100 c.c. blood.
,, *Cholesterol*	100—200 mgms. per 100 c.c. blood.
,, *Sugar (fasting)*	70—100 mgms. per 100 c.c. blood.
,, *Sugar*	Maximum after meals 180 mgms.
,, *Urea*	20—40 mgms. per 100 c.c. blood.
,, *Uric Acid*	2—4 mgms. per 100 c.c. blood.
,, *Sedimentation Rate*	*Males*
	Fall in 1 hour 3—5 mm.
	Fall in 2 hours 7—12 mm.
	Females
	Fall in 1 hour 4—8 mm.
	Fall in 2 hours 8—14 mm.
,, *Coagulation Time*	5—7 minutes.

Chapter Nine

ADMINISTRATION OF DRUGS AND MEDICINES

T he standard book on preparation of drugs in this country is the *British Pharmacopœia*. Prescriptions taken from it are marked B.P. Most hospitals with medical schools have their own pharmacopœia in which are prescribed the medicines and preparations in common use in the wards. The hospital pharmacopœia is usually a small book which the senior nurse finds useful in her work.

METHODS OF ADMINISTRATION OF DRUGS

1. **By Mouth.** Many drugs are prescribed orally, taking twenty to thirty minutes to be absorbed. They may be incorporated in a mixture or powder or pill, and examples are numerous.

2. **By Hypodermic Injection.** The advantages of this method are:

1. Quick absorption.

2. For patients who vomit.

3. For unconscious patients.

4. For the giving of drugs which are not absorbed by mucous membrane. These drugs must be prepared in a sterile form. Common examples are morphine and atropine.

3. **By Intramuscular Injection.** This method is used in case of drugs which would irritate the subcutaneous tissues. The needle is plunged deeply into the muscle. Examples are insulin, strophanthin.

4. **By Inhalation.** These drugs are usually prescribed to disinfect the respiratory tract. Examples: creosote, camphor.

5. **By the Rectum.** Drugs are sometimes given per rectum in cases of patients who are unconscious, or inclined to vomit. Basal anæsthetics are also given per rectum. Examples are: bromethol, paraldehyde.

6. **Into a Vein.** Drugs are given intravenously in urgent cases when immediate action is required. Examples: strophanthin, insulin.

7. **Inunction.** By this method drugs are rubbed into the skin in the form of oil or ointment. Examples: mercury, olive oil.

8. **Intrathecally,** that is, injected into the spinal canal by means of a lumbar puncture needle. Examples: spinal anæsthetics and sera.

9. **Ionization.** Drugs may be introduced into the body by means of an electric current. Example: potassium iodide.

CARE OF DRUGS AND POISONS

The rules regarding the care and administration of drugs in hospital wards must be kept conscientiously, both for the sake of the patients and also to safeguard the nurse herself. Great responsibility is placed on the nursing staff who handle drugs and poisons. Therefore, it is of the utmost importance that the most junior nurse in the ward should understand the rules regarding them, and the dangers involved:

1. All drugs and poisons must be kept in a locked cupboard, the key of which is kept on the person of the sister or the staff nurse. It is never left hanging on a nail or even in a drawer. There must be no loophole by which an unauthorized person can gain access to the drug cupboard.

2. Medicines should be kept separate from poisons, lotions, and dangerous drugs so that no mistake can be caused by the bottles being mixed together. Separate cupboards are best, but, if this is not possible, separate shelves in the same cupboard should be arranged.

3. All bottles and boxes containing poisons (that is, all except the ordinary prescribed medicines in common use), must be clearly marked 'Poison' with a red label. Poison bottles are usually of a different shape from those containing medicines. Instead of being round or rectangular they may be hexagonal, or fluted or made of blue or green coloured glass. Thus there is no excuse for the nurse not recognizing by look or feel that she has a poison bottle in her hand. The shape is an extra safeguard for night nurses who have to handle bottles in a dimmed light.

4. Labels, if they become smeared and illegible, must never be changed by the nursing staff. The bottle should be sent to the dispenser for re-labelling.

5. Medicines and lotion cupboards should be thoroughly turned out and cleaned once a week. Bottles which are nearly empty are sent down to the dispensary to be refilled. The nurse in charge of the cupboard is held responsible for keeping up the stock and advising Sister when new supplies are needed. The nurse should have a tray at hand and take out so many bottles at a time, wiping round the corks with a clean damp cloth. She should wash the shelf and return the bottles to exactly the same place in the cupboard. It is a great saving of time, and is also an extra safeguard against mistakes if the bottles are always kept in the same position.

DANGEROUS DRUGS

The *Dangerous Drug Act* was passed into law in 1919 and the nurse is closely concerned in its administration. The law controls the use of the following drugs:

1. *Opium and its derivatives.*
2. *Cocaine and its derivatives.*

3. *Heroin.*

4. *Indian Hemp.*

The reason for the inclusion of these drugs in a special act is that they are drugs of addiction, and in order to prevent addicts from obtaining them the act enforces the following rules:

1. Stocks of these drugs must be ordered in a special book. In hospital the order must be signed by a medical man, the sister or staff nurse of the ward. The book is sent to the dispenser and the drug is sent up to the ward in a sealed packet by special messenger. It is handed to a responsible person in the ward who must sign for its receipt. It is locked up immediately.

2. When the drug is ordered for a patient, one dose is usually prescribed, but as many as, but not more than, four doses may be ordered to be given at specified intervals. In each case the prescription must be signed by the doctor on the bed letter.

N.B. The nurse responsible for drugs and poisons makes an extra check on these drugs, noting the tablets and estimating her stock at frequent intervals so that she can see almost at a glance if more than a reasonable amount has been used.

3. In obtaining these drugs for a private patient the same rules apply. The prescription for each must be written and signed by the doctor and the chemist who dispenses the drug enters the prescription in a special ledger, together with the name, address of the patient, and doctor, and the date.

Hence a definite check is kept upon the supplies and use of the drugs coming into the country.

POISONS RULES 1935

Rules regarding what are known as 'Schedule I' poisons were passed by Act of Parliament in 1935. It was realized that many dangerous poisons, in addition to drugs of addiction, could easily be obtained by the public, and it was felt that these other poisons should also be controlled. So far as nurses are concerned except that other drugs and poisons are included, the working of the act is almost identical with that of the Dangerous Drugs Act. All poisons are ordered in a special book and prescribed and checked with great care. They all have a special label, 'Schedule I'. There is no need, however, for the house officer to sign each prescription as he orders it.

RULES FOR GIVING MEDICINES

Medicines are given by a senior nurse in the ward under the supervision of the sister or staff nurse. In some hospitals it is required that the nurse who is responsible for giving medicines shall have taken a course of lectures in pharmacology and simple dispensing.

ADMINISTRATION OF DRUGS AND MEDICINES

1. A medicine tray is prepared containing medicine glasses, minim glasses, oil cups, and teaspoons, a bowl of warm water; a jug of cold water and a clean medicine cloth (see plate 19).

2. The required medicines are taken out of the cupboard. The nurse takes the bottle in her right hand, reads the label carefully, shakes it and removes the cork with the third and fourth finger of her left hand, holding it there. She then smells the medicine and pours out the required dose holding the bottle with the label uppermost. The label is re-read before the cork is replaced. As she pours out the dose she holds the glass at eye level, taking care not to touch the rim of the glass with the neck of the bottle. She then hands the glass to the patient on a small tray. (It is unprofessional to carry medicine glasses, pills or powders in the hand.)

2. The dose of medicine is followed by a small drink of water.

3. The nurse washes the glass in the bowl of water or under a running tap, and dries and polishes it before using it for the next patient.

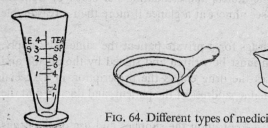 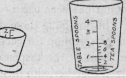

Fig. 64. Different types of medicine measures

The giving of minim doses. The required number of drops are measured by means of a drop bottle or pipette, or are measured into a minim glass. When the latter is used—and it is a more accurate measure—it is held up at eye level. It will be seen that the upper surface of the fluid falls in a shallow curve; the lower surface of the middle of the curve should coincide with the marking on the glass.

Powders and pills. Powders and pills should be handed to the patient in a clean teaspoon on a tray, or a powder is often put into a rice-paper cachet which is given with a drink of water. Certain powders and pills are less nauseating if given in a drink of milk. It is usual, however, to refrain from giving medicines in milk to small children in case they should take a dislike to it.

Castor oil. This is a very nauseating drug and needs giving with care otherwise it may cause the patient to vomit. The oil cup is first heated. Half an ounce of either soda water, brandy, or strong lemonade is put in the oil cup. The required ounce or half ounce of castor oil is then poured in. The dose is taken to the patient with either a slice of lemon or a piece of bread. If these precautions are followed the patient does not usually

aste the oil. The nauseating effect is caused by the oil sticking to the taste
buds at the back of the tongue.

Croton oil. Croton oil is a bowel irritant which is used occasionally as
a drastic purgative, chiefly for cerebral cases or unconscious patients. The
dose is one minim. A pat of butter is put on the handle of a spoon and a
small hole made in it. One minim is dropped into the hole and the butter
smeared over it. The pat of butter is then put to the back of the patient's
tongue; a gag may be inserted to do this. By the time the butter has
melted the croton oil will have reached the stomach.

Aspirin. This drug, so commonly used, is not easily dissolved. It should
always be crushed before it is given. At post mortem examinations aspirin
tablets have been found in the folds of the stomach wall, undissolved and
therefore unabsorbed.

THE ADMINISTRATION OF POTENT DRUGS

These are dangerous drugs and poisons and the precautions outlined
above have to be taken. In hospital the amount measured must be checked
by a state registered nurse who then assumes responsibility for the giving
of the drug. *The procedure is as follows:*

1. The prescription as written on the bed letter is read carefully and the
name of the patient and the number of the bed noted.

2. The drug is taken from the poison cupboard and the dose is carefully
measured, whether it be a dose of medicine, a hypodermic injection, a
tablet or a powder.

3. The bottle is kept out of the cupboard and the stopper, if a glass one,
is inverted to indicate that the dose has been taken out of that particular
bottle.

4. The nurse then shows the sister or staff nurse, who checks the amount,
the bottle, or box from which the dose has been taken, and the bed letter
on which it is prescribed.

5. The sister or staff nurse asks appropriate questions regarding the
patient, to make sure that no serious change has taken place in her condition which might alter the circumstances under which the drug was
originally prescribed. For instance, if there had been some serious change
in pulse or respiration since the dose was originally ordered, the state
registered nurse might think it advisable to consult the doctor over the
telephone before it is actually given. Hence the necessity for an experienced
person being finally responsible for the giving of dangerous drugs.

6. When the drug has been checked the bottle is put away and locked
up immediately.

7. The nurse takes the measured dose, with the bed letter, to the patient
at the time at which it is to be given. Before giving it she again verifies
the name and number of the patient. If this is not carefully done each

time, the drug can be given to the wrong patient quite easily, especially during the night when the lights are dimmed. It is only by the most careful adherence to these details that serious mistakes are avoided.

As soon as the drug has been administered the exact time at which it was given must be recorded on the bed letter.

8. Potent drugs ordered to be given in the night are measured by the night nurse whilst the doctor or sister is in the ward.

When some interval must elapse between the measuring and checking of the drug and its administration, the measured drug and bed letter are kept in the duty room or in some other place inaccessible to patients.

THE GIVING OF DRUGS BY HYPODERMIC INJECTION

A hypodermic outfit is kept in a locked cupboard in the ward with all the requisites for the giving of drugs by injection. On the tray are the following:

1. Two small record syringes, one marked in minims and one in units, several sharp needles and a small pair of forceps, in a jar containing methylated spirit.

2. Lint squares and methylated ether.

3. A bottle of carbolic lotion, 1 in 20.

4. A bottle of distilled water.

5. One small empty jar.

6. A file.

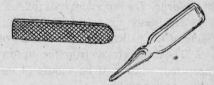

7. Bottles containing drugs in liquid form, and ampoules of drugs in tablet form.

FIG. 65. Ampoule containing drug (with file)

Method. The nurse washes and dries her hands. With the forceps she takes the syringe out of the jar and fits a needle on to it. She then fixes it firmly with her fingers at the hilt; she does not touch the shank or the point of the needle. The syringe and needle are rinsed in the distilled water. She

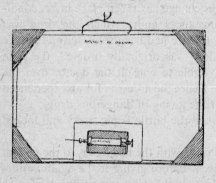
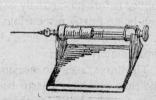

FIG. 66. Drug measured, ready to be given

ext draws up some of the drug in solution into the syringe through the needle. If the bottle is rubber-capped, the cap is cleaned with methylated ther before the needle pierces it. Holding the syringe in a vertical position, he piston is pushed upwards until the exact number of minims or units equired is measured. The vertical position will cause any air bubbles to ise to the surface and as the piston is pushed up they will be expelled.

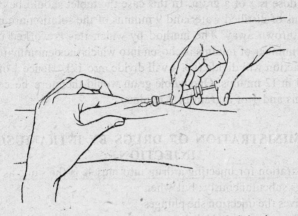

FIG. 67. Method of giving a hypodermic injection

The syringe is rested on a special stand or, if this is not obtainable, on a lint square in a dish. The dose is checked by a state registered nurse as described above. When the dose is due, it is taken on its stand or in the dish to the bedside of the patient, together with the bed letter, a lint square and methylated ether. A fleshy part of the body is chosen, usually the upper arm or the thigh. The skin is thoroughly rubbed with a swab soaked in methylated ether and the nurse then takes a fold of the flesh between the thumb and forefinger of her left hand. Holding the syringe firmly in her right hand, between the thumb and the first three fingers, she plunges the needle into the subcutaneous tissue in a slanting direction. Readjusting her fingers, she gets the right thumb behind the piston and presses it home. The syringe must be held very carefully so that there is no leakage at the point where the needle fits the syringe. The needle is then withdrawn and the puncture pressed with the wet swab for a few seconds. The nurse then writes on the bed letter the time at which the injection was given.

The syringe with needle is taken away and rinsed in the carbolic lotion which is expelled into the small empty jar. It is rinsed in distilled water and then methylated spirit and the parts are disconnected and replaced in the methylated spirit, not forgetting to put the stilette back into the needle.

When a drug to be given by injection is in tablet form, a teaspoon should be boiled. The tablet is shaken out of the phial into the teaspoon and checked by the sister or staff nurse. Six to eight minims of distilled water is measured in a syringe and then put into the teaspoon with the tablet, which is held over a methylated spirit lamp until the latter is dissolved. The drug, now in solution, is drawn up into the syringe and given as above.

N.B. Sometimes the exact dose prescribed is not contained in the tablet. For instance, the tablet may contain $\frac{1}{3}$ of a grain of morphia and the prescribed dose is $\frac{1}{4}$ of a grain. In this case the tablet should be dissolved in 12 minims of distilled water and 9 minims of the solution are used, the rest being thrown away. The method by which this is worked out is as follows: A number of minims is chosen into which the denominator of the required fraction will divide (i.e. 4 will divide into 12). Hence $\frac{1}{3}$ of a grain is dissolved in 12 minims. One whole grain would therefore be contained in 36 minims and $\frac{1}{4}$ of a grain in 9 minims.

THE ADMINISTRATION OF DRUGS BY INTRAMUSCULAR INJECTION

The preparation for injecting a drug into muscle is the same as that for giving drugs subcutaneously; but when the nurse gives the injection she plunges the needle deeply in a vertical direction into the muscle (usually the gluteal muscles) instead of in a slanting direction under the skin. If more than 1 c.c. of a drug is to be injected, the needle must be inserted into the muscle first, before the syringe is attached. The solution is given fairly slowly and again the needle is detached from the syringe before it is withdrawn. Sometimes this is a definite advantage as a little air leaks into the puncture as the needle is withdrawn. This seals the subcutaneous spaces, and prevents the solution leaking into the subcutaneous tissue in which it might cause irritation. After the in-

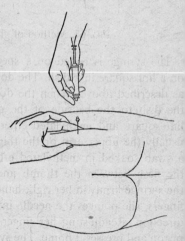

FIG. 68. Method of giving an intramuscular injection

jection has been given the swab soaked in methylated ether is put on the puncture and the area massaged very gently in a circular direction to aid absorption and dispersal of the drug.

TIMES OF GIVING MEDICINES

The usual times for the administration of medicines are as follows:
1. A.c. (ante cibos) medicines are given twenty minutes before food.

These are usually bitter drugs which stimulate appetite, such as quinine and gentian.

2. P.c. (post cibos) medicines are given twenty minutes after food, such as iron tonics.

3. T.d.s. medicines are given so that their effects last over twenty-four hours. In hospital 7 a.m., 1 p.m., and 7 p.m. are often found convenient times for their administration.

1. **Notes.** All instructions regarding medicines and drugs must be obtained in writing from the doctor. There is usually no trouble about this in hospital, but in private practice it is essential that the nurse should not get into the habit of receiving instructions by word of mouth. Notepaper should always be at hand so that the doctor can write them down without delay. Telephone messages concerning drugs for a private patient should be written on a piece of paper as the message is received and are read to the doctor before he leaves the telephone. On his next visit he should be asked to sign the prescription.

Difficulties may arise in hospital practice when a house officer rings up a ward to order a drug. The only person who is allowed to take a message regarding the drug over the telephone is a state registered nurse. She must write it down at once and see that it is written on the patient's bed letter on the doctor's next visit to the ward. If a message comes to the ward during the night, the nurse should refer the house officer to the night sister and give him her telephone number, or ask the night sister to get in touch with him.

2. If a mistake is made in regard to a drug, for example, if the wrong dose is given or the drug is given to the wrong patient, the nurse must notify the sister and the doctor without delay. There should be no hesitation, for, if the matter is reported at once measures can be taken to avert the danger. If time elapses while the nurse is considering what to do it may be too late. There is no argument or excuse for any other line of action and the nurse will have learnt her lesson. The authorities are likely to be lenient in such a case, whereas if the nurse is found not to have reported her mistake the matter will be regarded much more seriously by all concerned.

3. A nurse is not expected to learn the doses of dangerous drugs by memory. As she gains experience, however, she is bound to become familiar with the usual doses of drugs in common use. She should make a point of doing this so that she is an additional safeguard to the patient if drugs are ordered in emergency or under conditions where mistakes might be made. She is always within her right to question the dose of a drug if it appears to her excessive or unusual.

4. The nurse is in an exceptionally good position to observe the effects of drugs. By her observation on the length of time of their action and the response of the patient she can guide the doctor as to future modifications

of the dose. Patients vary so much in their reactions to drugs that this is largely an individual matter. What suits one patient will not suit another. The doctor is almost entirely dependent upon an accurate report from the nurse as to the effect of the drug. Not only must the nurse study the reactions of her patients but she should read up all she can on the subject so that she learns what results to expect. Thus some drugs are excreted from the body more slowly than they are absorbed. These are called cumulative drugs as their action accumulates unless the drug is carefully prescribed. Digitalis and mercury are good examples and also some of the barbituric group of sleeping draughts. Certain patients too are said to have an idiosyncrasy to a certain drug. This means that it has some undesirable action on the patient, even when given in small doses or quite usual ones. If the patient knows this and tells the nurse she should always take notice so that some other drug which is more likely to suit the patient may be substituted.

5. Sleeping draughts are usually ordered to be given at the nurse's discretion, no particular time being specified. She should remember that four or five hours of unbroken sleep are more valuable than a light sleep from which the patient wakes up frequently. The patient will then say that she has not slept well although the nurse may have found her asleep at every visit. Sleeping draughts, therefore, should be given at the beginning of the night if they are ordered and likely to be required. The patient should not have to wait for them until one or two o'clock. By this time she will feel that she has already had a bad night.

MEASURES

1 drop	=	1 minim—symbol (♏)
1 teaspoonful (small)	=	1 drachm—symbol (℈)
2 teaspoonsful	=	2 drachms or 1 dessertspoonful
4 teaspoonsful	=	½ ounce or 1 tablespoonful
2 tablespoonsful	=	1 ounce—symbol (℥)

Fluid Measure

60 minims	=	1 drachm—symbol (℈)
8 drachms	=	1 ounce ,, (℥)
20 ounces	=	1 pint ,, (O)

Solid Measures

20 grains	=	1 scruple—symbol (℈)
3 scruples	=	1 drachm ,, (℈)
60 grains	=	1 drachm ,, (℈)
8 drachms	=	1 ounce ,, (℥)

Other facts to be remembered

1 litre	=	35 fluid ounces (approx.)=1¾ pts.

1 gramme	=	$\frac{1}{30}$ part of an ounce (approx.)
1 kilogramme	=	$2\frac{1}{5}$ lb. (approx.)
1 fluid ounce	=	480 minims
1 ounce (apothecaries')	=	$437\frac{1}{2}$ grains
1 ounce (avoirdupois)	=	480 grains

N.B. The fact that $437\frac{1}{2}$ grains equals 1 ounce in Apothecaries' measure hould be remembered. This is because the fluid ounce (480 minims) is quivalent to $437\frac{1}{2}$ grains (solid). The practical application of this is met vhen percentage solutions are to be made up, and thus it is found that:

1 per cent solution equals 4·375 grains in 1 fluid ounce,

or 1 per cent solution equals 1 grain in 110 minims.

1 cubic centimetre	=	16 minims (approx.)
1 ounce (fluid)	=	30 cubic centimetres (30 c.c.)
1 pint	=	600 cubic centimetres

DILUTION OF LOTIONS

The nurse is often required to make up a solution for lavage, etc., in a weaker solution than the lotion she has in stock. To take two examples:

I. *To make up a pint of carbolic lotion 1 in 100 from a stock solution of 1 in 20 carbolic lotion.*

This is done by dividing the strength of the stock solution into the strength of the dilute solution required, e.g. $\frac{1}{100} \div \frac{1}{20} = \frac{1}{5}$. Hence the dilute solution is one-fifth of the strength of the stock solution. Therefore the quantity required, i.e. one pint, should be made up one-fifth stock solution and four-fifths water, or four ounces carbolic 1 in 20 and sixteen ounces of water.

II. *To make up 10 ounces of solution of perchloride of mercury, 1 in 10,000 from a stock solution of 1 in 2,000.*

$$\frac{1}{10000} \div \frac{1}{2000} = \frac{1}{5}$$

Therefore $\frac{1}{5}$ of the required $\frac{1}{2}$ pint should be of the stock solution and $\frac{4}{5}$ water, i.e. 2 ounces of perchloride of mercury solution and 8 ounces of water.

DOSES OF DRUGS

A useful estimate for normal dosage of drugs for children is Young's Formula. The age of the patient is divided by the age plus 12. Thus for a child aged 4 years the dose should be:

$$\frac{4}{4+12} = \frac{1}{4} \text{ of the adult dose.}$$

Normal doses in a pharmacopœia refer to adults, but towards the close of life comparatively smaller doses are usually sufficient.

The dose of some drugs (e.g. bromethol) is estimated according to the weight of the patient. The weight in stones is converted into kilogrammes and the dose is usually estimated per kilogramme of body weight.

ABBREVIATIONS

a.c.	ante cibos	before meals
ad lib.	ad libitum	to the desired amount
aa	ana	of each
alt. hor	alternis horis	every other hour
aq. dest.	aqua destillata	distilled water
b.d.	bis die	twice a day
b.i.d.	bis in die	twice a day
B.P.	British Pharmacopœia	
cat.	cataplasma	a poultice
c.c.	cum cibo	with food
c.m.	cras mane	to-morrow morning
c.n.	cras nocte	to-morrow night
comp.	compositus	compounded of
dieb. alt.	diebus alternis	on alternate days
emp.	emplastrum	a plaster
ext.	extractum	extract
Fahr.	Fahrenheit	
gutt.	gutta or guttæ	drops or drop
h.n.	hac nocte	to-night
h.s.	hora somni	at bedtime
inf.	infusum	an infusion
inj.	injectio	an injection
o.h.	omni hora	every hour
o.m.	omni mane	every morning
o.n.	omni nocte	every night
part. aeq.	partes aequales	equal parts
p.c.	post cibos	after meals
p.r.	per rectum	by the rectum
p.r.n.	pro re nata	as occasion arises
pulv.	pulvis	powder
p.v.	per vaginam	by the vagina
q.d.	quater in die	four times a day
q.h.	quartis horis	four hourly
q.l.	quantum libet	as much as is wanted
R.	recipe	take
rep.	repetatur	let it be repeated
rep. sem.	repetatur semel	let it be repeated once only
s.s.	semis	a half
sig.	signatur	let it be labelled
s.o.s.	si opus sit	if necessary

ABBREVIATIONS

stat.	statim	immediately
T.		temperature
t.d.s.	ter in die sumendum	let it be taken three times a day
ung.	unguentum	ointment

The Prescription

R Tinct. Ferri Perchlor.   ʒiii
   Quin. Hydrochlor.   Ʒss.
   Glyc.   ʒii
   Mag. Sulph.   ʒii
   Inf. Quas. ad.   ʒviii
Fiat mist.
   Sign Ʒ ss. t.d.s. p.c.
The translation of this is as follows:
   Take Tincture of Perchloride of Iron   ʒiii
      Quinine Hydrochloride   Ʒss.
      Glycerine   ʒii
      Magnesium Sulphate   ʒii
      Infusion of quassia to make the total quantity ʒviii
Let a mixture be made.
Label—One tablespoonful to be taken 3 times a day after meals.

METHODS OF PREPARING DRUGS

Liquors (*Aquae*)	Watery solutions of drugs.
Tinctures	Solutions of a drug in spirit.
Syrup	Preparation of a drug in sugar and water, generally with some flavouring agent added.
Inhalant	Preparation of a volatile drug.
Mixtures	Preparations of drugs in water containing some soluble agent to dissolve the drug if necessary; flavouring and colouring agents may be added.
Liniments	Drugs in oil or spirit for rubbing into the skin.
Lotions	Solutions of drugs for external application.
Powders	Finely powdered drugs.
Tablets	Compressed drugs.
Plasters	Drugs incorporated in various agents and spread on linen.
Ointments	Drugs incorporated in lard or soft paraffin wax.

CLASSIFICATION OF DRUGS

Anæsthetics	(1) General—depress the cerebrum and destroy consciousness, e.g. ether, chloroform.

159

	(2) Local—act on nerve trunks or nerve endings and thus have a local action only, e.g. preparations of cocaine such as novocaine, percaine.
Antipyretics	Reduce temperature, e.g. aspirin, quinine.
Anthelmintics	Are drugs which paralyse or kill worms, e.g. filix mas, santonin, quassia, and thymol.
Anodynes	Relieve pain, e.g. belladonna.
Antiseptics	Prevent the growth of germs, e.g. carbolic lotion, 1 in 100, lysol ½ per cent, and other disinfectants in weak solutions.
Aperients	Promote an action of the bowels.
Carminatives	Relieve flatulence, e.g. peppermint, cajuput, turpentine.
Diaphoretics	Induce perspiration, e.g. pilocarpine.
Diuretics	Increase the flow of urine, e.g. potassium citrate, organic mercurials such as mersalyl.
Ecbolics	Cause contraction of the uterus, e.g. pituitrin, ergot.
Emetics	Cause vomiting, e.g. mustard, ipecacuanha.
Expectorants	Loosen the bronchial secretions, e.g. squills, ammonium carbonate.
Hypnotics	Induce sleep, e.g. chloral, paraldehyde.
Mydriatics	Dilate the pupil of the eye, e.g atropine, homatropine
Myotics	Contract the pupil of the eye, e.g. eserine and cocaine
Narcotics	Induce sleep and relieve pain, e.g. opium preparation such as morphia and tincture of opium.
Tonics	Improve the general health, e.g. arsenic, iron.
Styptics	Contract the capillaries and arrest local hæmorrhage e.g. adrenalin, turpentine.

NOTES ON DRUGS IN COMMON USE

Digitalis. Prepared as a tincture, dose 5 to 15 minims. It is ordered i certain heart conditions such as auricular fibrillation and congestive heai failure. It slows, strengthens and steadies the heart beat and lessens th conductivity of the Bundle of His thus increasing the output of blood pe beat. It increases the flow of urine. Watch for and report (1) Slowing c the pulse below 70; (2) Nausea; (3) irregular or coupled beats (pulsi bigeminus).

Sodium Salicylate. Usually prescribed as a mixture, dose half to on ounce (10 to 15 grains in the ounce). It is prescribed in cases of acu rheumatism. It reduces temperature, relieves pain, but has no effect i preventing heart complications. It also has a diaphoretic action. Wato for and report: (1) Ringing noises in the ears and deafness; (2) Giddiness and (3) Depression.

Aspirin. (Acetyl-salicylic acid) belongs to the same group of drugs and has much the same action and effect.

Belladonna (Atropine). This drug is used:

1. As a pre-anæsthetic to inhibit the bronchial secretions.

2. As an anti-spasmodic to relieve spasm of plain muscle in renal or biliary colic.

3. In cases of gastric ulcer, to inhibit the gastric secretions.

4. In eye cases to dilate the pupil.

Belladonna is prescribed as a mixture or tincture, and atropine as an injection, dose 1/200 to 1/75 of a grain.

Watch for and report:

1. Dilated pupils.

2. Dryness of the skin and mucous membranes.

3. Scanty urine.

4. Pyrexia.

5. Scarlet rash.

N.B. Plenty of fluids should be given.

Opium (and preparations of opium, e.g. morphine tartrate, dose $\frac{1}{6}$ to $\frac{1}{3}$ grains; nepenthe, dose 5 to 30 minims; omnopon, dose $\frac{1}{3}$ grain).

Opium is the best narcotic drug known and is prescribed:

1. To relieve pain and induce sleep.

2. To lower the blood pressure and thus reduce the risk of hæmorrhage.

Watch for: (a) Slowing of the pulse, and respiration. (b) Pin-point pupils. (c) Cold clammy skin. (d) Drowsiness, deepening into coma.

N.B. Codeine is another alkaloid of opium and is used in soothing cough medicines, e.g. linctus codeinæ, dose 1 to 2 drachms.

Heroin (diamorphine) is a synthetic drug, whose action and poisonous effects are similar to those of opium. It is habit forming. The dose is $\frac{1}{12}$ to $\frac{1}{6}$ of a grain.

Bromide is a sedative drug. It makes the senses less acute and therefore quietens a restless and wakeful patient. It is often prescribed in conjunction with chloral in a mixture. The dose is usually 15 grains of each. Large doses of bromide may cause a rash, rather like acne, spots, pimples and pustules appearing, usually on the face.

Barbiturate Group. This group comprises a large class of hypnotic drugs. Some of the ones commonly prescribed are medinal, luminal, dial, evipan, nembutal, pentothol. They are very useful drugs for most types of sleeplessness. The doses vary according to the cause for which they are being used, the last three on the list being given as basal narcotics to induce a deep sleep before an inhalation anæsthetic is given.

Mercury. Mercury is a drug chiefly used in the treatment of syphilis. It may be rubbed into the skin by inunction. Organic mercurial drugs, e.g. mersalyl, are given intramuscularly (1 c.c.), to relieve œdema by increasing the flow of urine in chronic heart and kidney cases. Watch for excessive salivation, sore gums and a metallic taste in the mouth. Mercury should not be prescribed over a period of time for patients with dental sepsis.

Arsenic. Arsenic is a drug prescribed and given intravenously in cases of syphilis. The proprietary name for the most common preparation is novarsenobenzol (N.A.B.), but there are others. Many tonics contain small doses of arsenic. Liquor arsenicalis B.P. (Fowler's solution) dose 1 drachm, is a tonic of proved value. Watch for abdominal pain, diarrhœa, dermatitis and jaundice.

Strychnine. Strychnine is used as a nerve stimulant in cases of collapse and heart failure. Injection of strychnine hydrochloride, dose 1/60 to 1/12 of a grain, is given. Small doses of strychnine have a general stimulating effect and are prescribed in some tonics. Watch for: (1) Twitching of the muscles. (2) Restlessness; and (3) After large doses, convulsions.

Sulphonamide Group. These important drugs have been discovered in very recent years. The first of them, prontosil, was a German preparation and was put on the English market in 1936. This group includes:

(a) *M. & B. 693* (sulphapyridine). Particularly lethal to streptococci, meningococci, pneumococci and bacillus Welchii (gas gangrene bacillus).

(b) *Sulphanilamide* (prontosil album). Also of particular value in cases of bacillus coli infections, and lethal to streptococcus.

(c) *M. & B. 760* (sulphathiazole) is lethal to streptococci, meningococci, pneumococci, and is the only drug of the group which is thought to act on the staphylococcus (aureus).

(d) *Sulphaguanidine*. This drug is under trial for intestinal infections.

Drugs of the sulphonamide group are now extensively used for all cases of suppurating open wounds, pneumonia, meningococcal meningitis and gonorrhœa. The average dose is a gramme four-hourly for three or four days, then the dose is reduced. It is important that the full dose should be given regularly. The patient must be wakened if necessary when the dose is due, and plenty of fluids should be given.

Some of the toxic symptoms are: cyanosis (especially with sulphanilamide), nausea and vomiting (especially after M. & B. 693). Cyanosis, however, is not considered an indication for withholding the drug. It is to be expected and the nurse need not be unduly alarmed by it. Occasionally hæmaturia may occur where the kidneys are damaged. M. & B. 760 is much less toxic in its effects than M. & B. 693 and is proving equally efficacious in many conditions.

Saline purgatives and other drastic aperients should be avoided with patients having these drugs. Some authorities thought that sulphur-containing foods, such as eggs and onions, should be excluded from the diet, but this restriction is not now considered necessary by most physicians.

To avoid the nauseating effect of M. & B. 693 the drug can be given powdered in ʒi of milk, containing soda bicarbonate ʒi. It can also be given in fruit juice or in a mixture containing nicotinic acid. Although these drugs are miraculous in their effect it will be seen that they are by no means harmless. If the toxic symptoms persist or are very severe, blood tests are done. There have been some fatal cases due to agranulocytosis.

Hormone Preparations. Preparations made from the endocrine glands are now used extensively in medicine. Some of them are still in the experimental stage especially œstrogenic and progesterone preparations from the ovary. They are being used for various gynæcological disorders.

Insulin from the islets of Langerhans in the pancreas is used in the treatment of diabetes mellitus, dose from 20 to 100 units (prepared in four strengths).

Dried extract from the thyroid glands of sheep (thyroid sicca gr. ½ to 2) is used in the treatment of hypothyroidism. Preparations from the pituitary gland (pitocin and pitressin) are extensively used. They act on plain muscle and raise the blood pressure. Their chief use is to contract the uterus and thus prevent hæmorrhage after labour.

Adrenalin is a very important hormone preparation from the suprarenal glands. It is used for many purposes :

1. In cases of asthma to relax the bronchi. One minim a minute is given hypodermically until the attack subsides.

2. It contracts the capillaries and is therefore useful as a styptic in cases of nose bleeding or hæmorrhage from a tooth socket.

3. Because of its constricting effect it is used in conjunction with local anæsthetics to localize the drug in the part concerned.

4. Five to ten minims are given hypodermically in cases of serum shock (anaphylaxis). It has the temporary effect of raising the blood pressure, and therefore can be given in cases of shock from other causes.

5. It is combined with cocaine in treatment of the conjunctiva and nasal mucous membrane before operations on the nose. It is valuable in these cases for its constricting effect.

Aperients. The giving of aperients is frequently left to the discretion of the nurse. Therefore it is important that she should understand how long they take to act and in which cases the various types are most suitable. They are classified as follows :

1. *Simple lubricants.* The most valuable of these is liquid paraffin so commonly used. The dose is ½ to 1 ounce, once or twice a day. It should be given half an hour before meals so that the food particles are not surrounded by the oil, thus rendering them inaccessible to the digestive ferments. Paraffin is not digested nor absorbed, therefore it mixes with the intestinal contents and makes them soft. If too much is given or if the paraffin is of poor quality it defeats its own ends ; it makes the fæcal bulk

too soft and slippery and therefore the muscles become lazy and peristaltic movements slow.

2. *Bulk producers.* (a) Those containing seaweed preparations which swell in the intestine as they become saturated and warm. The presence of the bulk stimulates peristalsis. The ones in common use contain agar, e.g. petrolagar, agarol. The usual dose is one ounce given at night. These are safe aperients to use in cases of chronic constipation especially for patients ill in bed.

(b) Saline aperients. These produce bulk by the attraction of water into the intestine, thus a watery stool is produced. The common saline aperients are magnesium sulphate (Epsom salts); sodium sulphate (Glauber salts); magnesium carbonate. The usual dose of all these salts is one to two drachms, magnesium sulphate being the strongest in action. The various popular preparations on the market contain a mixture of these drugs, effervescing ones having magnesium citrate included in the prescription. They are all given in the early morning.

3. *Vegetable preparations*—known as anthracene purgatives. They stimulate peristalsis in the colon only, therefore they are given at night and produce an action about eight hours later. They are very commonly used and are not very harmful, except for the fact that they are habit forming in people who should not need them. They comprise pills, mixtures and powders, containing senna, rhubarb, cascara and figs.

If senna pods are prepared, it is best that they should be soaked overnight in cold water. Castor oil belongs to this class, but it is very drastic and is not for ordinary use. It has a value, however, for its sure effect as a pre-operative aperient, though it is not used nearly as frequently as in the past. Patients dislike it so much and the purging result from it is considered too drastic for weak or ill patients. It is certainly valuable in cases of food poisoning where the cause is known to be something eaten.

Drastic purgatives. These drugs begin their irritating effect in the small intestine and continue it through the colon. There is definitely a harmful inflammatory reaction on the mucous membrane, hence they are only prescribed in urgent cases. Drugs of this class are jalap, croton oil, colocynth, and calomel. The latter is a cumulative drug and is given in doses of $\frac{1}{2}$ to 2 grains at night always followed by a saline aperient in the morning.

Phenolphthalein is a useful aperient the action of which the nurse should understand. It is a white colourless pill, dose $\frac{1}{2}$ to 2 grains. It is also contained in some mixtures and is often found in very small doses combined with petrolagar preparations. Its particular value is that its effect lasts for two or three consecutive days. Therefore daily doses should not be given.

Chapter Ten

SURGICAL NURSING

It has been recently said that in the past the main problem was to make the operation safe for the patient. Now, however, the surgeon realizes that it is equally important to make the patient safe for the operation. During the last twenty years surgical technique has attained a high degree of safety and more recently the surgeon has been turning his attention to the general preparation before, and the care of the patient after, the operation. There have been many modifications in treatment recently. Patients' reactions have been studied, the methods of anæsthesia greatly improved, and, on the whole, nursing treatments are much simpler. Nurses, however, must understand the principles which underlie the treatments ordered, so that they themselves can vary the details in different cases.

We will take as a typical case for description the preparation of a patient who is to have an operation on the abdomen.

PRELIMINARY PREPARATION

The patient should be admitted two days before the operation if possible. The temperature, pulse, and respiration are taken night and morning. A specimen of urine is tested for albumen and sugar, as it is important that the kidneys should be functioning properly in order to excrete the anæsthetic. The presence of albumen in the urine is a sign of dysfunction. In a case of diabetes mellitus the anæsthetist chooses his anæsthetic with great care and chloroform is contra-indicated.

The nurse should talk to the patient and study her mental reactions. Nervous and excitable patients are much more likely to take an anæsthetic badly and to suffer from shock. If this is realized beforehand the patient can be saved much distress of mind by being given appropriate drugs and the difficulties can be realized and dealt with to some extent by a sympathetic and reassuring nurse. Fear is an important cause of shock.

The house surgeon will examine the heart and lungs. The nurse will report to him if the patient has a cough or cold. All these factors if they are known and treated previously contribute to the safety and success of the operation.

Sleep during the night before operation is important. The strangeness of a hospital ward and the apprehension of the patient naturally disturbs sleep. The nurse should see that some mild hypnotic is ordered and given at the beginning of the night so that a long uninterrupted period of sleep is obtained.

The atmosphere of the ward, the attitude of the nursing staff, should all be designed to give the patient confidence. As far as is possible she should be amongst other patients who are recovering from similar operations, and the nurse's attitude while being considerate and sympathetic should also convey the impression that there is nothing unusual in the treatments she is giving.

The patient must have a bath either in the bathroom or in bed. The mouth should be examined, the teeth cleaned and mouthwashes given. The patient has probably washed her own hair before coming into hospital. But if not, it should be washed if the patient is sufficiently fit. During the bath special attention should be given to the nails, umbilicus, folds beneath the breasts and the ears.

The patient should have a light ordinary diet during her first day in hospital, with the addition of glucose. This should be given liberally and in drinks; it is customary to give the patient glucose tablets to suck during the day. The giving of glucose helps to prevent shock and aids the liver to neutralize the anæsthetic toxins.

THE DAY BEFORE THE OPERATION

An aperient is given early in the day. In the past it was customary to give all operation cases at least one ounce of castor oil, the old-fashioned idea being to purge and starve the patient beforehand. Now it is realized that this drastic treatment is not necessary. The aperient chosen should give a satisfactory result without drastic purging, and if the patient can suggest what she knows will suit her, the nurse should give it when possible. It should be given early in the day or the patient's sleep may be disturbed.

The diet on the day before the operation should be light and contain little roughage. The main meal should be fish or chicken, potatoes and a pudding. Bread and butter and plenty of fluids may be given, and again, glucose in abundance.

The skin of the area of operation is shaved. Even the smallest hairs when seen under a microscope are covered with micro-organisms which penetrate into the hair follicles. A good lather is made with soap and a safety razor used if possible. In some cases if the patient's skin is very dirty ether soap may be used. (*N.B.* It is very inflammable.) Ether penetrates into the hair follicles and sweat glands dissolving fat and removing dirt, and the soap mixed with it makes an excellent lather.

ON THE DAY OF THE OPERATION

If the operation is to be early in the day, say at 10 a.m., the patient has a soap enema before breakfast or the previous evening. Tea only is given

'or this meal, say at 6.30 a.m. She then washes and may have a glucose
drink afterwards. If the operation is to be in the afternoon she is given a
breakfast of tea and toast, bovril for lunch at 10 a.m., and glucose drinks
up to noon. It is a bad plan to starve the patient for too long beforehand,
but it is a safe rule that no solid food should be given for four hours before
the operation.

The final preparation is left for thirty to forty-five minutes before the
patient goes to the theatre. Screens are put round the bed and a clean
strong sheet or stretcher canvas is rolled under the patient and a warmed
white theatre mackintosh is put under her buttocks. Long white woollen
stockings are put on and a clean bed-gown which must open down the
back, the top button being left undone. If the arm is to be operated upon,
it must be left outside the gown. All jewellery except the wedding ring is
removed. A clean blanket is folded over the patient and the top bedclothes
put back in position.

A pre-anæsthetic drug, usually atropine sulphate gr. 1/100, is given
thirty minutes before the operation. If there is delay before the patient goes
to the theatre, the time when the atropine was given should be reported by
the nurse. The dentures, if any, are removed, cleaned and put in a bowl
of cold water in a safe place. A mouthwash is given. Five minutes before
going to the theatre the bladder must be emptied. During all these preparations the nurse should be cheerful and reassuring in her manner.

The patient must be sent to the theatre comfortably warm, but in hot
weather it is important to see that she is not so warm as to perspire,
as a considerable amount of fluid can be lost by the skin in this manner.
Common sense should dictate how many blankets should be put over the
patient; the theatre is very warm and it is bad nursing to send her either
too cold or too hot. It may be necessary in the case of old people to send a
hot water bottle to the theatre to place between the patient's legs. If so,
it must only be warm and must be most carefully protected. If there are
long draughty corridors to be traversed on the way to the theatre, a blanket
should be well tucked round the patient's neck and a small one placed
round her head. The trolley should have a folded rug on the canvas
stretcher. The patient is lifted on to the trolley on the sheet or stretcher
canvas. The nurse helps and supervises the lifting and sees that the necessary case papers, X-ray plates, etc., go with the patient. It is desirable that
the patient's own nurse should prepare her, accompany her, stay throughout the operation and bring her back to the ward. This, of course, is not
always possible in hospital practice, but whenever it can be done it is
obviously the correct procedure. It gives the patient confidence to feel she
is in the charge of the person who is going to nurse her afterwards. From
the nurse's point of view, she will have seen the different stages of the
operation and will have heard the comments of the surgeon and the treat-

ment he orders. The case assignment method, by which nurses are given particular responsibility for special patients, is the ideal method of training nurses, both from the point of view of the patient and the nurse.

The fact that the nurse accompanies her own patient to the theatre instead of handing her over to strangers creates still another bond in the nurse and patient relationship. Anyone who has undergone an operation herself will appreciate the importance of this arrangement if it can possibly be managed.

PREPARATION OF THE SKIN

The methods of skin preparation advocated by different surgeons vary considerably. Usually all that he requires the nurse in the ward to do is to wash the part thoroughly, paying special attention to the nails if it is a limb, and shaving the site as above described. Occasionally for an operation on the trunk or soft tissues of the limbs the surgeon may also require a surgical 'compress', although this method of preparation is usually confined to bone cases. In this case after the skin has been washed and shaved, it is rubbed thoroughly well with swabs soaked in ether or methylated ether. The rubbing should be firm so that the ether penetrates into the sweat ducts and hair follicles, and each swab as used should be discarded, and not carried backwards and forwards over the skin. Even after thorough washing this method removes a great deal of dirt. The nurse then scrubs her hands and prepares as for a surgical dressing. With the aid of an assistant a sterile towel is put under the part, usually a limb, and the skin is painted with swabs soaked in methylated spirit or other sterilizing agent which the surgeon may order. (e.g. Liquor iodi 2 per cent, picric acid in spirit 1 per cent, Harrington's solution, etc.) The swabs are held with forceps and the area is treated with long sweeping strokes, the swabs being discarded frequently. The assistant then picks up the limb by finger or toe with a sterile swab (if the patient is unable to lift it herself), and the under-surface is treated in the same manner, care being taken that every part of the skin is painted. Finally the limb is wrapped in a sterile towel or compress cloth and bandaged securely.

The compress is not removed until the patient is in the theatre. The cloth or towel should be sent back to the ward to be washed and re-sterilized

Preparation in Special Cases

1. *Operations on the stomach.* Gastric lavage is usually required.

2. *Operations on the rectum.* Cleansing enemata on two successive mornings and a rectal lavage a few hours before the operation are given.

3. *Radical mastectomy for carcinoma of the breast.* The area of skin prepared is from beyond the sternum in front to the spine behind, well up into the neck and down to below the waistline, including the axilla on the affected side and the arm as far as the elbow.

4. *Preparations for operations on bones and joints*. The skin preparation must be specially thorough. Usually the surgeon requires the surgical compress to be repeated three times, twice the day before the operation and once on the morning of the actual day. The blood supply of bone is not so good as that of soft tissues and the surgeon incises deep structures in which sepsis would be serious. Hence the importance of very careful preparation.

If an elbow or knee joint is to be operated upon, the whole limb should be prepared, including the hand or foot. Special attention in the case of operations on the foot must be paid to cleanliness between the toes and to the nails. It may be necessary to soak the feet and scrub them daily for several days beforehand.

5. *Operations on the mouth*. Teeth should be examined and dental sepsis removed before the operation takes place, if possible. The tongue should be clean, teeth brushed and mouthwashes used frequently.

6. *Preparation for an emergency operation*. Instructions as to how far the preparation is to be carried out are usually given. In the case of a patient admitted for an emergency abdominal operation such as an appendix abscess or a perforated gastric or duodenal ulcer the minimum preparation is done. The patient's temperature, pulse, and respiration are taken, and she is undressed. The hands and face are sponged, dentures removed and a mouthwash is given. The hair, if dirty, is tied up in a clean towel. A specimen of urine must be obtained and tested for albumen and sugar; an enema is only given if ordered. Catheterization may be necessary. The skin preparation, including the shave, is usually done in the theatre with ether soap. If, however, the nurse is instructed to wash and shave the skin before the patient goes to the operation, she should do this very gently and carefully to avoid perforating the organ, if the diagnosis suggests this possibility. If perforation takes place before the diseased structure is removed peritonitis will result. For these cases the theatre staff will be prepared for blood transfusion or intravenous drip saline infusion.

IN THE THEATRE

The nurse must stay with the patient whilst anæsthesia is being induced. It gives her confidence if someone who knows her is present. She may like to grip the nurse's hand. In the second stage of induction, especially when ether is the anæsthetic used, the patient becomes excitable and restless. The nurse will help to restrain her, holding and controlling the limbs without using force. This stage soon passes into the third stage of complete relaxation, the condition known as 'surgical anæsthesia'. Absolute silence must be maintained whilst the anæsthetic is being induced. There should be no discussion or whispering. The doors of the anæsthetic room should be kept closed so that the patient 'goes under' in a quiet and peaceful atmosphere. Sometimes it helps to give the patient another mouthwash just before the anæsthetic is given, as atropine makes the mouth uncomfortably dry. The nurse attending the anæsthetist can learn a great deal by watching his technique. She should notice when he requires to use a mouth gag or airway, and should watch carefully how these are inserted, as she may later on have to do this herself when patients are recovering from anæsthesia. She should also see that the patient is kept well covered and warm whilst the anæsthetic is being given.

The temperature of the operating theatre should be between 68° and 70° F. and draughts should be excluded.

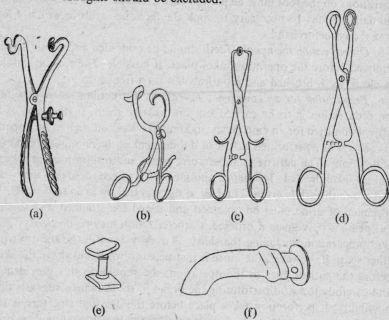

FIG. 69. Instruments required for unconscious patients. (a) Mason's mouth gag. (b) Doyen's mouth gag. (c) Tongue forceps (spike pattern). (d) Tongue forceps (ring pattern). (e) Dental prop. (f) Airway (Phillips)

THE RETURN OF THE PATIENT TO THE WARD

As soon as the patient has gone to the theatre the bed should be prepared for her return. This should be done at once, as it is not unusual for a patient, if any unforeseen complication arises, to return unexpectedly. The making of an operation bed has already been described, but again emphasis is laid on the necessity for the bed to be warm before the patient is put into it, hot blankets and gown ready, and all windows in the vicinity closed.

The patient is wheeled into the ward by 'dressers' or orderlies. A nurse always returns with the patient, either the patient's own nurse who has been present at the operation or otherwise a member of the theatre staff.

This nurse should be responsible for the patient being warm during transit. She should see that she has with her on the trolley a vomit bowl and cloth, a mouth gag, tongue forceps and sponge holder with sponge. The patient's head is kept to one side.

On arrival at the bed and before the patient is lifted off the trolley, the pulse should be taken. In most cases it will be found to be strong, regular but a little quicker than usual, say 100 to 110 beats per minute. The patient is lifted on to the bed, taking great care not to bump the shoulders or buttocks on the stretcher or bed-rail. Screens are put round the bed as dressers or orderlies remove the stretcher and two nurses deal with the patient. She is rolled from side to side while the stretcher canvas or sheet and mackintosh are removed. The head is kept turned to one side, the vomit bowl and cloth being placed under the chin. Some anæsthetists insist upon not only the head being turned to one side, but the whole body tilted also, by means of a pillow under the back. A hot blanket is put over the patient. If the gown is soiled or wet with perspiration, the skin is dried, and a clean warm gown put on, being left open down the back. The long woollen socks are removed if the body and legs feel comfortably warm, if not, they should be left on. The hot water bottles are left in the bed, under the bottom blanket and next to the mattress so that there can be no risk of the patient being burned while unconscious. If the bed is narrow, and the blankets thin, it is safer to remove all hot water bottles till the patient is fully conscious. The upper bedclothes which have been folded in a packet, are now unfolded over the patient, and the bed is completed. Accessories in the way of pillows, mackintoshes, bed cradle, sandbags, etc., are put in position as required.

CARE OF THE PATIENT WHILST UNCONSCIOUS

The patient is never left until consciousness is regained. In a hospital ward when several operations have taken place, it may be possible for one nurse to supervise several patients, but she must be in a position to see every movement and observe each patient separately. Her special observations will be the following:

1. *Pulse.* It is usual to record this every quarter-hour until the sister is satisfied with the patient's condition.

2. *Respiration.* It is in connection with breathing that an emergency may arise, if the nurse does not understand exactly what to do. The face may become blue if the patient stops breathing. The reasons for this is either that the tongue has fallen back, blocking the pharynx, or that the pharynx is blocked with mucus or vomit. The airway is thus obstructed, and treatment must be prompt. The nurse should:

1. Keep the head to one side so that the tongue will fall into the cheek, and mucus or vomit will trickle out of the corner of the mouth.

2. Press the jaw forward, thus drawing the tongue forward.

3. If the colour does not improve, a mouth gag may be inserted between the premolar teeth at the side of the mouth. The nurse should have learnt how to insert a mouth gag before she is entrusted with the care of patients recovering from anæsthetics.

4. The tongue may be pulled forward with tongue forceps and the mouth and pharynx thoroughly swabbed with sponges dipped in cold water held with sponge-holding forceps.

As soon as the airway is clear the patient will begin to breathe. The sister should be informed of the emergency as soon as possible. Oxygen may need to be administered, by putting the tube from the cylinder to the back of the mouth. It should be emphasized, however, that this emergency seldom arises if the nurse is careful to keep the patient well turned on her side. But if she allows her to roll on to her back, blocking of the airway may result. Some anæsthetists, as an additional safeguard, send the patients from the theatre with a rubber airway in the mouth. When the patient makes attempts to eject it, it should be removed, washed, boiled and returned to the operating theatre. Inhalations of carbon dioxide 7 per cent with 93 per cent oxygen are particularly useful for stimulating respiration after anæsthesia by bromethol, and after operations on the chest and upper abdomen in which there may be disturbance in the rhythm of the diaphragm.

3. *Dressing*. The bandage should be inspected for reactionary hæmorrhage although it is more likely to occur a little later on.

4. *Warmth*. The warmth of the extremities, especially of the feet, is a useful indication of the degree of shock. If the skin feels comfortably dry, the circulatory centres are functioning well; on the other hand, if the skin feels cold or clammy it is probable that the circulation has been disturbed by the effect of the operation on the nerve centres which control the vasomotor system.

RETURN TO CONSCIOUSNESS

As the patient recovers, and if her condition is satisfactory, that is to say, if there are no symptoms of severe shock, one pillow may be put under the head. The mouth should be swabbed with iced water containing a little vinegar. This is refreshing and takes away the taste of the anæsthetic. The face is sponged with cold water and the hair smoothed away from the face and nape of the neck.

When the effects of the anæsthetic have passed off, she is put in the position in which she is to be nursed. In the case of an abdominal operation, this is the Fowler position. The patient is sat up well with four or five pillows, arranged in armchair fashion. A knee pillow is inserted. A blanket should be kept next to the patient for twenty-four hours, unless the weather is very hot. After this it is convenient and comfortable for the patient to wear a woollen bed jacket with long sleeves, and a light chest blanket to cover the chest and shoulders. A stone hot water bottle—not too hot—is put at the feet, to prevent the patient from slipping down the bed. She usually sits on an air ring. There are many reasons why the patient should be nursed in a sitting-up position, the most important being for drainage. If there is any infection of the peritoneum, or if fluid or pus has leaked into the peritoneal cavity from a perforated ulcer or abscess, it is most important that the patient should sit propped up as high as possible so that the infection may drain downwards towards the pelvis and through the tube which the surgeon will have inserted. The pelvic peritoneum is more resistant to infection than that of the abdomen, and if the infection develops, it tends to localize and form a pelvic abscess which is comparatively easy for the surgeon to drain. A general peritonitis or an abscess high in the abdomen under the diaphragm, such as a sub-phrenic abscess, is much more serious. Other points in favour of Fowler position are:

1. The sitting-up position helps to avoid chest complications. The patient expands the lungs more fully and is able to cough up mucus from the bronchial tubes more easily.

2. The position reduces discomfort from flatulence which often follows an abdominal operation.

3. Flexing the legs over a pillow relaxes the abdominal muscles and is found to be more restful.

By the time the patient is comfortably sat up a hypodermic injection of morphia, gr. $\frac{1}{6}$ to $\frac{1}{4}$ is generally required. The effects of the anæsthetic are passing off and the patient begins to feel pain. Morphia should be given without hesitation if the condition is satisfactory, because at this stage sleep will do the patient more good than anything else. The pulse should be taken at frequent intervals. Every time the patient vomits the nurse should be at hand to hold the basin and support her head. The mouth should be swabbed when vomiting has ceased, or the patient may be given a mouthwash if she is able to use it. Eau-de-cologne put behind the ears, on the forehead and on the handkerchief is refreshing. Sips of cold water may be given in all but gastric cases unless instructions to the contrary have been received from the surgeon. The dressing should be examined periodically. The bed is kept screened while the patient is feeling sick and ill and is under the influence of morphia. During the first twelve hours the surgeon may order fluids to be given per rectum or by some other route. During the first night another injection of morphia or a milder hypnotic will probably be required and sips of water will be given when the patient is awake. The night nurse should give the patient a bedpan and encourage her to pass urine before morning. This point should be reported as there is often some temporary post-operative paralysis of the bladder after manipulation of the organs in the lower abdomen.

AFTER THE OPERATION

The First Day. In the early morning the patient is given a mouthwash and a cup of tea or coffee, if vomiting has ceased. Otherwise it may be wiser to continue to give water only a little longer. If the patient is feeling fairly fit the nurse washes her face, neck, chest, arms and axillæ. With the help of another nurse she removes all but two of the head pillows and turns the patient on to her side, washing between the legs and the bottom of the back. She rubs the buttocks thoroughly well with spirit and powder, the drawsheet is pulled through or changed if necessary and the air ring re-adjusted. A clean gown is put on and the bed made, arranging the patient comfortably in the Fowler position again. Each time the patient's position is altered she should be given some breathing exercises, being told to take six or eight deep breaths, using the chest muscles well. If this makes her cough, all the better; it will help to remove mucus from the respiratory tract. Some patients are afraid to cough or breathe deeply in case of rupture of the stitches. They should be reassured on this point. If they cough violently, they can be told to support the abdomen while they do so. The teeth are cleaned if the patient is able to do this, if not she should use a mouthwash.

The hair is brushed, and a clean handkerchief is given to the patient. It is important to change the pillow case or sheet, if they smell of vomit or anæsthetic. How much detailed attention can be given to the toilet on this first day depends on the condition of the patient and may vary considerably, but the wash and change of gown, etc., always make the patient feel fresher and better afterwards.

The temperature, pulse, and respiration are taken four-hourly. Quite often the temperature is slightly raised as a normal reaction to the operation. Surgical fluids in small quantities are given, bovril, clear soup, tea, coffee, soda water, fruit drinks, pineapple juice, jelly, etc. Urine should be passed at intervals, but the quantity will be small as fluids have been taken in limited amounts.

At midday or later the patient will probably feel restless and uncomfortable and some mild sedative drug may again be required. (e.g. Veganin, Tabs. 2.) Before this is given the hands and face should be sponged and the patient made thoroughly comfortable as before.

If a drainage tube was inserted at the operation, the dressing must be done according to the surgeon's instructions; probably the tube will have to be changed or shortened.

When the hands and face are washed again in the evening, the back should be well rubbed as before. If the patient is very thin or heavy or the ype in whom pressure sores might easily arise, this attention should be given every four hours at least. The bed should be stripped and re-made.

A hypnotic of a milder variety is usually required for the night, and liquid paraffin $\tilde{3}$i may be ordered as an intestinal lubricant.

The Second Day. The toilet may be done more thoroughly on the second day and the patient encouraged to move about the bed more. Breathing exercises should be continued including a few deep breaths while the patient is turned on her side. She should flex and extend her legs a few times, when the knee pillow is removed. The diet is given as on the previous day. There is usually no objection to the patient having a dry biscuit or a little toast if she fancies it. Liquid paraffin, $\tilde{3}$i is usually given in the morning and again at night. The dressing is attended to if necessary.

After abdominal operations the patient often feels more uncomfortable on the second than on the first day. The effects of the anæsthetic and drugs are wearing off and she begins to feel some flatulence, and altogether does not feel so well. Again some mild hypnotic may be required.

The Third Day. In the early morning the patient is usually given an aperient, cascara or senna, one which will ensure a result though it need not be too drastic. If the bowels are opened during the morning, the patient may be given fish and potatoes and a little milk pudding at lunch, and thus gradually proceed to a light digestible diet. Fluids are given freely. The knee pillow is removed; the dressing attended to if necessary. It may only be necessary to take the temperature, pulse, and respiration night and morning, if the chart shows no abnormality. If the bowels do not act during the day, the patient will be very uncomfortable and a soap enema should be given in the evening. This will nearly always make the patient feel much better.

Fourth and Successive Days. The patient should make steady progress, gradually doing more for herself, eating more and sleeping better without the aid of drugs. A daily action of the bowels should be encouraged, some mild aperient being required while the patient is in bed.

Two pillows may be taken away when she wishes to rest or to sleep. There is no objection to her turning on her side.

Removal of Stitches and Clips. Clips are usually removed on the fifth day, deep tension stitches on the tenth day and superficial sutures on the eighth day. The patient may get up on a couch on the eighth to tenth day, taking a few steps with assistance until she gradually walks un-aided. She should be ready to go home on about the fourteenth day. She is told to make a gradual return to her normal routine, and to rest each day as much as she can. In some cases she may be required to attend the out-patient clinic at some future specified date. If the out-patient department has a system by which appointments can be made, this can be arranged before the patient leaves and the necessary appointment card

175

given. She may be put in touch with the hospital almoner if necessary.

Other details of Nursing Treatment required after Abdominal Operations

Pain. Pain is usually a symptom after abdominal operation and patients vary considerably in the amount of pain and discomfort they can tolerate. Some patients are prepared for it and make no complaint at all, while others are alarmed and tend to exaggerate it. A good nurse does not rely upon drugs for the relief of minor degrees of pain. Lifting the patient up, arranging pillows, turning her on her side, placing an extra small pillow in the back, the use of rubber hot water bottles on the abdomen or under the back, gentle rubbing of the back, all these simple remedies may give the patient relief for a time and enable her to get little intervals of sleep. Brushing the hair often has a soothing effect, and it must not be forgotten that emptying the bladder often gives relief to vague abdominal discomfort even though the patient may not realize that this is what is wanted. If simple nursing measures fail, it is obvious that a drug must be given. The good nurse learns to know how long a sedative can be withheld without the patient being distressed by pain.

Thirst. This is a troublesome complaint. The pre-anæsthetic drug, atropine, inhibits the secretions and this is one cause of the thirst. It is not wise to give more than sips of water if the patient is inclined to vomit, as too much fluid only increases the vomiting. The patient may rinse the mouth frequently with iced water.

Vomiting. Modern anæsthetics do not cause vomiting to the extent that the older methods did. Vomiting, however, is a troublesome complication sometimes, especially after ether has been used. The following methods of relieving it may be tried:

1. Prohibit the giving of all fluids by mouth for twelve hours after the anæsthetic.

2. Give sips of water or soda water.

3. If vomiting is persistent give a tumblerful of tepid water, containing soda bicarbonate ʒi. The patient should not sip this, but take it as a long drink. It will probably act as a stomach lavage and help to get rid of the anæsthetic excreted by the mucous membrane and causing irritation. The long drink may be repeated.

4. Liquor iodi 2 per cent ♏i in milk ʒi, half-hourly, may be given for four doses.

5. A small cup of strong black coffee with glucose may be tried, or a small cup of thick Benger's Food to which is added an ounce of brandy.

6. A mustard leaf applied to the epigastrium is a method of counter-irritation which may help to relieve an irritable stomach.

Mouthwashes and swabbing of the mouth with water and vinegar should be done after each vomit, to remove the smell and taste; eau-de-cologne and smelling salts, cold compresses to the forehead often make the patient feel fresh and a little better.

7. Gastric lavage may be prescribed if the above measures fail, and this treatment should not be postponed too long, as it is often followed not only by cessation of the vomiting, but by a definite improvement in the general condition of the patient. Vomiting which continues more than twenty-four hours after the operation is not usually due to the anæsthetic. The surgeon should be notified and other causes sought for.

Flatulence. The low diet and the manipulation of the intestines, however carefully done, sometimes causes a slight degree of temporary paralysis. The contents of the stomach and intestines ferment, and the abdominal organs become distended with gas. The following methods should be tried to relieve this:

1. Keep the patient well propped up in the Fowler position.

2. A rubber hot water bottle may be applied to the abdomen; or a turpentine stupe, if the position of the dressing allows it.

3. A cup of very hot water containing four minims of oil of peppermint may be sipped.

4. Two drops of oil of cajuput on a lump of sugar may give relief.

5. A turpentine or treacle enema or a flatus tube may be prescribed.

The discomfort from flatulence is usually worse during the second or third day, before the bowels have been opened. Afterwards, when the patient is having a more generous diet, it gives no further trouble.

Hiccough. This symptom is due to spasm of the diaphragm. It can be so persistent as to be serious. It is particularly serious in cases of renal failure and peritonitis. Measures taken for its relief are:

1. A cup of hot water with 4 minims of oil of peppermint.

2. Two drops of oil of cajuput on a lump of sugar.

3. A long drink of soda bicarbonate, $\mathfrak{Z}i$ to Oss of warm water, or gastric lavage may be ordered.

4. The epigastrium may be sprayed with ethyl chloride. This sometimes relaxes the spasm.

5. Inhalations of carbon dioxide 7 per cent and oxygen 93 per cent or a mixture containing a higher percentage of carbon dioxide may be more effective.

The simpler methods of encouraging the patient to hold the breath and then to breathe deeply will have been tried in the first instance. But in some cases this symptom is very intractable.

Retention of urine. The muscles of the bladder may be temporarily paralysed after manipulation of the organs in the lower abdomen. It is important to overcome this difficulty, if possible, without resorting to catheterization. Suggested measures are:

M   177

1. Irrigation of the genitals with a measured amount of warm water while the patient sits on a bedpan.

2. Hot fomentations over the bladder area.

3. A change of position if possible.

4. The running of taps in the hearing of the patient may act by suggestion.

5. A few boracic acid crystals may be put on the tongue.

6. An injection of doryl or carbachol 1 c.c. may be given intramuscularly.

The psychological factor is sometimes a contributory cause of the inability of the patient to pass urine. Fear, the unusual position and the fact that the patient is wearing an abdominal bandage, tend to inhibit the reflex. The nurse can help by reassuring her, by placing her comfortably on the bedpan, and sometimes a little loosening of the bandage may help. Trying a bedpan of a different shape is sometimes successful.

COMPLICATIONS AFTER OPERATION

1. **Shock.** Shock is a clinical condition in which there is depression of the central nervous system. The medullary centres which control blood pressure are disturbed. Veins and capillaries are dilated and the blood tends to stagnate in them, causing a fall in blood pressure. The causes contributing to this condition are:

1. Long or difficult anæsthesia.

2. Extensive operations with considerable manipulation of the organs and consequent damage to nerve endings.

3. Loss of fluid (hæmorrhage, excessive sweating, vomiting and diarrhœa).

4. Cold and exposure.

5. Pain.

6. Fear or mental shock.

The symptoms of shock are most important. Every nurse should be able to recognize them in their various degrees, and realize their serious import. They are all due to failure of the circulation and are:

1. A cold and 'clammy' skin. (The lack of circulation to the surface of the body causes the sweat to accumulate, instead of evaporate.)

2. A subnormal temperature.

3. The pulse is feeble and of low volume. It is sometimes quick, irregular or thready, although it may be slow.

4. Respirations are shallow. Movements of the chest may be almost imperceptible.

5. The patient lies in a condition of complete muscular relaxation, quite still and limp. The muscles of the eyelids may be relaxed so that the eyes are half open, showing the sclerotics.

6. The extremities are cold.

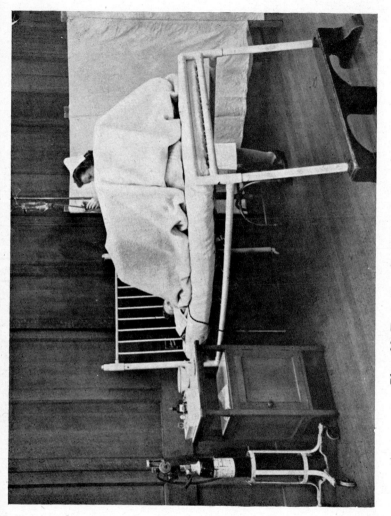

Plate 20. Treatment for shock. See page 178

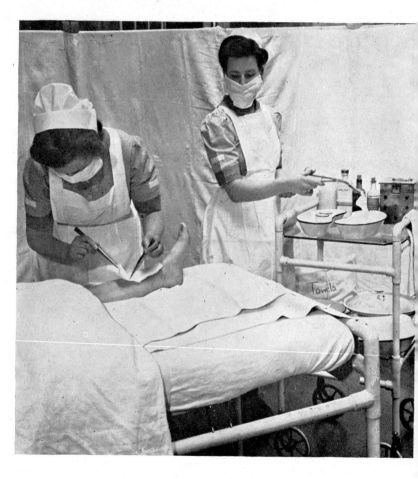

Plate 21. A surgical dressing. See page 185

Treatment. 1. The first and most important is rest. The nervous system needs time to recover. There should be limited movement and disturbance; To secure this, morphia is invaluable; it also relieves the pain. The patient should be kept quite flat with the head low, so that the blood is encouraged to circulate in the brain. The foot of the bed is raised on blocks.

2. Warmth is applied in every available form, such as hot water bottles, blankets, electric cradle. The perspiring skin is dried with a hot towel and a clean warm gown put on if necessary. Care should be taken, however, that the patient does not get too hot as this will make her restless and increase the risk of reactionary hæmorrhage.

Extra fluids should be introduced into the circulation in order to raise the blood pressure. After an abdominal operation it is not practicable to give them by mouth. The nurse should be prepared to give saline and glucose per rectum or subcutaneously. The house surgeon may wish to give blood, plasma, or saline and glucose intravenously in severe cases. Circulatory stimulants may be needed, e.g. injection of nicamide 1 c.c. hypodermically. This dose may be repeated.

Administration of oxygen may be required.

A careful record should be kept of the pulse which in favourable cases gradually improves, becoming stronger, of better volume and of more normal rate. The skin gradually gets warmer as the condition improves. Tone is restored to the muscles.

In cases of severe post-operative shock the symptoms may last for twenty-four hours, but often, marked improvement is seen in the patient after two or three hours (see plate 20).

2. **Hæmorrhage.** 1. *Primary hæmorrhage.* This occurs when the blood vessels are cut or damaged. There is always some primary hæmorrhage whilst the surgeon is operating.

2. *Reactionary hæmorrhage.* This is most important in post-operative care. It occurs within twenty-four hours of the operation and is due to the dislodging of the clots from the ends of small vessels which were not ligatured by the surgeon. Nature can be relied upon to seal up the ends by means of a clot. During the first hours after operation, however, as the patient recovers from shock and becomes restless, the blood pressure rises and some clots become dislodged. Occasionally a ligature may slip. If hæmorrhage is seen to be coming through the dressing the nurse should:

1. Report the fact to the sister.

2. Apply sterile wool pads over the dressing and bandage them firmly in position. The original dressing should not be touched.

3. A dose of morphia should be given if this has been prescribed. It will reduce the rate of the heart beat, and will keep the patient at rest. Clots will have a chance to reform at the cut ends of the vessels.

4. The pulse should be recorded quarter-hourly. A rising pulse is a sign of continuing hæmorrhage.

5. The dressing should be inspected frequently and if it 'comes through' a second time or in large quantity, the house surgeon should be notified. It may be necessary to take the patient back to the theatre and inspect the wound, and in some cases to ligature the bleeding vessels. Surgical technique is usually so good, however, that this is seldom necessary and the reactionary hæmorrhage is nearly always controlled by thorough packing, rest, and morphia.

3. *Secondary hæmorrhage*. This occurs from five to fourteen days after operation. It is almost invariably due to sepsis. Pus-forming organisms invade the wound, and erode the blood vessels, causing them to slough. Mismanagement of drainage tubes is sometimes a cause of secondary hæmorrhage. If they are kept in too long they may exert pressure against blood vessels and erosion may occur. A warning that a secondary hæmorrhage may be imminent is the appearance of a little fresh blood on the dressing seen when the latter is removed. This may indicate that a small vessel has broken down and that a more serious hæmorrhage may soon occur. If the chart shows a rising temperature, this may be an indication of sepsis. The dressing should be shown to the surgeon who may think it necessary to explore the wound in the theatre to see to what extent the sepsis has progressed. Thus the hæmorrhage might be avoided.

Secondary hæmorrhage is not common after abdominal operations.

Signs of Internal Hæmorrhage. It may be that the patient is bleeding into the abdominal cavity, although there is no sign of blood on the dressing. The symptoms of internal hæmorrhage are as follows:

1. A rising pulse.
2. Restlessness.
3. Coldness, clamminess, and sweating.
4. Fall in temperature.
5. Air hunger as the patient begins to feel the lack of oxygen owing to loss of blood. She gasps for air, and if the hæmorrhage continues, sighing respiration, showing exhaustion, will follow.
6. Giddiness and fainting due to exhaustion of the medullary centres; this is called syncope.

It will be clear that the signs of internal hæmorrhage are very similar to those of shock. It is by no means always easy to differentiate between the two. Perhaps the most outstanding difference is the fact that in hæmorrhage the patient is restless, anxious and suffering from air hunger, whereas in shock she lies limp and still. Also most cases of shock tend to improve, whereas if a hæmorrhage continues the symptoms get worse, especially the pulse.

COMPLICATIONS AFTER OPERATION

Treatment of Internal Hæmorrhage

1. Notify the house surgeon.
2. Put the patient flat, block the foot of the bed and apply warmth.
3. Record the pulse at fifteen-minute intervals or oftener.
4. Keep the patient very quiet and if conscious reassure her.
5. The patient, if in hospital, may be taken to the operating theatre at once and the bleeding vessel found and ligatured.
6. Morphia may safely be given to a patient who has been under observation and when the cause of the hæmorrhage is known; but in accident cases with internal hæmorrhage, morphia may mask the symptoms and confuse the diagnosis. This difficult point, however, may be left to the judgment of the surgeon.
7. If surgical aid is not forthcoming, in a severe case of internal hæmorrhage the legs may be bandaged firmly from the ankles to the groins, using firm calico or flannel bandages to encourage the blood to return and stay in the vital centres.
8. Fluids and circulatory stimulants are not indicated in hæmorrhage. They would only serve to raise the blood pressure and increase the bleeding. When the bleeding point has been found and ligatured, blood plasma or saline may be put into the circulation to replace that which has been lost.

3. **Acute Dilatation of the Stomach.** Post-operative vomiting which persists for more than twenty-four hours suggests that the muscular wall of the stomach has lost tone and become dilated. This is caused by manipulation of the stomach and the surrounding viscera. The patient is critically ill, the pulse is rapid, and vomiting is profuse. The surgeon must be notified of any case in which this condition is suspected. All fluid by mouth should be avoided. The stomach must be washed out and kept empty until the muscles have regained their tone. Some method of continuous suction such as a Sprengel's pump may be attached to a tube in the stomach, in order to keep the organ empty, or the stomach tube may be left in position and the contents aspirated half-hourly by means of a syringe. If treatment is prompt the patient soon begins to show signs of improvement.

4. **Paralytic Ileus.** This is a similar condition to the above, but in this case it is the intestines which are involved, being toneless and paralysed. It is a very serious condition which develops from twenty-four to forty-eight hours after operation. The symptoms are:

1. Vomiting.
2. Rapid pulse.
3. Distension of the intestine with gas.
4. Inability to pass fæces or flatus. Peristalsis is temporarily stopped and the contents of the bowel ferment. The condition is often associated with peritonitis.

The nursing treatment is:

1. Keep the patient at rest and warm.
2. Withhold fluids and food by mouth.
3. The stomach is washed out and kept empty as described above.
4. A turpentine or treacle enema may be ordered and a flatus tube passed.
5. Injections of pituitrin, $\frac{1}{2}$ c.c. and eserine $\frac{1}{2}$ c.c. are given at four-hourly intervals alternatively to stimulate peristalsis. Acetyl-choline is a drug which is also used to stimulate the plain muscle in the wall of the intestine to contract. Some surgeons however, are averse to prescribing treatments which cause over-stimulation of the muscle, and think that the tone will be regained better if the intestine is allowed to rest and take its own time to recover.

The main thing is for the nurse to understand the condition and the dangerous symptoms; to measure the vomit and to record the pulse at regular frequent intervals; and to notice particularly if flatus is passed. She should be prepared to give, or help to give, gastric lavage. The patient's condition is usually so critical that fluids are given intravenously to counteract shock which accompanies this complication.

5. **Peritonitis.** General infection of the peritoneum is usually a complication of abdominal conditions in which there has been perforation of an organ or rupture of an abscess (e.g. perforated duodenal ulcer, perforated appendix abscess). In these cases drainage tubes are inserted into the abdominal cavity to drain away the infected fluid, and to minimize the risk of peritonitis spreading.

Symptoms

1. A rapid, thready pulse, with a rise in temperature.
2. Distended, rigid and painful abdomen.
3. Vomiting.
4. Hiccough.
5. Shallow breathing in which the thoracic muscles only are used.
6. The patient appears very ill with increasing pallor and a typically anxious expression. This appearance was described by Hippocrates centuries ago, and is known as the 'Facies Hippocratica'.
7. The patient is constipated, passing neither faeces or flatus.
8. It is a bad sign if the pulse continues to rise without a corresponding rise in temperature.

Treatment. The treatment is similar to that of paralytic ileus. The surgeon, of course, ensures that drainage is efficient and generally orders one of the sulphonamide group of drugs to counteract infection. If the infection in the peritoneum localizes and forms an abscess it is most likely to be either in the pelvis or under the diaphragm. The treatment is incision and further drainage.

6. Chest Complications. A variety of chest conditions may follow anæsthesia and abdominal operations. They are:

1. *Bronchitis* which may develop into *broncho-pneumonia.* The type of patient who most often develops this complication is the elderly thick-chested, short-necked patient who suffers from attacks of bronchitis. The mucous membranes of the respiratory tract are very liable to infection and soon become irritated. In addition, these patients usually have a rigid chest wall and do not breathe deeply. Inhalation anæsthetics are very likely to light up an attack of bronchitis which may spread into the bronchioles.

Treatment. The nurse is warned of the onset of the bronchitis by a cough, a rise in temperature, a 'tight' pain in the chest and cyanosis. The patient must be well propped up and deep breathing encouraged. Expectorant mixtures containing squills and ammonium carbonate are prescribed. In elderly subjects there is likely to be a strain on the heart. Brandy and four-hourly injections of strychnine are often ordered and all the nursing care required by a patient who has developed a serious chest condition. Fluids are given freely.

Babies are also likely to develop bronchitis after anæsthesia. They must be kept very warm and out of draughts, as they cannot stand changes of temperature. The cot must be screened and the windows near by kept closed, and, if necessary, the baby's head kept covered with a shawl or bonnet. The pillows must be arranged so that the child is propped up; some change of position from time to time, from one side to another, helps the child to cough up the secretion.

2. *Massive collapse of the lung.* It is not uncommon for a patient, especially the type of adult described above, to have a portion of the lung collapsed owing to a plug of mucus blocking a bronchiole leading to the area. The tight chest and the abdominal condition prevent the patient from coughing vigorously and so the mucus is not expectorated. The symptoms are: (a) cyanosis; (b) rise in temperature, pulse and respiration; (c) pain in the chest. The patient must be encouraged to breathe deeply and cough. Drugs are given to help the patient to expectorate. Inhalations of carbon dioxide and oxygen help the expansion of the lungs, and breathing exercises while the patient is turned on the side may dislodge the mucus. Brandy and stimulants are often required.

3. *Pulmonary embolism.* An embolism is a foreign body circulating in the blood stream. It may be a blood clot, air bubble or septic material detached from some focus. In the case of pulmonary embolism after abdominal operations the embolus is almost always a clot of blood. It is thought that the clot forms in the pelvic veins from which it reaches the lungs lodging in a vessel too small for it to pass through. The factors which cause the formation of the clot in the vein are not fully understood, but they are thought to be:

1. Sepsis entering at the time of operation.
2. Poor circulation due to lack of movement.

Death from pulmonary embolism is one of the tragedies of surgery which cannot be foreseen. It occurs at about the ninth or tenth day. Up to this time the patient has been making normal progress and may even have been sitting up out of bed. She complains of sudden pain in the chest, is unable to breathe and appears very distressed and cyanosed. She may have a desire to defæcate and ask for a bedpan. Death sometimes occurs before anything can be done. The patient should be screened, the position altered as little as possible, apart from adjusting the pillows. A window may be opened while the surgeon is summoned. The drugs which are given in this emergency are: nicamide, 1 c.c., morphia gr. ¼, or an ampoule of amyl nitrite, 5 minims given by inhalation. If the clot is a large one no treatment is of any avail. If, however, the patient presents less urgent symptoms, that is, if there is a sudden pain in the chest with mild distress and dyspnœa, it may be that the clot is only small and will block a terminal vessel supplying only a small area of the lung. This portion will collapse and fail to function. Such a condition is called a *pulmonary infarct*. With good nursing the patient will recover as the clot is reabsorbed in the course of a few weeks. *The treatment* is to nurse the patient in a comfortable position at complete rest. The chest on the affected side may be painted with liquor iodi 2 per cent and sedative drugs are employed. The temperature may be raised. Fluids and a light diet are given. The patient should be moved carefully by two nurses when nursing treatment is done.

Although the nurse should learn to recognize the symptoms of chest complications and know how to deal with them, it is far more important when nursing surgical cases that she should know how to *prevent* them. The following nursing details cannot be over-emphasized in this respect:

1. Observation before the operation; the type of patient; history of respiratory disease; and postponement of the operation if the patient has a cold or cough. If this is impossible, the anæsthetist will choose his anæsthetic with great care.

2. The patient must be kept warm and guarded from draughts in transit from the theatre to the ward. The temperature of the theatre should be 68° to 70° F., as the patient is particularly susceptible to cold whilst exposed and under the anæsthetic. The windows round the bed when the patient returns should be closed, and care taken that the patient does not get a chill through lying in a gown wet with perspiration.

3. The sitting-up position should be adopted whenever possible, the chest being kept well covered. Deep breathing exercises should be encouraged, both before and after the operation; a few deep breaths several times a day at intervals, including exercises given whilst the patient is

urned on her side for bedmaking. The
legs should be moved up and down the bed
freely after the first twenty-four hours and
the knee pillow removed on the third
morning. All this movement helps to improve the circulation and prevent irritating matter accumulating in the bronchial
vessels, and the patient is more likely to
cough it up.

4. Tight bandaging of chest or abdomen
should be avoided as this constricts the
movements of the chest muscles and diaphragm. It is the practice of many surgeons
to secure the dressing on an abdominal
wound by means of strapping.

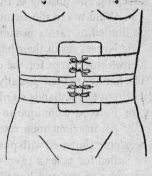

FIG. 70. Dressing held in
position by strapping corset

7. **Femoral Thrombosis.** This is the formation of a clot in one of the femoral veins. The causes are the same as those which cause the clot in the case
of pulmonary embolism, that is, sepsis and stasis in the vessels. Another
predisposing cause is the use of hard lumpy knee pillows, left in the bed too
long. These press on the veins and impede the circulation. On about the
tenth day the leg becomes swollen and painful. The clot may be felt if it
is in a superficial vein. The temperature is raised, 100° to 101° F. The leg
must be put on a soft pillow and immobilized by sandbags. A cradle
should take the weight of the bedclothes. Hot or cold applications may
be prescribed, or the part may be treated with glycerine and hot fomentations applied; antiphlogistine poultices, or glycerine and belladonna dressings are also used. Sometimes an evaporating lotion containing lead and
opium may be applied as a compress. Fluids are given freely. Rest is
required for four to six weeks until the clot is reabsorbed. Great care must
be taken when changing the position of the patient. Two nurses are required. Sometimes the surgeon orders the leg to be fixed comfortably on a
wooden back-splint with footpiece.

Again preventive measures are important:

1. Perfect asepsis in the operating theatre.
2. Care in the use of knee-pillows.
3. Leg exercises to maintain the circulation.

DRESSING THE WOUND

General Rules for Ward Dressings

1. Two nurses are required: (a) The dresser. (b) The trolley assistant.
2. Properly fitting masks to be worn. (Arrangements must be made for
the disinfection and washing of these; they must not be kept in the nurses'
pockets.)

3. Dressings should not be done till one hour has elapsed after th sweeping and dusting of the ward.

4. Windows in the vicinity of the patient are to be closed and traffic t be limited as far as possible.

5. Nurses scrub their hands with soap and hot water and dry them o a *clean* towel kept for the dressers only (this may be kept on the trolley The hands are then 'socially clean' but not sterile. No amount of scrubbin will render the hands sterile. Nails are to be cut short.

6. Forceps technique to be used throughout.

7. All instruments are to be boiled for two minutes (unless they hav been contaminated with pus or fæcal matter, etc., in which case they shoul be boiled for at least twenty to thirty minutes.) Sharp instruments may b wrapped in lint and boiled. Instruments should be used dry and kept i *covered* dishes all the time.

8. The dressing is to be exposed for the shortest possible time.

9. Receptacles for soiled dressings and used instruments must b covered.

10. Materials for each dressing should be made up in individual packets wrapped in lint or linen. This wrapping may be used as a towel for th purpose of doing the dressing and may be washed and resterilized. If th dressing is a large one, a full sized towel is required.

These rules are devised to limit as far as possible infection of wound from: (a) droplet infection from nose and mouth. (b) hands. (c) dust.

Note

1. Wet hands and instruments are more likely to carry infection tha dry ones.

2. Methylated spirit and alcohol are not reliable disinfectants. Instru ments, syringes, etc., which *have been sterilized* may be kept sterile i spirit.

3. Syringes, needles, etc., should be kept for their special purposes onl (e.g. hypodermic needles for hypodermic injection—aspirating needles fo aspirations only, etc.). Needles, etc., which have been grossly contaminated by pus, infected fluid, etc., must be thoroughly dealt with (either auto claved or boiled for thirty minutes). It is comparatively safe to replace hypodermic syringes and needles in spirit if they are kept for hypodermi use in clean cases only.

A Simple Dressing

Requirements

1. Mackintosh.
2. Receiver for soiled dressings (covered).
3. Receiver for used instruments (covered).
4. Receiver for used, but clean, top dressings (salvage).

5. Lifting forceps.
6. Hand towel.
7. Two face masks.
8. Sterile dish (covered) containing three pairs of dressing forceps.
9. Two sterile dishes; gallipot.
10. Methylated spirit.
11. Drum of sterile towels (if required).
12. Drum of sterile dressings.
13. Bandage and safety pin.
14. Elastoplast strapping.

Method. Masks are put on and both nurses scrub their hands and dry them on a clean towel. The trolley assistant prepares the patient. She puts her in a comfortable position. If it is a limb to be dressed, a pillow should be put underneath it. The mackintosh is put in position. Using the lifting forceps, the trolley assistant then takes out of the drum, a packet of dressings and a towel if necessary. She puts these in a sterile bowl. She pours spirit into a gallipot. She then removes the bandage.

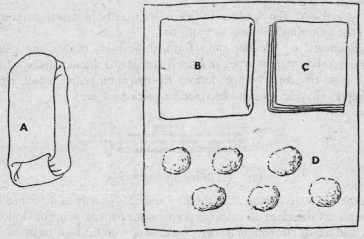

FIG. 71. Ward Dressing packet. (a) Dressing folded in square lint or linen which may be used as towel. (b) Wool pad. (c) Gauze squares. (d) Wool swabs

She next lifts a pair of dressing forceps out of the covered dish (using lifting forceps) hands them to the dresser and replaces the cover. With the dressing forceps, the dresser removes the top dressings. If these are clean she places them in the receiver for salvage, otherwise they are put into the covered receiver. She then discards her forceps, putting them into the covered dish for used instruments. With the lifting forceps the trolley assistant hands the other two pairs of dressing forceps to the

dresser, who opens the packet of dressings and then proceeds to remov
the dressing next to the wound. This is placed in the covered receiver, th
trolley assistant lifting the lid. The dresser then proceeds to clean and dres
the wound as required, using the same forceps. The trolley assistant fixe
the wool and bandage, makes the patient comfortable and tidies the bed
The instruments used by the dresser must come in contact with nothing bu
the last layer of soiled dressing over the wound, the wound itself, and th
clean dressing put on the wound. Thus no infection other than that alread·
present in the wound should gain entry. The whole aim of careful surgica
technique when doing ward dressings is to prevent cross infection from
complicating the existing condition. The instruments and dishes are re
boiled and the trolley reset. If another dressing is to be done at once, it i
convenient if two sets of instruments are available. The gallipot containing
spirit should be covered so that it may be used again, if it is quite certain
that it has not been contaminated. Soiled dressings are emptied into a
covered bucket in the annexe as soon as dressings are finished. They are
burnt in the incinerator (see plate 21).

Dressing of Septic Wounds

Requirements. The dressing trolley is set exactly as described above
with the following additions as required:

Instruments: e.g. Probe; sinus forceps; scissors; rubber and gauze
drainage tubes, various types and sizes; corrugated drains; sterile safety-
pins; glass irrigating syringe; lotions for irrigation (saline, eusol, etc.);
antiseptics (flavine, gentian violet, iodine, picric acid, etc.).

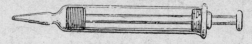

Fig. 72. Glass irrigating syringe

Method. The technique of doing the dressing is exactly as described for
a simple dry dressing; the assistant prepares the patient, pours out lotions,
etc., and hands all requirements to the dresser with lifting forceps.

The nurse whilst doing the dressing should judge of its progress. She
must be able to report the amount of discharge, its character and the
appearance of the wound. She will note if it is draining satisfactorily, or
if the discharge is scanty and if the sinus leading to the wound is healing.
She must make sure, if the sinus forceps or probe do not penetrate
as far into the wound as she expected, that the pus is not 'pocketing' at
the bottom. If she suspects this, she inserts the sinus forceps, closed, deeply
into the wound. She then opens the forceps in order to release any pus
which may have collected at the bottom. When the wound begins to heal,
the amount of granulation tissue must be noted. This should form from

ie bottom and is recognized as new pink velvety tissue, which bleeds
isily when touched with an instrument. Granulating tissue should not
row too quickly before the wound is clear of pus, nor should it be allowed
) grow too exuberantly on the edges of the wound, or an ugly scar will
:sult. The granulations may be touched with a silver nitrate stick to
mit excessive growth.

Lotions used for irrigating are prepared at a temperature of 100° F.;
iey must be made up in an accurate strength—antiseptics used in too
rong solution do more harm than good by devitalizing the tissues. The
iges of the wound and the skin surrounding it must be cleaned with
iline to remove dried discharge and debris, but it must be well dried,
therwise it will become sodden and liable to secondary infection.

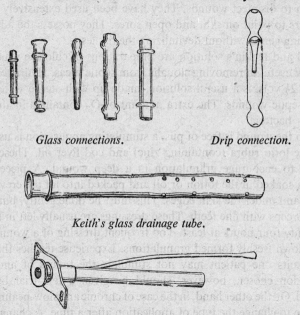

Glass connections.   *Drip connection.*

Keith's glass drainage tube.

*Tudor Edwards's empyema drainage tube with catheter incorporated for
irrigation.*
FIG. 73

Drainage of wounds. Wounds are drained if there is likely to be much
ozing of blood, serum or pus. Various methods are used: e.g. rubber or
lass tubes, gauze drains, corrugated rubber, or pieces of soft rubber cut
·om old gloves, may be put into the wound to keep it open. The drain is
:moved or changed according to instructions received from the surgeon.
t is most important that rigid tube drains should be shortened, turned,
r removed frequently, to prevent them eroding blood vessels. Erosion
iay lead to sloughing and secondary hæmorrhage.

A septic wound may be immersed four-hourly in a saline bath or water containing some other disinfectant, such as calcium hypochlorite (eusol) The bath should be at a temperature of 100° F. and the bowl or bath itself must be disinfected before use, by mopping with pure lysol. The lysol must be rinsed off carefully with sterile saline or boiled water. The thermometer used for testing the temperature of lotions is itself kept in antiseptic

Lacerated or dirty wounds are sometimes dusted or sprayed with sulphonamide powder before the dressing is applied. Tablets are crushed to powder and put into small gauze bags which are sent to be sterilized in a dressing drum. The powder is sprinkled on the wound by shaking the bag or tapping it with forceps, as the dressing is being done. Aniline dyes such as gentian violet, mercurochrome, malachite green, acriflavine are used in solution to disinfect wounds. They have been used extensively in the last few years to paint on skin and open sores. They possess the advantage of destroying germs without devitalizing the tissues.

Eusol and Dakin's solution are preparations of chlorine which are particularly useful in removing sloughs from septic areas. Hydrogen peroxide (H_2O_2) $2\frac{1}{2}$ vols. is a useful solution, made up with sterile water, for irrigating septic wounds. The extra amount of O_2 contained in the solution oxidizes bacteria.

When the wound is free of pus, a stimulating application is used. Useful ones are lotio rubra (containing zinc) and cod liver oil. These are often applied to encourage granulation in a deep wound. A piece of sterile gauze is soaked in the lotion or oil and packed into all the crevices of the wound and under the skin edges. This must be done gently, but precisely using forceps with fine teeth. These dressings are usually left in the wound for twenty-four hours at least. Too frequent dressing of a wound tends to break down freshly formed granulations. Experience teaches that a lotion which suits one patient may not stimulate the tissues of another. The application chosen, however, should be given a fair trial before it is changed. On the other hand, in the case of chronic and slow-healing wounds it is wise to change the type of application after a time. A change seems to have a stimulating effect on the cells.

Elastoplast and zinc ointment strapping are very useful dressings for superficial cuts and lesions. The same dressing can be kept on for several days, even if the wound is septic. The healing process is stimulated by the zinc contained in the plaster.

Ointments and dressings containing strong antiseptics must be cut to the size of the wound and applied only to that area. A gauze dressing of a large size can be applied over it. The whole is then bandaged in position. If a dressing is to be kept in position by strips of plaster, the strips should be secured at a reasonable distance from the wound on to healthy skin.

It is important that the skin area in the region of the wound should be
ept healthy and dry by frequent washing and rubbing to maintain the
rculation.

A hæmatoma is an extravasation of blood into the tissues. It sometimes
ccurs in the neighbourhood of the wound. It appears as a hard painful
urplish mass under the skin. If it is very painful, a hot fomentation should
e applied. The surgeon usually evacuates the fluid without delay.

Rupture of the wound. The superficial stitches may give way and the
ound burst open. This sometimes happens in fat patients who have put
rain on an abdominal wound by coughing or vomiting. In a patient whose
bdominal wall is very fat and flabby, careful attention should be paid to
e method of applying the dressing, in order to ensure that the stitches have
dequate support. If the stitches should rupture, the patient should be put
the dorsal position, with the knees flexed, whilst a sterile towel or
ressing is put over the gaping wound and a supporting bandage applied.
he house surgeon must be notified at once and the patient will go to the
perating theatre to have the wound resutured. In the meantime, she
ould be reassured and encouraged to lie still.

emoval of Stitches

Requirements: as for a simple dressing, with the addition of a pair of
arp-pointed scissors.

Method. The part is prepared as for a surgical dressing. The skin is
wabbed with spirit and the dresser picks up each stitch in turn with a pair
f forceps held in the left hand. With the scissors in the right hand, she
uts the suture between the knot and the skin. The cut should be as near

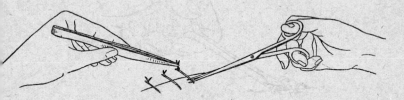

FIG. 74. Removal of stitches

the skin surface as possible. The stitch is pulled out from the other end
that none of the external portion is drawn through the tissues. The
ound is then cleaned with a swab soaked in sterile saline or spirit to re-
ove dried skin and blood. It is dried with another swab and painted with
ethylated spirit. Forceps technique is used throughout. Sometimes it is
ot necessary to apply a dressing after stitches have been removed.

To remove a continuous suture. This may be of fine salmon gut, horse
air, or silk. The technique for removal of a continuous suture is almost
e same as described above, remembering that each stitch must be re-

moved separately, to avoid any of the
external part of the suture being drawn
through the skin. Each stitch is cut near
the skin and withdrawn from the further
end.

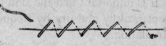

FIG. 75. A continuous suture

Removal of Clips

Requirements. The requirements are as above. The extra instrument
required are Michel clip removers.

Method. The curved blade of the clip removers is inserted under the
middle of the clip. The upper blade is pressed home over the clip, in order
to bend it in the middle. This releases it at either end and it comes away
quite neatly (see diagram).

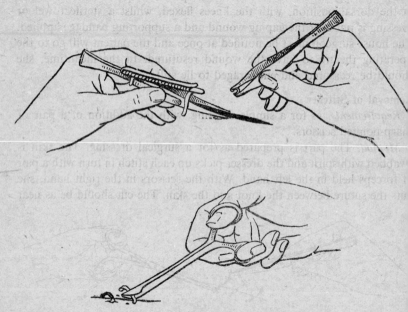

FIG. 76. Insertion and removal of Michel clips

Stitch Abscess. It is not uncommon for pus-forming organisms (usually
staphylococci) to invade the superficial tissues. This often occurs at the
side of a stitch. The area becomes inflamed and sore, and a little pus may
be seen at the point where the stitch enters. As soon as this is obvious the
stitch is removed, causing the wound to gape a little. This affords an exit
for the discharge. It should be well cleaned up with saline and a hot
boracic fomentation applied four-hourly to the wound generally brings
the inflammation to the surface. The other stitches must be watched carefully and it may be necessary to remove a second one.

DRESSING THE WOUND

The house surgeon must be asked to inspect the dressing. He may examine the wound, using probe or sinus forceps to make sure that the trouble is not deepseated. Usually it is very superficial and clears up in a few days. When the sepsis has been cleared up by fomentations, the part is kept dry with spirit.

All scars should be massaged lightly with lanoline as soon as they have healed. This renders the scar supple and prevents it from adhering to the underlying tissue.

Chapter Eleven

BURNS AND SCALDS

Burns are caused by dry heat; scalds by moist heat. The treatment is the same in both cases.

Burns are described as of three degrees, according to the depth of skin tissue which is involved:

First degree. Reddening of the skin. The superficial layer of the epidermis only is damaged. The reddening is termed erythema. No scars result.

Second degree. The epidermis is separated from the dermis and lymph collects between the two. The result is blistering. Healing generally takes place without scar formation.

Third degree. The dermis is destroyed. The deeper tissues may also be involved. The result is severe pain and shock as the nerve endings are exposed. Scars result. Third degree burns are very serious.

Burns vary in severity according to:

1. *Extent rather than depth*. A large superficial burn is more serious than a smaller deep one. This is because of the number of nerve endings involved and the shock which results from depression of the nervous system.

2. *The age of the patient*. Burns in young children are very serious because the nervous system is unstable and consequently the child's resistance to shock is poor.

3. *The site of the burn*. Burns of the chest and abdomen are more serious than burns of the limbs. This again is due to the extent of the nerve injury.

TREATMENT OF BURNS

First Aid Treatment. This is directed to two ends:

1. The treatment of shock.
2. The prevention of sepsis.

The patient is put flat on a couch (if available) and covered with warm rugs and blankets or coats. If possible, an assistant should prepare a hot drink; sweet tea is very good or a stimulant such as brandy or whisky. As exposure of nerve endings is the cause of the shock, immediate attention to the burnt area is necessary. The clothing over the burn is removed as soon as possible, though if it is stuck to the skin it should not be pulled away as the pain of doing this would increase the shocked condition. If the affected part is a limb, the best thing to do is to immerse the part in a bath of warm water, temperature 98° F., containing a tablespoonful of oda bicarbonate to the pint. If it is not possible to put the part in a bath, ieces of clean lint or linen should be soaked in soda bicarbonate solution nd put on the part whilst very wet. They should be kept soaked all the me. If the patient is a child and the burns are extensive, the clothes should e removed as quickly as possible and he should be sat in a bath. A blan-et may be put over the bath to keep the child as warm as possible. Weak ailky tea with plenty of sugar is a suitable drink to give him.

If soda bicarbonate is not immediately available, compresses soaked in trong tea or normal saline can be applied. Tannafax jelly is now found in 10st first aid sets. This, if applied thickly, is a very good first aid treatment. 'ormerly it was usual to apply some oily solution such as olive oil or •araffin or carron oil (a mixture of lime water and olive oil). The modern reatment, however, discourages the use of oily preparations as all the •il has to be removed before tannic acid or other coagulating agents are sed.

In cases of burns of any severity, the patient should, if possible, be aken to hospital immediately. If this is not possible, a doctor should be etched at once. In the meantime the above measures should be taken to :eep the burn covered and clean and the patient as warm and free from •ain as possible. As soon as medical aid is available a narcotic drug will be •rdered, in all severe cases; the usual one is injection of morphia, gr. $\frac{1}{6}$ to $\frac{1}{4}$.

Treatment of Severe Burns. As already stated, these should in all cases •e treated in hospital. The surgeon will decide at what stage the patient's ;eneral condition makes it safe for an anæsthetic to be given. It may be •ossible for the patient to be taken to the theatre immediately on admis-ion. The anæsthetic is given in an ante-room, and the patient undressed vhilst unconscious. This will avoid unnecessary pain and therefore will educe shock. In many cases the patient will be first taken to a ward. A take-in' bed will be prepared, and all pillows except one will be removed. Hot blankets and bottles will be applied and the foot of the bed raised on •locks. An electric cradle is helpful in the treatment of shock. The pulse is ecorded frequently. The patient should not be undressed at once as the :xposure and change of clothing is likely to induce further shock. If, however, it were a case of scalds, or if the flames had been extinguished by means of water, the wet clothes should, as far as possible, be removed quickly. A warm dry gown is then put on. Before the patient goes to the ward she will have had an injection of morphia in the casualty department. If shock is so severe that fluids must be given, they are given intravenously or subcutaneously, or possibly per rectum. Blood plasma 1 to 3 pints may be given and inhalations of oxygen. The surgeon is usually anxious to proceed with the treatment of the burn as soon as possible, knowing that the sooner the appropriate treatment is given the sooner the general condi-tion will improve.

BURNS AND SCALDS

Before the patient goes to the theatre, dentures should be removed, bedpan given and a pre-anæsthetic drug, as prescribed. Under the anæsthetic all fragments of clothing and debris are gently cleaned away and the burnt area cleansed thoroughly with sterile saline. Every trace of dirt which may lead to infection of the wound must be carefully removed; some of the damaged tissue may be excised. When this has been done some solution is applied which will exclude the air and encourage healing. The following may be used:

1. *Tannic acid*. In 1926 the treatment of burns and scalds was revolutionized by the introduction of the tannic acid treatment. Tannic acid powder is made up fresh in distilled water to the required strength. This may be $2\frac{1}{2}$, 5, 10, or 20 per cent according to the surgeon's instructions. The solution is put into a scent spray insufflator and is sprayed on the wound in the theatre. A compress of lint soaked in the solution is put on the part. The patient is then taken back to the ward. Here the treatment by spraying may be continued at fifteen-minute intervals up to twelve hours or until a sufficiently thick coagulum is formed. On the other hand, the compress may be left in position and kept moist with the tannic acid solution.

The *advantages of tannic acid* treatment are many:

1. It coagulates the proteins in the tissues and thus forms a coating over the whole area. This coagulum excludes the air and covers up the nerve endings, thus relieving pain.

2. It prevents the entry of germs and loss of fluid from the area.

3. Toxic substances produced in the damaged tissues by the injury are fixed in the coagulum and thus prevented from entering the circulation. This last factor is important in preventing toxæmia.

After ten to fourteen days the thick brown coagulum begins to peel off and healing is found to have taken place successfully underneath it. It was thought until recently that tannic acid treatment was the perfect treatment for burns and scalds for the above reasons. It reduced the mortality rate from shock and infection to a comparatively low figure. During the last year or two, however, the treatment has been further improved upon. There are *certain disadvantages* in using tannic acid:

1. If the treatment is delayed and the wound in the meantime becomes infected, pus forms under the coagulum and is difficult to deal with.

2. If used in the neighbourhood of a joint, for example, on the hands, the coagulum becomes dried and rigid as the healing process begins, and unless great care is taken the joints become contracted. In some cases it has taken months for the full use of the hands to be regained.

Tannic acid treatment for burns of the hands is now considered quite unsuitable by all authorities.

2. *Triple solution*. The improved method and one which is now being

sed is to apply, either by spray or compress, a solution containing tannic
.cid (10%), silver nitrate (10%), and gentian violet (1%). This applica-
ion is a coagulant as it contains tannic acid; the silver nitrate is a strong
antiseptic, and the gentian violet, in addition to being antiseptic, is an
aniline dye which encourages healing and counteracts devitalization of the
issues. Triple solution forms a coagulant which is not nearly so rigid or
ikely to cause contractions in the neighbourhood of joints.

3. *Saline baths*. The coagulating
methods described above are not used
n the case of burns of the hands.
The hands are immersed for twenty
to thirty minutes at four-hourly intervals in a bath of sterile saline solution, temperature 98° F. The bowl or
bath being used must have been
boiled or mopped out with a strong
disinfectant such as pure lysol, to
render it aseptic, and rinsed with
sterile saline. The dressings are removed whilst the hands are in the
bath. Forceps are used for this purpose, the nurse must not put her
hands in the bath. If this is absolutely
necessary sterile rubber gloves must
be used. The saline baths are very
soothing and the patient appreciates
this. When they are taken out, the
wounds are gently dried. The drying
may be done near an infra-red lamp;
if the area is a large one, the lamp
helps to counteract the effect of the
exposure. The areas may then be
quickly sprayed with sulphonamide
powder, after which the wounds are
dressed with tulle gras.

This consists of a coarse-meshed
gauze, sterilized and impregnated
thickly with sterile vaseline containing balsam of Peru. The tulle gras
dressing is covered with saline compresses and wool; the saline compresses must be kept moist.

If other parts of the body are

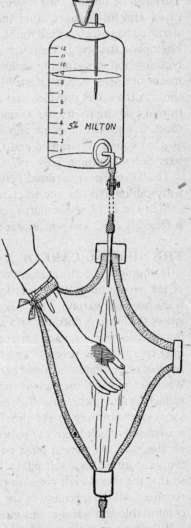

Fig. 77.
Bunyan-Stannard Envelope

involved, the patient may be wholly immersed in a full-sized saline bath
It is essential that two nurses should do the treatment and that everything
should be prepared methodically beforehand, so that the dressings are
done very quickly; with good team work large areas should be dressed
and covered in two or three minutes.

4. *Bunyan-Stannard Envelope*. This method has been introduced and a
large measure of success has been claimed for it. The envelopes or bag
are made by certain manufacturers of strong oiled silk specially coated
They can be obtained for treatment of any part of the body. In the case
of an arm for instance, after initial cleansing, the limb is put into the
sterilized bag which is fixed round the upper part of the arm by means of
elastoplast strapping. Thorough irrigation of the wound by an electro-
lytic solution of sodium hypochlorite 5 per cent (100° F.) is carried out by
means of a glass nozzle inserted into one of the inlets. The solution drains
through the outlet provided and oxygen may be admitted into the bag
from a cylinder to dry the wound. Hence the wound does not need to be
touched when dressings are applied. Granulations of the epithelium grow
as the wound is cleansed and the limb may be moved freely within the
bag. See illustration, page 197.

The envelope is sterilized before and after use by thorough flushing
with sodium hypochlorite solution 20 per cent.

Many cases of severe burns require skin grafting when the wound is
sufficiently clean and where large areas of epithelium have been destroyed.

THE NURSING CARE OF A PATIENT WITH SEVERE BURNS

In addition to the local treatment above described, the general condition
of the patient needs expert nursing care, and the first thing to emphasize
is the need for warmth. This is not always easy to apply on account of the
site of the burn. A difficulty also arises from the fact that a blanket should
not be put near a tanned surface whilst the coagulum is forming, as it
interferes with the process. An electric cradle should be made use of in
suitable cases. Windows should be closed and screens kept round the patient.
Wherever possible the patient should be placed in a sitting-up position;
bronchitis and pneumonia often result from extensive burns, owing to the
shock and exposure at the time of the accident. The position must be
maintained which keeps the patient off the injured part. If the burns are
on the back, the patient must be nursed in the prone position with the
arms supported on a soft pillow. A small pillow is put under the ankles
so that the toes do not press on the bed. A bed cradle will, of course, be
required. All the ingenuity of the nurse must be used to keep the patient
comfortable and warm in this most difficult position.

If the burn is in the neighbourhood of a joint, care must be taken that
it does not become flexed. The limb must be fixed in an extended position

whilst the tissues heal. Areas in which this precaution must be taken are the axillæ and the flexor surfaces of the knees and elbows. For cases of burns of the neck, the nurse must see that the head is kept in a good position, bent slightly to the opposite side to over-correct the tendency to flexion.

If the patient is a child or very restless, precautions must be taken that the wounds are not touched. It may be necessary to tie the hands to the side of the bed until the restless stage is passed.

Sedative drugs are required during the first twenty-four to forty-eight hours after the accident, after which the patient is usually much more comfortable.

A nourishing diet with extra fluids is essential to build up the patient's resistance, and counteract the shock resulting from the accident. Fluids are particularly important, as the blood volume will have been lessened by the loss of fluid from the burnt surface, and the loss from sweating during the period of shock. The amount of fluid lost in this way is always considerable. Quite often, too, the patient has had a period of acute vomiting which again means loss of fluid. The drinks given must be measured and plenty of glucose should be put in all feeds. The amount of urine passed must be measured. Retention sometimes results from the shock and suppression of urine from the depletion of the volume of fluid.

If the buttocks or the pubic areas are burnt, it may not be possible for the patient to use a bedpan, and a shallow kidney dish is often useful instead. A padding of wool should be put round the edges so that the hard rim does not hurt the patient. In these cases an enema should be given every other day, and if it is not possible for the patient to use a well-padded bedpan, a rubber one can be tried. The nurse must use her ingenuity to fix up the patient comfortably when the bedpan is required, otherwise the pain and discomfort will make her unable to use it. The urine should be tested for albumen.

Burns of the face. The eyes may need irrigating and the lids should be smeared with lanoline if they are stiff or if the skin is damaged.

COMPLICATIONS OF SEVERE BURNS

1. *Primary shock.* This occurs at the time of the accident due to depression of the nervous system, caused by the exposure of nerve endings. Pain and fright also contribute to this. In some cases primary shock results in death within a few hours. Otherwise with efficient treatment the condition gradually improves.

2. *Toxæmia.* Symptoms occur from twenty-four to forty-eight hours after the patient has recovered from the primary shock. It is most often seen when there has been delay in the treatment of the burnt area. Toxic substances are formed and enter the circulation. The temperature rises and albumen appears in the urine. Abundant fluids and glucose should be given.

3. *Sepsis*. This occurs when there has been delay or lack of thoroughness in the treatment of the burnt area. The burn may result in a septic wound. The infection prevents the formation of fresh epithelium and, when the wound is clean, skin grafts may be necessary.

4. *Chest complications*. Good nursing, warmth, fluids and early treatment for a cough or a cold should prevent them. The most serious is broncho-pneumonia.

5. *Deformity due to contraction of scar tissue*. This is particularly likely to occur in deep burns where the fascia and muscles have been involved.

1. **Treatment of Small Burns. First degree burns** involving a small area can be treated with a soothing ointment such as lanoline or vaseline. Sunburn is a good example of this type.

2. Small *second degree burns* with blisters of raised epthelium. The blisters should be removed with sharp-pointed sterile scissors. The raw surface underneath can be treated with various applications, suitable ones are: Tannic acid 5 per cent applied as a compress; tannafax jelly; equal parts of tannic acid 5 per cent, and perchloride of mercury, 1 in 1,200; equal parts of tannic acid, silver nitrate, and gentian violet; acriflavine in paraffin; sterile paraffin or vaseline; zinc and castor oil ointment (ung. zinc et ol. ric.); and picric acid 1 per cent in water.

Wax dressing for burns. This is only used for burns which are quite clean. Paraffin wax is heated until it melts and all preparations are made as for surgical dressing. The raw area is cleaned very gently with normal saline and is then covered with a coating of wax, using a sterile camel-hair brush. A layer of gauze or a very thin layer of wool is put on the wax before it sets. A second and third coating with gauze or wool are applied and the part is covered with a pad of sterile wool. The dressing is renewed in forty-eight hours' time. The wax covering can be lifted off by inserting forceps under the edges. No antiseptics must be used.

Chapter Twelve

SPLINTS, EXTENSIONS AND PLASTERS

THE USE OF SPLINTS

Splints of various kinds are used for immobilizing different parts of the body. Splints may be made of: (1) Wood. (2) Aluminium. (3) Celluloid. (4) Iron. (5) Wire. (6) Plaster of Paris.

1. *Wooden splints* are generally used for temporary immobilization of limbs or joints. They are usually straight, angular or guttered. They are cheap, easy to renew and clean, but they do not fit sufficiently accurately to secure perfect immobilization. Nurses are often required to keep a stock of padded wooden splints for emergency and first aid work.

To pad a wooden splint. First scrub the splint with soap and water. Cut a piece of smooth, old linen or calico three times the width of the splint and allow three inches at either end. In the middle of this, place a smooth piece of soft brown wool, which should have been heated to 'fluff it out'. It should be at least one inch in thickness and should overlap the splint at sides and ends by one inch. On top of the wool tease some tow, avoiding hard, stringy pieces. The padding, when prepared, should be at least four inches high before it is made into the pad. Make the pad by loosely herringboning the linen, leaving the ends free. Secure the pad to the splint by firm cross stitches of strong linen thread. Turn down the ends and stitch them neatly. When finished, the padding should be very full and soft, so that when the whole weight of the limb is put on the splint the wood is not felt by the patient. Cover the splint with gutta-percha tissue, sealing it in place with chloroform. Finally bandage the splint neatly with a muslin bandage of suitable width.

When the splint is discarded, remove the bandage, wash the gutta-percha tissue with antiseptic solution and re-cover with bandage. After a certain amount of usage, the padding needs to be renewed.

2. *Aluminium splints* are frequently used. They are lined with elephant felt, which adheres to the surface of the splint. Besides being light in weight, they possess the advantage of being easily moulded to fit the part. They are easily cleaned by washing with soap and water. Fresh elephant felt is then applied.

3. *Celluloid splints* are also very light and very comfortable for patients in whom the limbs or trunk have to be immobilized for any length of time.

4. *Iron splints* are heavy, but they consist only of a firm iron framework

201

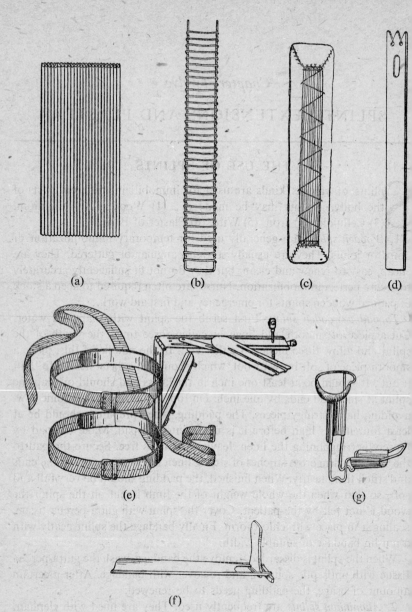

Fig. 73

(a) Gooch's wooden splinting.
(b) Cramer wire splint.
(c) Padded wooden splint.
(d) Liston's long splint.
(e) Bohler's aeroplane splint for humerus abduction.
(f) Back splint with footpiece.
(g) Robert Jones's humerus extension splint.

in which a limb can be slung by means of flannel strips. They are mainly used as a support to which extension apparatus can be fixed.

5. *Wire splints* are light and can be bent and cut to fit the part. They are useful where heavy or firm splinting is not required.

Splints may be used internally as well as externally. In difficult cases of fracture, the bone itself is splinted by bone grafts, pegs, steel plates, pins, screws or silver wire. An open operation is required for the insertion of such splints.

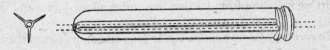

Smith-Petersen pin for fractures of neck and femur.

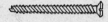

Screw.	*Bone plate.*

FIG. 79. Internal Splints

GENERAL RULES FOR THE APPLICATION OF SPLINTS

1. The splint must be of a suitable size. It is most important that a variety of splints should be kept in the store cupboard of wards where they are likely to be required.

2. Splints must be adequately padded.

3. In cases where it is possible, the limb should be washed before the splint is applied, the bony prominences being well rubbed with spirit and powder. In fractures and other injuries, it is usually impossible to do this, but in others this treatment should not be forgotten. For instance, for orthopædic patients who wear splints and appliances for a period of months or years, the skin should be treated each time the apparatus is reapplied.

4. Where wooden splints are used, sufficient wool should be put round the limb, especially in the region of bony prominences, to prevent them from getting rubbed.

5. If a splint has to be bandaged in position, the type of bandage must be selected with care; a strong calico or crêpe bandage is usually best. In applying the bandage, turns of sufficient tightness should be used to secure the splint in position; at the same time watch should be kept that the distal end of the limb, e.g. the hand or foot, does not swell or become cold or blue, due to too tight bandaging. This is particularly important in the case of the fore-arm. *Volkmann's ischæmia* is a type of paralysis which

may be caused by the cutting off of the blood supply by too tight splintage and bandaging.

Extensions. Extension or traction is applied for the following reasons:

1. *To reduce fractures* by a continuous pull on a broken bone. In some cases this is the best way to overcome strong muscle spasm. Extension method of reduction is nearly always used in cases of fracture of the shaft of the femur.

2. *To immobilize inflamed and infected joints.* The continuous traction on the limb keeps the inflamed joint surfaces apart, thus preventing pain and further irritation from friction. e.g. tuberculous joints and infective arthritis.

3. *To correct joint deformities.* e.g. In long-standing cases of rheumatoid arthritis, in which the knees have become flexed, the flexion can be overcome by extension.

There are two methods of extension:

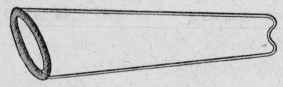

FIG. 80. Thomas's knee splint

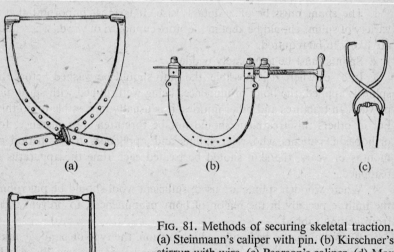

(a)   (b)   (c)

(d)

FIG. 81. Methods of securing skeletal traction. (a) Steinmann's caliper with pin. (b) Kirschner's stirrup with wire. (c) Pearson's caliper. (d) Max Page's stirrup with pin. Traction is obtained by weights attached to the stirrup or caliper

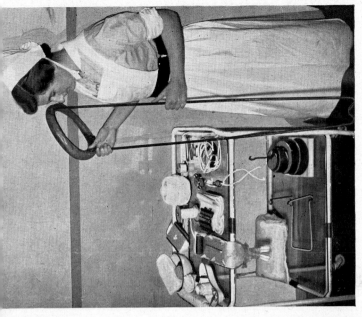

Plate 23. Requirements for extension.
See page 205

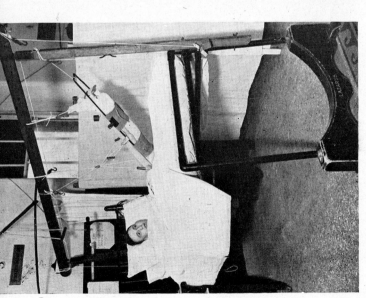

Plate 22. Sliding extension with Thomas's splint
—showing counter extension by means of blocks.
See page 205

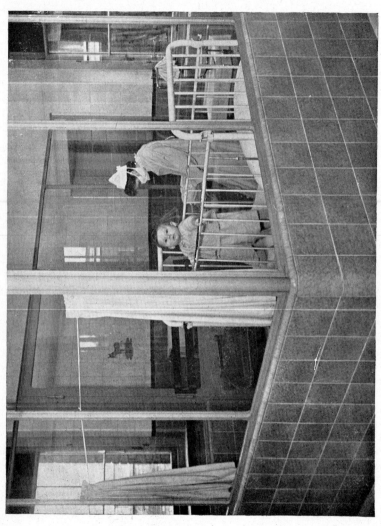

Plate 24 Cubicle in children's ward. See page 242

EXTENSIONS

1. Exerting a pull on the skin by means of adhesive strapping, i.e. *skin traction*.

2. Exerting the pull on the bone, by means of steel pins or wire driven through the bone, i.e. *skeletal traction*.

Extension cord is attached, either to strapping, pin or wire, and the actual traction is made by means of the cord. The nurse should understand the difference between:

(a) *Fixed traction*.
(b) *Sliding traction*.

(a) **Fixed Traction.** The limb is supported in an iron frame splint, e.g. a Thomas's knee splint for a fractured tibia. The rim of the splint which must fit perfectly is pushed into the groin until it rests on the ischial tuberosity. The cord attached to the strapping or wire is tied firmly to the end of the splint, exerting a continuous pull on the bone while the limb is completely immobilized.

(b) **Sliding Traction.** The limb is supported in a Thomas's knee splint, applied as above. The cord is taken over a small pulley fixed to the bar at the bottom of the bed, and weights are attached. This arrangement would tend to pull the patient down the bed and therefore counter extension must be applied to pull him in the opposite direction. This can be done by placing the bottom of the bed on six inch or nine inch blocks.

A more elaborate method of extension and counter extension can be secured by attaching a system of weights and pulleys to an overhead beam. The idea in any method of sliding traction is that sufficient pull should be exerted on the bone in both directions, and, by a knowledge of mechanics, the surgeon arranges this in such a way that the patient can move about in bed without altering the extension (see plate 22).

The nurse must be able to help the surgeon to put up an extension and when she has done this a number of times, she will learn the principles involved and will understand exactly how the patient may be moved for nursing treatment.

Requirements for skin extension (see plate 23).

1. Soap and water, towels, methylated spirit and powder. Nail brush and scissors. Razor. (The amount of preliminary preparation of the skin varies with the condition being treated and thorough washing and cleansing may not be possible.)

2. Good adhesive strapping, either Holland's soap strapping or zinc oxide adhesive strapping three inches wide; cord, wooden stirrup (or spreader), cleats and pulleys; weights, and bed blocks.

3. Thomas's knee splint (or Braun's splint, or, if an arm, Robert Jones's splint); foot piece; straps of flannel eighteen inches by four inches; safety pins, strong paper clips.

An overhead beam may be required, according to the method used.

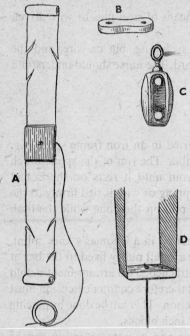

FIG. 82. Skin Traction. (a) and (d) spreader with strapping ready for application; (b) cleat; (c) pulley

Method (for fractured femur). A piece of strapping about thirty inches long is cut and placed on a table with the adhesive surface uppermost. In the exact middle of this a wooden spreader is placed. Another piece of strapping, about twelve inches long, is placed over the spreader, to keep it in place and adhering to the strapping on either side. A hole is made in the strapping over the spreader and through it the cord is threaded and knotted. The strapping is then applied from well above the knee down to the malleoli, the bony prominences of these being protected by a piece of lint. The strapping must be of good quality so that it adheres to the skin securely. The limb is bandaged very firmly from the malleoli upwards with a gauze bandage. The only thing that remains to be done is either to tie the cord to the splint (fixed traction) or to attach weights over the pulley as already described.

If the limb is to be slung in a Thomas's splint, the flannel strips are pinned or clipped to the splint to provide support. A foot piece may be attached so that while the foot is kept well supported a reasonable amount of movement at the ankle joint is allowed for. The toes must be kept warm by means of a sock, and the leg covered with a small blanket tied in position with tapes. The bed is made in divided fashion.

THE NURSING OF A PATIENT IN A THOMAS'S SPLINT, WITH SLIDING EXTENSION

The patient may sit up in bed, the leg may be moved up and down from the hip joint and, in some cases, the knee can be flexed. He can lift his buttocks off the bed, by putting his weight on his arms or by pulling on an overhead pulley. None of these movements will alter the arrangement of the extension. The nurse must not touch any of the weights, as this will at once alter the traction; the weights must hang free and not touch the bedstead. She should inspect all knots and cords at frequent intervals, to see that they are tight and not wearing thin. She should tighten up and djust the flannel slings in which the leg is supported. *The most important ne to keep tight is the one under the site of fracture.*

The foot and toes and nails must be washed and powdered. The areas ound the malleoli and heel should be inspected, to make sure that no oreness is developing, and to prevent this they should be rubbed with pirit and powder three times a day. The skin in the groin must also be well nassaged with spirit and powder. The discomfort of the leather ring may)e overcome by placing an air-ring under the buttocks, in such a position hat the ring of the splint comes over the edge of the air-ring.

The patient can soon wash the upper part of his body himself and it s all to the good that he should move himself about to do this, but the iurse must see what parts of the body he cannot reach, and help him to vash his back and the lower part of his good leg. The patient must be vashed all over every day, except the leg which is in extension. The giving)f bedpans and the treatment of his back is made quite easy, because the)atient can raise himself off his buttocks.

As in all cases of bony disease or damage, the diet should be generous with extra milk and vitamin D. Occupational therapy and other means of nteresting the patient are of great psychological value in nursing these patients.

In those cases where skeletal traction is applied, careful surgical prepara- :ion of the skin is required before operation. Afterwards there may be ome slight moistness or discharge where the pin punctures the skin. These areas should be treated with a spirit dressing.

PLASTER OF PARIS SPLINTS

Plaster of Paris splints are used more than any other type of splint in orthopædic and fracture cases and for immobilizing wounds. For example, in cases of osteomyelitis, the old method of daily dressings and irrigations, the limb being immobilized on a wooden splint, is a thing of the past. The limb is now encased in plaster of Paris, and the surgeon trusts nature to carry on the healing process under the plaster, as long as the bone has been widely opened up, so that septic material can escape. The wound granulates from below upwards. The plaster may become soaked with discharge and very offensive; the patient is nursed out of doors if possible and as long as the temperature remains normal and the general condition of the patient is satisfactory the plaster is left unchanged anything from two to six weeks ('Winnet-Orr' treatment). The plaster may be enclosed in a loose absorbent felt bag which prevents the escape of unpleasant odours.

To make Plaster Bandages. Bandages should be six yards in length and four inches to six inches in width. Plaster muslin is prepared and rolled loosely into bandage form. The bandage is placed on an even base of plaster on a wooden tray. It is unrolled six inches to eight inches at a time. Plaster is sprinkled on to it and the surface wiped off with the ulnar surface of the hand, leaving an even layer of plaster in the meshes of the gauze. There is no need to rub it in, but the important thing is to use a firm smooth stroke of the hand. The bandage should not be rolled tightly or the soaking process is interfered with.

Application of Plaster. A bowl of tepid water is used for hand-made plaster bandages, but, if the proprietary makes (e.g. cellona bandage) are used, the water should be cool or even cold. Hot water makes the plaster set more quickly, cold more slowly. Salt added to the water hastens setting; borax slows down the setting of the plaster.

When the surgeon is ready to apply a plaster, the bandage is carefully placed in a bowl and left until all bubbling has ceased. Hand-made bandages take about two minutes to soak and proprietary ones a few seconds. When the bandage has ceased to bubble it should be lifted out horizontally and squeezed firmly at both ends, in order to express excess moisture and also to squeeze water into the centre of the bandage. The bandage should never be wrung out as it makes it too dry. The loose end is then unrolled for a few inches and the bandage handed to the surgeon.

There are two types of plaster casts, padded and unpadded.

Padded plasters. In this case the limb is wrapped in plaster wool before the application of the plaster. This method is indicated for any part of the body which is subjected to constant pressure, and when the patient has to wear the plaster for any length of time. Plaster wool, before use, must be sterilized in the autoclave, as it sometimes contains considerable numbers of tetanus spores. There are quite a number of cases of tetanus on record caused by infected plaster wool.

Unpadded plasters. Unpadded plasters are in very common use in most ordinary fracture work. First, a plaster slab is applied and it is fixed on by circular turns of plaster bandages. The length of the plaster slab required is first measured by the surgeon with a gauze bandage. The slab is usually made with six

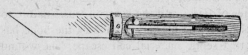

Fig. 83. Plaster Knife

layers of bandage. The bandages must, of course, be soaked and it is made with the wet bandages.

For a limb two lateral slabs are used. The circular turns are applied fairly quickly. This is important because it is essential to finish the application of the plaster before it sets. The plaster is then moulded to the leg with the hands so that it fits accurately around the bony contours and prominences. In this way plaster sores are avoided. In most cases the knee is kept slightly flexed at an angle of 15°. The moulding of the plaster to the imb must be done with a very firm touch, avoiding undue pressure in any one spot. It is not necessary to shave the limb before the application of plaster.

In orthopædic work the limb is usually washed with soap and water before the plaster is reapplied, and some surgeons like the skin, especially over the bony prominences, to be rubbed with spirit and powder. In cases where joints are involved, the assistant holding the limb is required by the surgeon to hold it in extension, that is, to exert a slight pull on the limb the whole time, so that the plaster itself is a means of keeping the joint surfaces apart.

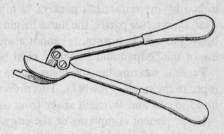

FIG. 84. Plaster Shears

Drying the Plaster. A plaster sets in about ten minutes, but it takes thirty-six to forty-eight hours for it to dry completely. During this period it is very easy to crack a plaster by improper handling. The limb should be supported on a soft even pillow and not suspended from a cradle. A free circulation of air should be arranged round the plaster by means of a cradle, the bed being left open at the bottom. It may be possible to arrange the limb on top of the bed without any covering at all. Radiant heat is sometimes used, but it tends to dry the plaster too quickly and causes cracking. Casts made from proprietary bandages dry more quickly than those made from hand-made bandages. No weight should be taken on the cast for thirty-six hours after application. It is very easy to make a dent in a plaster by resting it against a hard surface whilst it is drying. In this respect special notice should be taken of the heel, and the leg should be raised on a soft pillow to keep the heel off the bed and off the trolley during transport from the plaster room to the ward.

Patients are instructed by the surgeon and masseuses to exercise the muscles within the plaster in order to keep up their tone by contraction exercises. The plaster, of course, prevents movement of the bony structures.

The bed to which the patient returns should be warmed with hot water bottles, as the patient feels chilly with the dampness and exposure. The bedding needs to be protected by an extra mackintosh and drawsheet placed over the part where the plaster will rest. Pillows supporting the plaster should have mackintosh covers under the pillow cases. Hot water bottles should not be placed near the plaster while it is still wet, to avoid cracking. Loose pieces of plaster should be removed from the bed at once. Sheets on which plaster has dried should be soaked in cold water before being sent to the laundry.

Nursing. All splashes of plaster on the toes, fingers, etc., should b removed at once before they set hard.

Patients in plaster jackets and shoulder spicas will have to be bathed in bed by the nurse; but patients in hip spicas and long leg plasters ca wash themselves partly, the nurse helping with the inaccessible parts of the body. Patients in hip spicas cannot always clean themselves well after th use of the bedpan and generally need help.

Patients wearing hip spicas are made more comfortable if a soft pillov is put in the small of the back. This prevents the edge of the plaster pressin into the ribs and stomach at the front and sides.

If the patient complains of the edges of the plaster being tight, extra pieces of wool should not be pushed under them, as these only make the plaster fit more closely. The nurse should get her fingers under the edge and move the skin as much as possible, massaging it with methylated spirit. If the plaster is padded, a little of the wool may be drawn out and smoothed over the outside edge of the plaster. It is permissible to cu away a v-shaped piece from the edge and this often relieves the pressure. Raising the limb also relieves the discomfort of a tight plaster by limiting the swelling.

Careful watch must be made for: (1) Swelling. (2) Coldness. (3) Discolouration.

The toes are usually cold at first but should soon become warm i covered with a woollen sock. The nurse should try and distinguish between the patient who complains of general and vague discomfort when a plaster has been applied and one who is complaining of definite pain at a certain spot. She should realize that if the plaster is exerting damaging pressure on one area the patient will complain of pain; if nothing is done to relieve it the pain will disappear within twenty-four to forty-eight hours. This generally means that the skin has become necrosed and when the plaster is removed at a later date a plaster sore will be seen. It is most important that the nurse should not hesitate to report if a patient in plaster complains of persistent pain. It may be necessary for the surgeon to remove the plaster. Most surgeons would support the nurse who, if she could not obtain advice within a few hours, removed the plaster herself, rather than run the risks associated with too tight plastering; but it needs experience to know when this course of action would be justifiable.

Patients in plasters should get up and walk about, if possible. It is important to remember that patients who lie immobile in the dorsal position for long periods of time are particularly liable to urinary complications (e.g. renal calculi). High blocks put at the head of the bed help to prevent this by encouraging the flow of urine by gravity.

Spinal cases are sometimes nursed in plaster beds which enclose the whole body. The plaster is made in two halves which fit the contours of

he body perfectly. The patient lies in the posterior shell; it is not usually
necessary to turn him for treatment of the back more often than once a
week or even longer. When this is done the anterior shell is strapped in
position and the patient turned on to the face by at least six nurses. The
plaster bed is placed on wooden supports; this arrangement facilitates the
use of the bedpan, etc.

Chapter Thirteen

THE NURSING OF GYNÆCOLOGICAL CASES

Gynæcology is the study of diseases of women. These are concerned with the generative organs in the pelvis, and the anatomy and physiology of these parts should be revised by the nurse who is nursing gynæcological cases.

Gynæcological Cases Include:

(a) Operations necessary for the following conditions: Cancer, fibroids, polypi of the uterus, and cysts of the ovary.

(b) Disorders resulting from abnormal positions of the uterus, e.g. retroversion and prolapse.

(c) Injuries to the vagina, perineum and cervix, from tears during labour.

(d) Accidents of pregnancy, e.g. abortion, ruptured ectopic gestation.

The nurse should understand what is done in the following operations in order that she may intelligently carry out the preparation before, and the treatments after, the operation.

1. Hysterectomy

(a) *Subtotal hysterectomy*, is removal of the body of the uterus; the cervix is left intact. It is done in cases of fibroids and uterine polypi.

(b) *Panhysterectomy or total hysterectomy*. The whole of the uterus is removed, both body and cervix. The fallopian tubes may or may not be removed at this operation. It is performed for carcinoma of the body of the uterus.

(c) *Wertheim's operation*. This is the removal of the uterus, tubes, ovaries, upper third of the vagina, together with the pelvic lymphatic glands. It is one of the most extensive operations performed and is done in cases of carcinoma of the cervix.

2. Repair Operations

These are done for tears resulting from childbirth. The tears involve the vagina and the pelvic floor, and result in prolapse of the uterus. The names of the operations are:

(a) *Perineorrhaphy*—repair of the perineum.

(b) *Colpo-perineorrhaphy*—repair of the vagina and perineum.

If the anterior wall of the vagina is stretched or torn, the bladder may bulge into the vagina, causing difficulties of micturition (*cystocele*).

212

If the posterior wall is stretched or torn the rectum herniates into the vagina (*rectocele*). The operation for the repair of these conditions is called an anterior or posterior colporrhaphy, according to which wall is repaired.

(c) *Fothergill's operation*. This is repair of the vagina and perineum, together with amputation of the cervix. It is done in severe cases of prolapse of the uterus (*procidentia*).

Oophorectomy is removal of the ovary. It is usually performed for cysts.

Salpingectomy. Removal of the fallopian tubes. It may be performed for abscess in the tube or tubo-ovarian abscess, or in cases of repair of a tubal pregnancy.

Dilatation and curettage. The cervix is dilated by bougies, and the lining of the uterus is scraped with a curette. It is performed for some cases of painful menstruation (dysmenorrhœa) and in cases of incomplete abortion, where fragments of the ovum have been retained, in the uterus. Curettage is also necessary if fragments of placenta or membranes are left behind during the third stage of labour. Such retained products lead to puerperal sepsis.

Tubal insufflation. The cervix is dilated and air is injected into the uterus. If the tubes are blocked by scar tissue, the air cannot escape into the peritoneal cavity. Therefore tubal insufflation is a treatment done under anæsthesia to investigate cases of sterility.

PREPARATION OF A PATIENT FOR EXAMINATION BY A GYNÆCOLOGIST

Requirements
1. A good light.
2. Mackintosh and two receivers.
3. Footstool.
4. Right-hand rubber gloves and powder.
5. Vaginal specula (Sim's and Ferguson's), vulsellum forceps, Playfair's probe.
6. Dry wool swabs, lint squares.
7. Vaseline or dettol cream.

Method. The bladder must be empty, and the examination will not be a success if the patient is constipated. In some cases, if the nurse has time and opportunity to prepare the patient beforehand, an enema should be given, if it seems necessary. No preparatory cleansing or shaving is done, as it is important that the surgeon should examine the parts before they have been treated in any way. The patient is told beforehand what the surgeon is about to do. The nurse should take particular care to reassure the patient and tell her that the examination will be uncomfortable but not painful, and that she can help a great deal by trying to lie still and relax.

The examination should be postponed if the patient is menstruating, unless the condition needs urgent treatment.

The nurse arranges the patient in the Sims' position, that is, an exaggerated left lateral position, the patient semi-prone, the right knee drawn up towards the chin, the left arm behind her and the buttocks well to the edge of the bed. Bedclothes are arranged in divided fashion, so that the blanket over the buttocks can be turned back with the minimum of exposure. A warm mackintosh is placed under the buttocks, and the light and footstool and other requirements are placed in position, while the surgeon scrubs his hands. The requirements (instruments, etc.) listed are not necessarily sterile for a routine examination. They are washed and boiled immediately after use, and put in covered dishes ready for the next case. If, however, the examination is done post-operatively, all requirements should be sterile.

Catheterization

Requirements

1. Warm mackintosh and receiver.
2. A good light.
3. Lifting forceps in antiseptic solution.
4. Sterile towel.
5. Sterile wool swabs in warm dettol solution 2 per cent.
6. Dry sterile wool swabs.
7. Two sterile catheters, rubber or glass, in covered sterile dish.
8. Measure bowl.
9. Sterile bottle for specimen, if required.
10. Powder.

Method. The patient is screened and put in the dorsal position with the knees flexed, removing, if possible, all but one pillow at the head. The bed is arranged in divided fashion, so that the lower blanket can be pulled down at the level of the groin. The warm mackintosh is put under the buttocks and the electric switch is arranged to give a good light. The trolley containing the requirements is placed at the side of the patient, so that the nurse can conveniently use her right hand for passing the catheter.

The nurse scrubs her hands with soap and water and immerses them in a bowl of dettol 2 per cent. She goes to the bedside and the trolley assistant hands her a sterile towel on which to dry her hands. She next arranges the sterile towel under the pubic area and drapes it over the thighs. She then swabs the vulva, parting the labia with the left hand and swabbing from above downwards, using each swab only once and then discarding it into the receiver. The swabbing must be very thorough, to prevent organisms being carried into the bladder when the catheter is inserted. The sterile dish is placed in position and the nurse then takes one of the catheters and arting the labia directs it into the urethral orifice just above the vagina. A swab may be placed in the entrance to the vagina. If, by accident, the catheter becomes contaminated by touching another part, it must be discarded and the second one used. It is sufficient to insert it one and a half inches, until the urine begins to flow into the dish. When the bladder is empty, the catheter is removed and put into the receiver. The dish of urine is put safely on the under shelf of the trolley and the patient is once more swabbed with dettol solution, after which the vulva is carefully dried with the dry wool swabs. The towel is removed, the patient turned on her side, the mackintosh withdrawn and the buttocks dried. The vulva is powdered, the patient is arranged comfortably with a warm blanket and the bed is remade.

If catheterization is being done to prepare the patient for an operation the catheter may be left in position and clipped or spigotted.

If a sterile specimen of urine is required for bacteriological examination, boracic lotion or saline should be used for swabbing.

VAGINAL DOUCHE

A vaginal douche is ordered for the following purposes:

1. To cleanse the vagina before operation.

2. To remove offensive discharges.

3. To apply heat for certain infections high in the genital tract, e.g. salpingitis.

4. After radium has been used. (Plain water or saline douche.)

5. For haemorrhage.

Lotions used

Dettol ½ per cent.

Lysol ½ per cent.

Iodine 6 per cent solution ℨi to Oi.

Normal saline.

Boracic lotion, saturated solution with an equal quantity of water.

Perchloride of mercury, 1 in 8,000, followed by plain water or saline.

Potassium permanganate, two crystals to the pint.

One quart of solution is prepared. The temperature for an ordinary douche is 105° F. A hot douche, in cases of salpingitis, is prepared at 110° F., and in cases of hæmorrhage, the temperature should be 118° to 120° F.

Requirements

1. Warm mackintosh and bedpan.

2. Receiver.

3. Bowl of wool swabs in warm dettol solution 2 per cent.

4. Dry wool swabs.

5. Douche can containing lotion, rubber tubing and douche nozzle

clip. The nozzle is put into the lotion while the patient is prepared.
6. Thermometer.
7. Powder and vulval pad.

Method. The bed is screened and the patient, if possible, is put in a recumbent position with one or two pillows. A warm mackintosh is arranged under the buttocks and the bedpan is placed in position. The 'Perfection' type is most satisfactory for this purpose. Bedclothes are arranged in divided fashion separated at the groins so that the patient is kept warm and exposed as little as possible. The nurse washes and dries her hands. She then parts the labia with her left hand and swabs the vulva from above downwards with dettol solution, using one swab only once and discarding it into the receiver. The patient holds the douche can if she is able to do so, while the nurse slips the nozzle in a backward direction into the vagina. It should be inserted three or four inches. The clip is removed and the nurse then holds the douche can in her left hand and steadies the nozzle with her right. The douche can is held six inches above the level of the bed, unless a high-pressure douche is ordered, in which case it is held two or three feet above the patient. High-pressure douches are not prescribed in cases of infection of the vagina, as the organisms might be driven higher up the tract; they are most often ordered in cases of salpingitis, when there is little danger of further spread. There is no need to move the douche nozzle whilst it is in the vagina; the holes at the end of the nozzle allow the solution to irrigate the passage quite sufficiently.

When the douche is finished, the nozzle is disconnected from the tubing and put into a receiver. The bedpan is removed, the vulva dried and powdered and the pad put in position. The patient is turned over on her side, the mackintosh is taken out and the buttocks are thoroughly dried, and powdered, and the drawsheet pulled through and straightened. She is then given a warm blanket and the bed is tidied. The contents of the douche pan should be examined and shown to the sister, if they appear abnormal in any respect.

Vaginal douching is not a sterile procedure, except after vaginal operations, or in rare instances when it is ordered after childbirth. In these cases the technique is similar to that of catheterization, the hands being dried on a sterile towel, the swabs and pad used being sterile. The douche can and tubing should be boiled. When the technique is not strictly sterile, however, the douche nozzle must be dealt with very carefully after the douche. It is rinsed in cold running water, then in warm water and boiled for twenty minutes. Each patient in a gynæcological ward should have her own douche nozzle, kept in a glass jar and labelled with the patient's name. Special precautions should be taken in cases of salpingitis or other cases of infection, the bedpan being kept for the one patient's use only.

PLUGS

Vaginal tampons or plugs of various types are used after gynæcological operations to keep the vaginal walls apart and to absorb serum and blood. Plugging is also used for arresting hæmorrhage, and wool plugs impregnated with antiseptics are used in some cases of vaginal discharge. Plugs are made of gauze, two yards long and eight inches wide. Kite-tailed tampons are sometimes used. They consist of wool swabs strung together with thread, rather like the tail of a kite.

When plugging the vagina, a long pair of ovum forceps should be used. The patient is arranged on her left side, and the plug is first directed into the posterior fornix and packed tightly. The anterior fornix is then packed and the remains of the plug are used for the vagina itself. Unless plugging is tight, all the crevices and folds will not be reached by the antiseptic. In cases of hæmorrhage, the pressure exerted by the tight packing helps to arrest bleeding. A loose plug is often put into the vagina after the application of radium, so that the plaque or tube shall not be lost. After operations the plug is removed twelve to twenty-four hours later, and the removal is followed by a sterile vaginal douche.

The removal of a plug is quite a simple procedure. The external end of gauze or wool is grasped with dressing forceps and the plug is gently pulled into a receiver placed in position.

PESSARIES

Pessaries are rubber or vulcanite appliances used to correct mal-positions of the uterus. The three commonly used types are:

1. *The Hodge* chair-shaped pessary for retroverted uterus.
2. *The vulcanite ring pessary* for prolapse of the uterus.
3. *Rubber watchspring pessary* for cases of prolapse.

Insertion of a pessary. A cleansing douche is given and the patient is then turned on to the left side. The pessary, which should have been boiled, is dipped into a lubricant such as olive oil or paraffin, and is then slipped in position, round the cervix. With a little practice it is quite easy to feel if the pessary is in the right place. The insertion of a pessary is not a sterile procedure, but the nurse's hands should be well washed before and after treatment.

Vaginal and Cervical Smears
Requirements
1. Mackintosh.
2. Good light.
3. Sims' or Ferguson's speculum
4. Platinum loop.

5. Wool swabs (in kidney dish).
6. Lubricant.
7. Spirit lamp.
8. Glass slides in covered kidney dish.
9. Receiver.
10. Pathological report form.

Vaginal and Cervical Swabs

Requirements
1. Mackintosh.
2. Good light.
3. Sims' or Ferguson's speculum.
4. Wool swabs (in kidney dish).
5. Lubricant.
6. Receiver.
7. Swab sticks in tubes.
8. Pathological report form.

Method. (1) *Vaginal Smear*. The patient is arranged in the left lateral position. A Sims' duckbill speculum is passed into the vagina. The platinum loop is sterilized in the spirit flame, and when cool some of the discharge from the vaginal wall is picked up in the loop. The nurse can generally see the area where the discharge is most profuse. It is smeared on the slide which is then taken immediately in a covered dish to the bacteriological laboratory with the appropriate pathological form.

(2) *Cervical smears*. The Ferguson's speculum is used and the smear is taken from the cervix in exactly the same way as described above. A Sims' speculum is often used however as it is more easily passed. Care must be taken not to touch the vaginal walls with the platinum loop.

(3) *Vaginal and cervical swabs*. These are taken in the same way, but a prepared swab stick is used (instead of a platinum loop) and the swab is returned to the sterile test tube in which it is sent to the laboratory.

PREPARATION OF A PATIENT FOR A GYNÆCOLOGICAL OPERATION

Abdominal. The preparation of a patient for an abdominal hysterectomy varies little from that of a patient for any other abdominal operation, except that in some respects it must be more thorough. In addition to the preparation described in the chapter on surgical nursing, the following additional treatments are required:

1. The rectum must be empty. An aperient is given two days before the operation and a soap enema on the morning of the day before the operation and another on the day itself.

2. The whole pubic area must be shaved as well as the abdomen. The

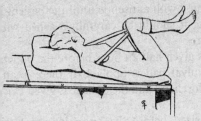

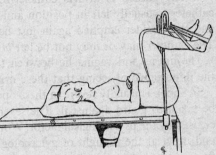

*Lithotomy position maintained by
use of Clover's crutch.*

*Lithotomy position for vaginal
and perineal operations.*

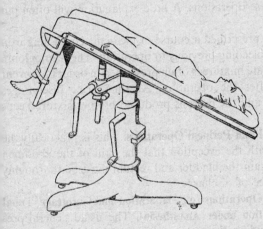

*Trendelenburg position
for pelvic operations.*

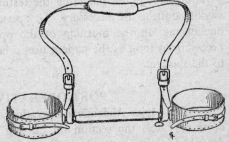

Clover's crutch.

Fig. 85

219

pubic area and perineum is not painted with antiseptic until the patient is under the anæsthetic. After shaving, it should be carefully washed with warm soap and water and powdered.

3. An antiseptic vaginal douche is given half an hour before the patient goes to the theatre, and a sterile vulval pad is applied. If there is any discharge, it must be investigated beforehand and the douche is given twice daily.

4. The patient is always catheterized before the operation, and the catheter is usually left in position and clipped. The clip will be released and the bladder emptied again just before the patient leaves the ward. The catheter may or may not be left *in situ*.

The uterus and vagina lie between the rectum and the bladder hence the importance of seeing that these organs are empty.

5. Shock is usually severe in these operations so extra precautions must be taken to guard against it. The severity of the shock is sometimes increased by the psychological factor. Women are often particularly sensitive and upset at the thought of gynæcological operations. The nurse should find time to talk to the patient who may be ignorant and have exaggerated ideas of the results of these operations. A little explanation will often put her mind at rest.

6. The patient is often prescribed a course of medicine containing iron if there has been uterine bleeding previous to operation. The hæmoglobin is tested. A potassium citrate mixture is often prescribed in order to prevent urinary complications after the operation. Alkaline urine discourages the growth of organisms and the diuresis produced by the mixture keeps the urethra well flushed.

Preparation for Vaginal and Perineal Operations. This is practically the same as for the above with the exception that the skin of the abdomen need not be prepared. Again the bladder and rectum must be thoroughly empty and the vagina free of discharge.

Preparation for Minor Operations (e.g. Dilatation and Curettage, Tubal Insufflation and Examination under Anæsthesia). The usual general preparation is required including the testing of urine. A pubic shave and vaginal douche are necessary. An aperient is given the day before and one enema on the morning of the operation. Catheterization is not necessary as long as the patient uses a bedpan immediately before going to the theatre.

POST-OPERATIVE CARE

1. **After Major Abdominal Operations.** In connection with the nursing of these cases, the section on nursing after abdominal operations as described in the chapter on Surgical Nursing should be studied carefully. Shock is usually severe, especially after a Wertheim's operation. The foot

f the bed is blocked and the patient is kept flat until her condition is atisfactory. After four to six hours she is sat up in the Fowler position. n injection of morphia, gr. ¼ is given and fluids are withheld twelve hours r longer if vomiting is troublesome. The routine with regard to diet and btaining an action of the bowels is the same as that in other abdominal ases. There is likely to be difficulty in the passing of urine. Sometimes the urgeon leaves a catheter in the bladder. The spigot is released at intervals nd the catheter removed after twenty-four to forty-eight hours. Special ursing measures must be taken to avoid femoral thrombosis. The legs re exercised by bending and stretching them in bed and the patient is ncouraged to turn on her side, breathe deeply and move herself about a ittle. The knee pillow is removed on the third morning. The dressing is ooked at, the sponges changed, and the bandage readjusted on the second lay. Vaginal douches are not given unless ordered. If a gauze plug has een put into the vagina it is removed after twenty-four hours. Stitches re removed on the tenth to twelfth day or clips on the sixth day. The oatient gets up after three weeks and goes home at the end of a month.

Complications associated with these operations are:

1 Shock.

2 Bladder complications.

3 Thrombosis of the femoral veins.

4 Pulmonary embolism seems to be more common after operations on the pelvic organs than after other operations.

2. **After Minor Gynæcological Operations (e.g. Dilatation and Curettage).** When the patient has recovered from the anæsthetic she is given two pillows and lies in the position which is most comfortable. A sedative drug is required the first night after operation. In the morning the night nurse removes the vaginal plug and gives an antiseptic vaginal douche. Micturition may be a difficulty due to the manipulation in the region of the bladder. It is dealt with in the usual way and catheterization should not be necessary.

A mild aperient such as an ounce of mist. senna co. is given the day after the operation. A light diet can be given as soon as vomiting has ceased. The patient gets up on the sixth day and goes home after ten days. Vaginal douches are given if ordered. If a dilatation only has been done, or insufflation of the tubes, the patient gets up on the second day and goes home on the fourth day.

3. **After Plastic Repair Operations of the Vagina and Perineum.** The patient is put to bed with the knees strapped together and flexed over a soft pillow. When she has recovered from the anæsthetic she is given one pillow under the head. In a few hours' time she is allowed a second pillow and should always be given an air-ring. The knee strap can be removed as soon as the patient is well enough to understand that too much

movement will be harmful. An injection of morphia will be required as soon as the patient is fully conscious and if she suffers great pain another injection will be required during the night, and on the following night milder sedatives are given until the patient is more comfortable.

A catheter may have been left in the bladder. It will be removed after forty-eight hours. If the surgeon has not left a catheter in position, the nurse must be prepared to overcome difficulties in the passing of urine. The vaginal plug is removed twenty-four hours after the operation and a vaginal douche is given with *all aseptic precautions*. At intervals the nurse may lift the patient on to her side and maintain this position by the use of a pillow in her back. A third pillow at the head can be used if it makes the patient more comfortable. The knee pillow is removed on the third morning.

Each time the bedpan is used the vulva and perineum are irrigated or swabbed with warm antiseptic solution, dettol 2 per cent or iodine 6 per cent ʒi to Oi water. For irrigation, the nurse scrubs and dries her hands on a clean towel, parts the labia with the left hand while she pours the irrigating lotion from a sterile jug over the vulval area while the patient is still on the bedpan. A convenient method of irrigating is to put the solution in the douche can which the patient holds. The nurse then directs the lotion over the area through the rubber tubing. At least one pint of solution should be used for a thorough irrigation. The bedpan is removed and the patient dried carefully and gently with sterile wool swabs. She is turned on her side and the buttocks are carefully dried and the drawsheet attended to. The stitches are then powdered generously with an antiseptic powder, or they may be swabbed with methylated spirit. Thin long stitch pads or pieces of lint are put under the ends of the sutures so that they do not scratch the skin. A large sterile vulval pad is fixed in position with a T-shaped bandage. The air-ring is replaced and the patient made comfortable.

For the first three days the diet should contain little residue as it is undesirable for the patient to have the bowels opened until the wound has started to heal.

A suitable diet consists of abundant fluids with only a little milk; tea, coffee, fruit juices and glucose, bovril, clear soup, jelly and toast. On the second evening one ounce of liquid paraffin is given and this is repeated on the third morning. One ounce of mist. senna co., or some similar aperient may be given on the third or fourth evening and a soap enema on the fourth or fifth morning, according to instructions given by the surgeon. The first act of defæcation after these operations is very painful and the nurse should prop the patient up as comfortably as possible with pillows and stay within call in case the patient feels faint. After the bowels have been opened, the diet can be more liberal, fish, chicken, milk puddings, fruit, etc. Liquid paraffin, one ounce every evening, is given and mild doses of stronger aperients, as required. It is important that normal habits of micturition and defæcation should be resumed as soon as possible. Swabbing after each bedpan is required until the stitches (if salmon gut) are removed on the twelfth to fourteenth day. The patient is allowed up on a couch on the eighteenth to the twenty-first day and goes home after four weeks. A daily douche may be ordered to be given from the tenth to the seventeenth day.

No surgical case needs more detailed and patient nursing than these operations. If the repair is a success, a great measure of the credit is due to the care and attention given by the nurse.

4. **After Radium Implantation.** In certain cases of cancer of the cervix the Stockholm method of applying radium is used, if more radical treatment by operation is not advisable. The patient is prepared as for a perineal operation and plaques containing the radium are inserted, one being put in the cervix and one in each of the fornices. A vaginal plug is inserted and the patient is nursed with one or two pillows. She may be more comfortable with a soft knee pillow. After twenty-four hours the plug is taken out and the radium removed. Tapes are usually attached to the plaques, so that they can easily be removed by forceps. A douche of sterile water is given and the nurse should note carefully the amount of discharge on the pads during the next day or two. The temperature should be recorded four-hourly. All proper precautions must be taken with the radium, so that it cannot possibly be lost (see chap. 20).

THE NURSING OF PATIENTS WITH INOPERABLE CARCINOMA OF THE UTERUS

These cases demand the utmost nursing skill and care, if the last few weeks of the patient's life are to be made tolerable. There is usually much offensive vaginal discharge from the growth and there may be fistulæ into the bladder from erosion. The pain increases due to pressure on nerves and the patient suffers from cramp and neuralgia in the legs and back. There may be ascites and gross œdema of the legs. The patient is cachectic and her condition gradually deteriorates. The end may come gradually from exhaustion and toxæmia. Bladder and kidney infection may increase the toxæmia and hasten death. A sudden hæmorrhage may occur.

The nurse must endeavour to obtain good supplies of bed linen, and pads. Douches of formalin, 1 in 1,000, potassium permanganate, six crystals to the quart, are given two or three times a day, according to the amount of discharge. The pads are changed very frequently and generous use should be made of talcum powder and eau-de-Cologne. Fumigating cones are often helpful to counteract unpleasant odours. If the bladder is infected, lavage may be necessary, and if fistulæ are present measures must be taken to deal with incontinence. The skin of the groins, vulva,

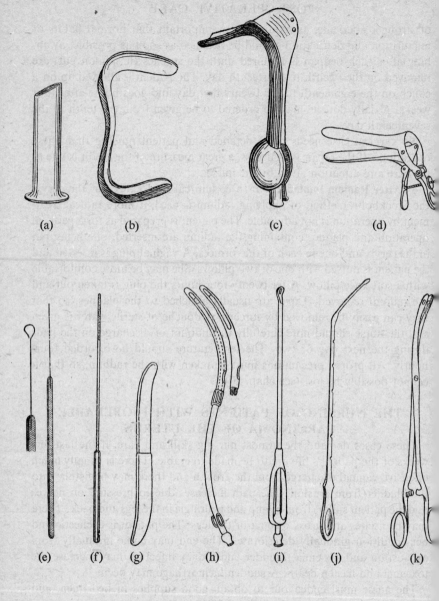

FIG. 86. Gynæcological instruments

(a) Ferguson's speculum.
(b) Sims' vaginal speculum.
(c) Auvard's vaginal speculum.
(d) Cusco's vaginal speculum.
(e) Platinum loop.
(f) Playfair's probe.
(g) Hegar's dilator.
(h) Intra-uterine douche nozzle.
(i) Flushing curette.
(j) Uterine sound.
(k) Uterine dressing forceps.

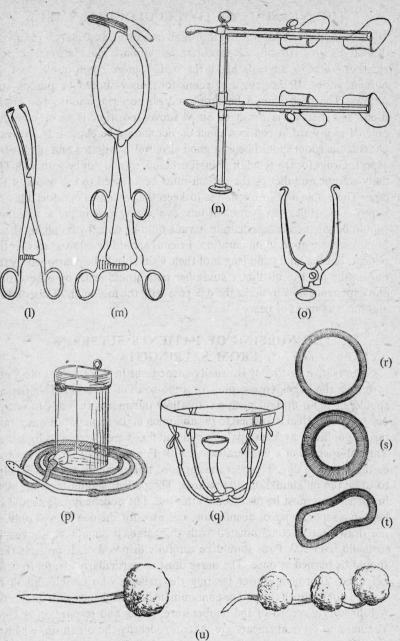

(l) Vulssellum forceps.
(m) Berkeley and Bouney's vaginal forceps.
(n) Berkeley's abdominal rectractor.
(o) Perineorraphy rectractor.
(p) Douche apparatus.

(q) Cup and stem pessary.
(r) Ring pessary.
(s) Watchspring pessary.
(t) Hodge pessary.
(u) Kite-tailed tampon.

and back needs very careful and thorough treatment, as urinary and vagina
discharges are irritating. Paracentesis abdominis may give relief. Ai
rings or water or air beds make the patient more comfortable, and th
nursing easier. If the legs are œdematous, they should be put on so
pillows. The heels should be supported on heel rings and a bed crad
used. The patient is arranged in whatever position is most comfor
able. If in a ward, a bed in a quiet corner should be chosen. If a privat
patient, the room should be of a good size, well ventilated and of cheerf
aspect. Drugs for the relief of pain, if ordered, should not be withheld. Th
daily routine and diet of the patient must be adapted to the needs of th
case. The whole aim in nursing is to keep the patient as comfortable an
happy as possible. Any particular fancies she may have in the way of foo
should be satisfied unless definite harm would be done by indulging then
Stimulants are good in moderation. Friends should be allowed to visit th
patient, but the hours and length of their visits should be controlled by th
nurse. She must in all things study her patient and learn by observatio
and experience how to make the day pass with the minimum of discomfo
and the maximum of peace.

THE NURSING OF PATIENTS SUFFERING
FROM SALPINGITIS

Conservative treatment is usually carried out in these cases unless pu
forms in the tubes (pyosalpinx or tubo-ovarian abscess). The patier
should sit in an upright position to allow inflammatory fluids to escap
per vaginam. Heat is applied to the abdomen in the form of hot water bot
tles or poultices, to relieve pain. Abundant fluids are given and a light die
Vaginal douches at a temperature of 110° F. are ordered to be given tw
or three times a day. The heat thus applied to the vagina and cervix help
to draw the inflammation downwards. The patient should have her ow
bedpan which must be disinfected after use. The douche nozzle should b
kept in a separate jar of disinfectant and used for the one patient only. I
the drawsheet is contaminated with discharge, it should be soaked i
formalin, 1 in 500. Pads should be carefully disposed of. If possible the
should be burned at once. The nurse must be particularly careful to was
her hands thoroughly after treating the patient, who herself should b
warned not to touch the pad or contaminate her own hands with discharg
A four-hourly record of the temperature, pulse, and respiration is kep
Vaginal and cervical smears are taken to identify the organism, which i
usually a gonococcus or streptococcus. Medicated pessaries containin
antiseptics are sometimes inserted into the vagina, but the modern us
of sulphonamide therapy causes the inflammation to subside quickl
without further treatment.

VAGINAL DISCHARGES

A patient troubled with what she considers is an abnormal amount of discharge from the vagina will often ask a nurse for advice, before she can be persuaded to consult a doctor. Normal vaginal discharge is white and glairy. It not uncommonly increases in amount (leucorrhœa) before a menstrual period, or if the patient is constipated. The nurse should inquire how many pads per day are used and should inspect them. She should advise the patient as to her general hygiene, emphasizing the necessity for thorough washing with a non-irritating soap. The parts must be carefully dried as the skin is particularly sensitive in the vulval area. A good talcum powder should be used and the pads changed very frequently. The underwear should be loosely fitting and not made of irritating woollen material. Bed clothing should be cool as irritation and discharge is often worse at night. The nurse should test the urine for sugar and should inquire whether the patient suffers from constipation, hæmorrhoids, or intestinal worms. As a result of her investigations, the nurse will know whether she should persuade the patient to consult a doctor. She should not delay in doing this as many cases of excessive vaginal discharge are due to infection (gonococcus, or trichomonas vaginalis), or growths, and the sooner they are dealt with the better.

The diet of these patients should be light, with plenty of fruit, vegetables, and fluids. Condiments, pastries, pickles and stimulants should be avoided if the discharge is very irritating.

THE NURSING OF CASES OF ABORTION

Abortion may be inevitable or threatened, and it is important that the nurse should know what to do in each case, if the doctor's advice is not immediately available.

In the case of inevitable abortion, the ovum detaches itself from the lining of the uterus and is expelled, generally before the third or fourth month of pregnancy. If the patient complains of abdominal pain of a spasmodic type and has a little vaginal hæmorrhage, she should stay in bed quietly. The nurse will seek medical help, and, in the meantime, will save all pads and discharge. The pulse should be recorded and sterile pads applied to the vulva. There should be no attempt to examine the patient or to interfere in any way. If the miscarriage is complete, that is to say, if the fœtus and membranes come away whole, the uterus contracts and the patient soon recovers. If the abortion is only threatened, attempts should be made to save the pregnancy. The patient is kept quietly in bed for a week after the hæmorrhage has ceased. She is advised to lead a quiet life, and, as it is in the early stages of pregnancy, it is advisable that she should go to bed for a day or two when the next menstrual period is due. Hot

227

stimulating fluids should be avoided in cases of abortion. If the abortion is incomplete, fragments of the ovum which are not expelled from the uterus may be recovered by curettage. Preparations of ergot are also given to stimulate uterine contractions.

MATERNITY NURSING

Every trained nurse should know sufficient about labour and its complications to be able to cope with an emergency and look after mother and baby, if a trained midwife is not available.

The Three Stages of Labour. Labour consists of muscular contractions of the uterus which expel the fœtus. A 'labour pain' accompanies each contraction.

First stage terminates when the cervix is fully dilated and the head enters the vagina.

Second stage is the passage of the baby through the vagina and terminates when it is born.

Third stage consists of the expulsion of the placenta and membranes (afterbirth). It occurs ten to thirty minutes afterwards in normal cases.

In a *primipara* the first stage lasts anything from twelve to thirty-six hours; the second stage, one to two hours. In a *multipara* the first stage may last three or four hours and the second stage be a matter of minutes. Hence it is not unusual for the actual birth to be sudden and unexpected.

A Vertex presentation (that is, the head presenting first), is the normal method of birth and abnormal presentations are not likely to be emergencies. However unexpected the birth may be, the nurse should, if possible, scrub her hands thoroughly and rinse them in disinfectant. Asepsis is of great importance. The patient may lie on her side or back, and as the head distends the perineum the nurse should try to guard it from tearing. Soon after the head is born, the shoulders rotate and the rest of the body slips out with the next pain. The nurse should notice if the cord is round the baby's neck, and if so, she should remove it quickly. As soon as possible she should wipe the child's eyes to prevent discharge entering. When the cord ceases to pulsate it is tied with two ligatures of sterile thread, two inches from the umbilicus, and cut with sterile scissors. The baby is wrapped up warmly and the mother, lying on her back, is watched until a further pain expels the placenta. There should not be more than one or two ounces of blood lost at a normal birth, and an emergency birth is likely to be quick and normal. The less the nurse interferes the better. After the delivery of the placenta, the external genitals should be swabbed with antiseptic solution, such as dettol 2 per cent or lysol $\frac{1}{2}$ per cent or perchloride of mercury, 1 in 4,000. A clean pad should be applied and the mother made comfortable with one pillow under her head. The baby is then bathed and dressed (see chapter on the nursing of children).

If the nurse has to continue to look after mother and baby, the following are her responsibilities:

1. To prevent infection entering the placental site.
2. To establish lactation.
3. To look after the baby.

General Nursing. All pads used should be sterile. Every time a bedpan is used the nurse scrubs her hands and swabs the patient down, using sterile swabs. The bedpan should be kept for the one patient only and should be cleaned and disinfected after use. The nurse should wear a mask when doing this treatment; some schools insist upon gloves being worn for all vulval treatments and they are boiled each time after use. After the first few hours, the patient should sit up in bed with several pillows to promote drainage from the uterus. It consists of blood from the placental site, bright red at first, gradually becoming less profuse and brownish in colour. It should cease by the seventh to tenth day. The discharge is called the 'lochia'.

The patient's temperature, pulse, and respiration should be taken night and morning. She should be well fed, being given plenty of fluids and at least half a pint of extra milk a day to keep up her supply of calcium while she is feeding the baby. Visitors, except the husband, should be forbidden during the lying-in period. This should be at least ten days to a fortnight. If she is allowed to get up too soon, before the uterus has returned to its normal size and position (involution of the uterus) prolapse of the uterus may result.

The method of putting a baby to the breast and the bathing of the infant will be described in the next chapter.

Chapter Fourteen

THE NURSING OF CHILDREN

I t is desirable that student nurses should have as much knowledge and understanding of the normal child as possible, in order to guide them in their observation and handling of the sick child. Until comparatively recently the intimate connection between the child's physical and psychological needs has not been recognized and nurses have not therefore been alive to the great psychological harm which may arise from faulty nursing. For this reason it may perhaps be useful to try to give very briefly some of the more important factors in the development of the normal infant, and to show the psychological reactions to physiological conditions.

Feeding. The infant is born with his instincts and his senses, and although he has as yet no knowledge or understanding, his wants and wishes, fears and angers, likes and dislikes are present from the beginning. Very intimately connected with his feelings of like and dislike is the question of feeding, and in this respect breast feeding is all important. To the tiny infant, the breast represents not only food as such, but essentially mother's love and security—which are his by right. Because of his lack of knowledge and experience, any delay in feeding (i.e. appeasing his hunger) is to him absolute denial of all that is vital to him : and he should never be allowed to reach the stage of crying till he is exhausted. In the rush of the hospital ward it is difficult for the nurse, striving to feed so many babies in a given and often limited time, to remember the infant's point of view, but unless she does so, she is only helping to produce a nervous and unstable adult.

Bottle feeding is at best a very poor substitute for the breast, both from a psychological and physiological point of view, and it is a very serious reflection on our teaching of mothercraft and nursing that so many babies still come in to hospital with a diagnosis of 'malnutrition due to wrong feeding, mismanagement', etc.

Training in Cleanliness. The young child is quite naturally interested in his excretions, and, if he is dealt with in a sensible way, he can generally be trained in habits of cleanliness quite quickly. If, however, the mother or nurse adopts a scolding or superior attitude and expects too much of the child, feelings of guilt and fear will soon creep in ; in the case of a nervous,

230

highly-strung child these may lead to serious complications in his up-bringing.

Play. Until recently far too little importance was attached to this activity. Play is the child's right, and the means by which he learns and grows. A children's ward without toys is indeed a sad place, and while it is a trial of patience to the nurse to have a 'comic' torn up and toys strewn over the floor by a toddler, just when she has tidied the ward, the whole situation takes on a very different aspect when she realizes the child's point of view. He is exercising his instinct of curiosity and constructiveness and is making all sorts of exciting discoveries through his play.

Handling. The emotion of fear plays a large part in the tiny child's life. The chief fears of infancy are those of falling and loud noises, and while no nurse would wilfully allow a baby to fall, many are thoughtless and jerk or bump him up and down in the scales when he is weighed. This gives him the feeling of being dropped and terrifies him. He can only know us by what we do to him. His other chief fear is of loud noises, and in this respect banging doors (usually due to thoughtlessness) and rattling trays and trolleys are probably the chief sources in hospital. The young child is extremely intuitive and readily picks up the mental attitude of his mother or nurse. For this reason a nervous, fussy mother has a nervous, restless baby, and a nurse (especially on night duty) who may for any reason be feeling irritable or over anxious will quickly transmit these feelings—all unconsciously—to the children in her care. It is impossible to overestimate the advantage to the nurse of the possession of a quiet mind.

IMPORTANT CONSIDERATIONS

1. Children cannot adapt themselves to sudden changes of temperature. The nursery or ward should be kept at a temperature of 65° F., fresh and well ventilated. The heat regulating centre is not fully developed, so the child must be well wrapped up when taken out of its cot. It is equally important to remove excess clothing when the child is indoors or in bed. A baby cannot complain that it is too hot and depends on the nurse to keep its cot comfortably warm. Very often a baby is restless, fretful, and sick because it is too hot, especially if the temperature is raised. A warm sponge, change of clothing and the use of a bed cradle will often soothe a restless, ill baby to sleep.

2. Children cannot stand loss of blood or fluid. Diarrhœa and vomiting quickly become serious conditions in the young baby for this reason. Prompt measures must be taken to deal with them. Adults can afford to have diarrhœa and sickness for a day or two, but a baby soon shows signs of collapse. Medical advice should be sought without delay. In the meantime any baby who is vomiting its food should be given boiled water only

to drink. It is no exaggeration to say that this may be the means of saving the baby's life.

3. A baby cannot stand excitement. The nervous system is unstable, and continuous over-excitement causes a rise in temperature and vomiting in the highly strung child. This type of child does not quickly recover from fright. In the child guidance clinics many difficulties in later years have been traced by the psychiatrists to errors of management in the early years. Threats and frightening stories make more impression than one imagines on the sensitive mind of the nervous child.

4. A positive attitude should be adopted to the active and intelligent child at the toddler stage and later. The word 'don't' should not be used. Substitute the word 'do' and give the child something to attract his attention from the forbidden line of action. Nagging and constantly saying, 'Don't do this,' 'Don't do that,' leads to the negative type of child who always wants to go the opposite direction to authority. They become very difficult to manage when they are a little older. Non-interference and 'watchful neglect' while the child follows his own pursuits is a good policy to follow. Left alone, a well-managed child will amuse himself to a great extent and a wise mother or nurse lets him find his own interests in his new world, only interfering to guard him from harm.

THE DEVELOPMENT OF A NORMAL CHILD

A child weighs six to seven pounds at birth. During the first week he loses half a pound, but by the twelfth to fourteenth day he has regained his birth weight. By the age of six months he should be 7 lbs. heavier than his birth weight, and at the age of a year 14 lbs. heavier than his birth weight. At about four months the head is held erect, and the baby generally can sit up in his cot at about six months of age. When he is fifteen to eighteen months old, he stands up and begins to walk. The anterior fontanelle of the child closes at the age of eighteen months to two years.

The teeth begin to erupt at the age of six months, the lower central incisors coming first. By the age of a year the child has seven or eight teeth, and by the age of two the first dentition of twenty teeth is complete. The permanent teeth begin to displace the milk teeth at the age of six or seven years. By the age of twelve the child has twenty-eight permanent teeth; the last four molars (wisdom teeth) erupt between the age of eighteen and twenty-five years.

There is a great difference in the rate at which babies develop and the fact that a baby appears to be backward in teething, walking or talking, is of no serious importance, provided that the child is healthy, eating and sleeping well, and making some progress each month. The biggest babies are by no means always the healthiest.

A nurse working with sick infants and children is liable to lose her sense

f proportion and forget what normal, healthy children are like. It is
most valuable if she takes every opportunity of studying normal children
t all ages, asking questions as to their age and development, so that she
an at all times compare her own patients with them. The behaviour and
ymptoms of sick children are difficult to assess unless one is familiar with
those of the normal child.

BREAST FEEDING

There should be no argument as to the advantages of breast feeding
he infant. Mother's milk is the natural food and cannot be improved
upon. During the first forty-eight hours after the baby's birth, the breasts
secrete a dilute milky fluid, called colostrum. It is of correct composition
o educate gradually the baby's digestion before it has to deal with milk
of a richer quality which comes into the breasts when lactation is established by the third day. The colostrum contains mild aperient substances
which stimulate peristalsis in the bowel of the child. It is also rich in anti-
bodies from the mother's blood. Thus the baby makes a perfectly scientific
start in life, unless it is interfered with by ignorant or over-anxious mothers.
The psychological value of breast feeding is of great importance also.

To put a Baby to the Breast. *First Day.* The first day after birth three
minutes to each breast, three- or four-hourly according to the size of the
child. Babies weighing over six pounds generally do well on four-hourly
feeds, the smaller babies require three-hourly feeding at first.

Second day. Five minutes at each breast.

Third and subsequent days. Ten minutes at each breast.

Ten minutes before a feed is due the baby is taken out of his cot and
changed. Before each feed the mother is encouraged to drink a glass of
water. She sits up with her pillows comfortably arranged, and is given a
dish in which are two gallipots, one containing boracic lotion and wool
swabs and the other empty. She is shown how to swab the nipples with the
boracic lotion, discarding the used wool into the empty gallipot. The baby
is put into her arms, and, if it is her first child, the nurse helps the mother
to get the baby into a comfortable position. Some mothers need no help
at all, while others are very clumsy and inept at feeding their babies. The
baby's nose should not be pushed up against the breast, otherwise it cannot
breathe and will be restless and uncomfortable while it is satisfying its
hunger. It will become exasperated and will probably take large gulps of
air (aerophagy) and the feed will be followed by indigestion. The mother
should give her whole attention to the baby while it feeds. If she gossips
or reads, the child is likely to lose the nipple and drop asleep before the
feed is finished. He will then wake up unsatisfied before the next feed is
due. Half-way through the feed, when the baby is changed from one breast
to the other, he is sat up and patted on the back. This is done because all

babies swallow a little air as they feed from the breast. Putting a baby in the upright position causes the air bubble to rise to the cardiac end of the stomach and to be expelled. This is also done again when the child has finished. Afterwards the mother washes her nipples and dries them carefully. The baby is now satisfied and drowsy. He is changed again if necessary and put back in his cot, slightly on his side, being most careful that he cannot possibly roll on to his face if he becomes restless, the cot blanket and quilt being firmly tucked in to maintain his position. It is advisable not to have a too large and soft down pillow; tragedies have happened from babies being smothered in their cots through not being carefully placed.

A breast-fed baby is often weighed daily for the first fortnight; after this it can be weighed every fortnight or month. In some cases it is better not to encourage the mother to weigh the child regularly, as slight variations tend to worry her unnecessarily. Any intelligent woman will know whether a baby is progressing satisfactorily or not, without resorting to the scales every week. If breast feeding is satisfactory the child will grow, will be contented and sleep well.

After the first three days the baby should have one or two soft yellow inoffensive stools per day. During the first two days he will pass a little greenish-black, sticky material called meconium. This is a natural lubricant which stimulates peristalsis.

Difficulties in Breast Feeding. (a) *The Mother*. The breasts may be underdeveloped and insufficient milk be secreted. In this case breast feeding should be persevered with and supplementary feeds given. To ascertain how much the baby gets from the mother, he is weighed in his clothes before and after each feed for twenty-four hours. It is no use weighing the baby after one feed, as the amount of milk in the breasts varies at different times of the day. The sucking of the baby is the best stimulus for the secretion of milk, and if the mother is persevering, the milk supply will, in most cases, improve and become sufficient.

Hot and cold douching of the breasts four hourly is helpful in improving the secretion of the milk. Large bowls of hot and cold water are required. The bed is protected with a mackintosh and the nurse helps the mother to douche each breast first with hot and then with cold water, using a large sponge.

N.B. A good supplementary feed for a new-born baby is made up as follows. The milk should be boiled for five minutes.

1st Strength (for the first 3 or 4 days)		2nd Strength (after 5 days)	
Milk	ʒi	Milk	ʒifs. (1½ oz.)
Water	ʒii	Water	ʒifs. „

Cream	$\mathfrak{Z}i$		Cream	$\mathfrak{Z}i$
Lactose	$\mathfrak{Z}i$		Lactose	$\mathfrak{Z}i$
Sodium citrate	gr. 1		Sodium citrate	gr. 1 fs.
Soda bicarbonate	gr. 1		Soda bicarbonate	gr. 1 fs.

The soda bicarbonate counteracts the slight acidity of the cow's milk and the sodium citrate reduces the denser curd to one of a more flocculent and more easily digested type.

Depressed nipples. These should be noted by the nurse who examines the patient during pregnancy, otherwise successful breast feeding is very difficult. The nipples are pulled out with the fingers and massaged with lanoline until they are a better shape. If they are inverted there is little chance of breast feeding being successful.

Cracked nipples. Cracked nipples complicate breast feeding. They should not occur if the toilet of the nipples is attended to before and after feeds. A small crack is best treated by taking the baby off the one breast for twelve hours, expressing the milk and painting the crack with friar's balsam whilst it is still small. When the baby is put back to the breast the mother must endure the pain of the sucking. After the feed she must wash the crack and paint it with friar's balsam. A neglected crack may lead to a breast abscess.

An over-anxious mother. An over-anxious mother is not usually a successful breast feeder. The psychological element is strong and if she is anxious and nervous of carrying out her function or worried about her supply of milk the glands are inhibited and secretion fails. On the other hand, if the mother does not wish to feed her baby and tries to find excuses for not doing so, the supply of milk may fail. The best mothers are those who look upon the whole function in a natural and philosophical way and carry it out without worry and excitement.

Open tuberculosis in the mother is always a contra-indication to breast feeding. The close contact with the mother's breath as she bends over the baby is likely to give him massive doses of tubercle bacilli by droplet infection. Apart from this disease and serious illness which may complicate the lying-in period, there is no other argument against breast feeding.

(b) *The baby.* The premature baby is drowsy and a feeble sucker. Small feeds should be given two-hourly and if necessary milk must be expressed from the breasts and given by bottle or small spoon. The baby with slight jaundice is sleepy and a lazy feeder. The mother must endeavour to keep it awake and see that it gets a full feed until the symptoms of jaundice have passed off.

The lusty and hungry baby often makes difficulties for himself by feeding too hungrily and rapidly. This may cause indigestion. In these cases it is a good plan when the feed is due to give the baby a bottle containing boiled water, so that he can work off a little of his surplus energy on the bottle before he goes to his mother. It may be that the baby is hungry because he is not getting sufficient milk. This must be looked into.

If the baby has a cold and his nose is blocked, feeding is difficult as he cannot suck and breathe through his mouth at the time. A little alkaline lotion dropped into the nostrils with a pipette, or a wisp of wool, just before the feed is due will probably keep the nose clear for a time, while the baby sucks.

The proper establishment of lactation is one of the most important parts of the work of the maternity nurse and experience and patience often overcome difficulties. Even a few weeks' breast feeding is worth while although it may not be possible to continue it longer. It gives the baby the best start in life.

ARTIFICIAL FEEDING

Food Requirements. To cover the minimum protein requirements, a baby requires 45 calories per pound of body weight per day up to the age of six months.

It requires 40 calories per pound of body weight per day over the age of six months.

It requires $2\frac{1}{2}$ ounces of fluid per pound of body weight per day.

It requires $1\frac{1}{2}$ ounces of cow's milk per pound of body weight per day.

Example: A baby weighing eight pounds requires 8 x 45 = 360 calories daily.

He requires:

$$8 \times 2\frac{1}{2} \text{ oz. of fluid} = 20 \text{ oz.}$$
$$8 \times 1\frac{1}{2} \text{ oz. of cow's milk} = 12 \text{ oz.}$$
$$8 \times 1 \text{ drachm of sugar} = 1 \text{ oz.}$$

Therefore a twenty-four hours' feed would consist of:

12 ounces of milk

8 ounces of water

1 ounce of sugar

This will be divided into five four-hourly feeds of four ounces each giving the last feed at ten o'clock at night and the first at six a.m. Boiled water can be given during the night if necessary.

CALORIFIC VALUES

One ounce of cow's milk yields 20 Calories.

One ounce of sugar yields 120 Calories.

Therefore the calorific value of the above feed would be:

Milk   12 x 20 = 240 Calories

Sugar   1 x 120 = 120 ,,

Total = 360 ,,

N.B. Cow's milk of good quality (accredited) is considered the best
substitute for breast milk. The tinned milk preparations, e.g. Cow and
Gate, are very good, especially for mothers who have not the advantage
of a good kitchen, clean saucepan and pantry.

It is not always possible to work out a feed on the weight and calorific
basis. In district work scales may not be available. Until the feeds can be
adjusted to the standard requirements their average size at different ages
is somewhat as follows:

Up to 1 month of age	..	3 oz., four-hourly
,, 2 months ,,	..	3 to $3\frac{1}{2}$ oz. four-hourly
,, 3 ,, ,,	..	$3\frac{1}{2}$ to $4\frac{1}{2}$ oz. four-hourly
,, 4 ,, ,,	..	$4\frac{1}{2}$ to 5 oz. four-hourly
,, 5 ,, ,,	..	5 oz. four-hourly
,, 6 ,, ,,	..	6 oz. four-hourly

The feed consists of two parts of milk and one part of water up to the
age of six months, after which the child can take whole milk. For healthy
babies the milk should never be weaker than two parts of milk to one of
water. It is safe to say that when a baby can take thirty ounces of whole
milk per day it is time to give additions to its feeds.

The addition of vitamins is required for all artifically fed babies. Two
minims of halibut liver oil are given twice daily (vitamins A and D);
two teaspoonfuls of orange or tomato juice (vitamin C) are given night
and morning. Healthy babies do not usually need additional vitamin B,
but babies who are or have been ill should be given a quarter of a teaspoonful of marmite in water daily. It is inadvisable to put it in the milk as the
baby may not like the taste.

It is not always as simple to work out the amount of feed on the calorific
basis as the above example would show, as babies seldom weigh an exact
number of pounds. Feeds must therefore be worked out as nearly as possible to the above figures. The tests as to whether the feed is satisfactory are:

1. Is the baby satisfied?
2. Does the baby finish the feed?
3. Does he sleep to within half an hour of the next feed?
4. Are his stools normal?—soft, yellow, inoffensive and containing no
undigested milk curds?
5. Is he gaining weight satisfactorily?

Most babies thrive well on a balanced artificial feed. It is the difficult
cases which are met with in the babies' wards. Experience will teach
how to adjust the feeds day by day until one is found which suits the
individual child. General rules for adjustment are:

1. Addition of more sugar if the stools are constipated.
2. Giving less sugar if the stools are too loose.

Dextri-maltose is a valuable form of non-fermenting sugar which can be given in large quantities without causing diarrhœa. It is most useful in enriching the feeds of sickly babies and increasing their weight. Although constant weighing of babies is to be discouraged, daily weight charts in the case of ill babies are essential. It is safe to say that if an ill baby is putting on a little weight each day, its general condition is improving and it is probably on the road to recovery.

THE MILK KITCHEN

In a children's ward a special room should be kept for the preparation of feeds, and the sister usually makes up the feeds at the beginning of the day, having one or more nurses to help her. In this way each nurse in turn learns the science of infant feeding. The kitchen should contain one or more gas rings or a small stove. A large fish kettle or other apparatus such as the Soxhlet sterilizer must be available for sterilizing bottles. Several saucepans, a sufficiency of jugs, bottles, teaspoons and tablespoons strainers, forks, etc., are required; a food thermometer standing in a glass of boiled water. There must be a refrigerator, a cupboard for stores and a sink.

The kitchen must be kept well ventilated and scrupulously clean. The sink and drains should be maintained in perfect condition, and the door of the kitchen always kept closed. The windows should be fitted with a fine gauze curtain to keep out dust and flies.

It is safer for ill babies that all milk should be boiled for five minutes before the feeds are prepared. The saucepans must be scrupulously clean and scalded with boiling water before the milk is put in. Spoons should be boiled before use and dried with a clean towel. Clean towels should be put out two or three times daily as required. Bottles, when they have been used, are rinsed in cold water, cleaned with a bottle brush, rinsed in warm water and boiled. Teats are cleaned under the cold tap and then rinsed in hot water and boiled twice daily. A different mop should be kept for cleaning the sink.

The best type of bottle to use is the Soxhlet bottle. It has a special shaped rounded end so that there are no corners or crevices to which milk may cling. They are bought in a round stand which accommodates these bottles and fits into a container in which the feeds can be sterilized. The amount prepared in the morning is divided into the number of feeds required for the day, each is put straight into a separate stoppered bottle. When the feed is due one bottle is stood in hot water; the stopper is removed and a teat fitted on when the feed is ready.

To give a baby a bottle feed. Unless there is any good reason against it the baby should be taken out of his cot to be fed. In hospital, however special precautions should be taken when doing this, to prevent cross infection from one baby to another. The nurse should wear a mackintosh apron and over it a gown which is kept for the one baby only. She should wear a mask. The baby should be changed before he is taken out of his cot. The nurse then washes her hands thoroughly and collects the feed. She sits on a low chair with the child comfortably in her arms with the head slightly raised and gives him her whole attention. He should be well wrapped up in a blanket, his arms fastened down to his sides so that his fists do not get in the way. A bib is essential. The feed should be given warm, 98° to 100° F., and if for any reason it is interrupted the bottle should be kept standing in a bowl of hot water. Sometimes at the end of a feed a baby regurgitates some of it; this is called posseting and should not be confused with vomiting. It merely indicates that the baby has had rather more milk than the stomach can deal with. The nurse should always report if a baby has not taken the whole feed. Ill babies are seldom hungry for their feeds and the nurse requires patience and persistence in encouraging the child to take an adequate amount. It is very important because the child is not likely to get better if he is constantly getting a smaller feed than he requires.

BATHING AN INFANT

The baby should be bathed in the morning at about 9.30, as he will usually be due for a feed at 10 a.m. The feed should be prepared beforehand so that when the bathing is finished the bottle can be given at once. The bathing should be done before a fire or in a warm corner of a heated room. The windows are closed.

Requirements
1. A mackintosh and flannel apron or gown.
2. Screen, low chair.
3. Bath, one-third full of water, temperature 100° F.
4. Clothes-horse containing the baby's clean clothes and napkins well aired.
5. A tray or basket containing a rectal thermometer; wool swabs in a small bowl of disinfectant and a small receiver; a bowl of warm water, and dry wool swabs.
6. A large bath towel.
7. A good simple soap such as Knight's Castile or White Windsor.
8. A sponge or washing flannel.
9. Talcum powder.
10. Hair brush.
11. Receivers for soiled napkins and soiled clothes.

Method. The child is undressed. The temperature is taken per rectum keeping the napkin under the buttocks meanwhile. Patterns of modern babies' clothes vary, but they usually all fasten down the back or down the front, so that turning is avoided. The baby is then wrapped up in the towel. The face and ears are washed with wool swabs and warm water, no soap is required. The nostrils are cleaned with little wisps of damp wool.

The face is then dried with wool, special attention being paid to the drying of the ears. The head is held over the bath with the left hand, and the hair is soaped with the nurse's right hand. She rinses it with the flannel, still holding the head over the bath. It is then dried. With well-soaped hands she next washes the neck, arms, trunk and legs, half turning the baby over to do the back and buttocks, special attention being paid to the cleanliness of the folds in the groins. If the cord is not yet separated this area is kept dry; if it has separated the umbilicus is thoroughly washed. Taking the child in the crook of her left arm, and holding the baby's left arm with her left hand, and both legs with the right hand, she lowers him into the water and rinses off the soap with the sponge. After a minute or two he is taken out of the bath, put on his face on the nurse's knee and carefully dried, again paying careful attention to the folds of the skin, the groins behind the ears, the neck, between the toes. He is then turned on his back and the chest is dried. The groins and buttocks are powdered and the napkin and vest and other garments if they fasten down the back are put in position before the child is turned over again. The napkin is then adjusted comfortably and the rest of the dressing is completed. The hair is brushed. The baby is wrapped up warmly in a shawl and given his feed before he is put back in his cot.

In the case of a new-born baby, the face and eyes should not be touched with the bath water.[1] At birth the baby is covered with a fatty material called *vernix caseosa*. It lubricates the mother's vagina during the birth, and if any infection should be present the eyes of the baby might become contaminated. For this reason it is wise to wash and dry the face and eyes of the child with wool as described above. The towel used for the first bath should be sent to the laundry and not used again. Before the cord separates care must be taken that the umbilical area does not get wet. A few inches of water only are put into the bath and the child rinsed carefully. A 'keyhole' dressing (see diagram, p. 293) is put round the cord, which is generously sprinkled with astringent powder (pulv. starch, boracic and zinc in equal parts is a good powder for this purpose), and the dressing is then folded as a packet round the cord. It is kept in position by a flannel binder which is stitched. The cord separates at about the eighth day.

To Change a Baby

Requirements

1. Hot water.
2. Soap and flannel.
3. Towels.
4. Wool swabs.

[1] Some authorities recommend that for the first few days, the eyes, ears, and buttocks only should be washed. This is to avoid minor abrasions of the delicate skin, thus minimizing the risk of infection.

5. Receiver.
6. Pail.
7. Powder.
8. Napkins.

Method. See that all requirements are ready near the cot and within
ach. Fold the clean napkin. Fold down the top bedclothes tidily, and
over the baby with a small blanket or shawl. Take out the pin from the
oiled napkin, and if the baby's temperature has to be taken, do so before
moving the napkin (if it is not soiled), as the presence of the thermometer
the rectum so often stimulates bowel action. Slip out the napkin and
ut it straight in the pail provided, and put the towel under the baby's
uttocks. Clean off any fæcal matter with damp wool swabs, and then
ash and dry the buttocks thoroughly with soap and water, paying
articular attention to the groins. Take out the towel, and place the clean
apkin under the buttocks; apply a little dusting powder, and fasten the
apkin securely, with the pin lying horizontally and not vertically. Tuck
p the baby comfortably, put away soap, flannel and personal belong-
gs, empty the used water. Leave the bowl clean and ready for the next
aby. The hands must be washed at once after changing a napkin. If the
aby is well enough to be lifted from his cot the nurse may change him on
er lap. She must wear a special apron or gown kept for the one child only.

Cleaning a Baby's Mouth. This must be done with the utmost gentleness,
r it will do far more harm than good. Glycerine boracis is generally used,
xcept in severe cases of stomatitis when Bowman's solution or monsol
—800 or some other preparation is ordered.

Requirements. Small tray containing:

1. Gallipot for glycerine; fairy Spencer Wells forceps; cut pieces of
   gauze about 1½ inches square; small paper bag or receptacle for
   soiled dressings; or
2. Wooden wool carriers; small thin squares of best quality white
   wool. The wool carrier must be dressed in the same way as for
   mopping an ear, but the tuft should be larger. (See p. 277.)

Method. The mouth is usually cleaned before and after feeds. Dip the
ressed wool carrier into the glycerine and *very gently* mop round between
he baby's gums and cheek. Then with another carrier, gently touch the
ront of the baby's tongue and let him suck off the glycerine. Watch care-
ully at this point. The wool carrier must be very firmly dressed, or the
aby might suck off the wool. Three moppings are usually sufficient. On
o account should the nurse touch the back of the baby's tongue, as this
ould cause him to vomit. Where Spencer Wells forceps are used, they
ust be well protected by the gauze, and the forceps firmly locked. All
tensils must be kept for the use of one baby only and boiled up at least
wice daily.

Babies' Napkins. The nurse may be required to wash wet napkins. soon as they are taken off they should be put into a bucket of cold wat They are rinsed and wrung out in this and then washed with a good soa or soap flakes. Strong soaps, soda or ammonia are never used. The di napkins are put in a separate pail. The fæcal matter is removed by thorou rinsing in several changes of water under the tap, a mop may be used help clean them. They are sent in a separate bundle to the laundry. T private nurse who has only one baby to look after generally washes the napkins herself.

Babies' Woollies. These should never be sent to the laundry. Th should be washed in a good soapy lather and should be squeezed rath than rubbed. They are then well rinsed in warm water, not hot. They m not be soaked beforehand. After washing they are thoroughly dried squeezing them rather than wringing, being well shaken and stretched their normal shape. They should never be put on a heated radiator to d They are usually put on a clothes horse and dried quickly in the open or before a fire, if a proper drying-room is not available They must well aired.

Wards in a modern children's hospital are built in cubicle style; ea baby is nursed in a glass cubicle, with its requirements kept separate. some cases an overall is kept for all nursing treatments, and this is ke hanging in the cubicle. There is a washing sink which is used as a bath a a nursing chair and a trolley containing all requirements for bathin changing, etc.; also a radiator for airing napkins (see plate 24).

Other equipment includes: Thermometer; adequate supplies of pap towels for drying the hands; receptacle for soiled towels; nail brush ar soap.

For older children suitable toys and games must be provided and cloth suitable for all ages. All crockery of the toddlers who take meals togeth should be boiled after each meal. All children must have intervals of sle during the day. The time varies according to their age.

THE NURSING OF COMMON CONDITIONS

Nervous Unrest. This condition is usually the result of mismanageme on the part of an unintelligent or over-anxious mother. The nervous syste of a child reacts to that of the mother in an incredible way, the tiniest chi will feel an atmosphere of anxiety and uncertainty and will become restle and sleepless. Under such conditions its digestive system soon becom deranged. It refuses its feeds, suffers from flatulence and indigestion becau it never takes its food in a calm and peaceful way. Thus a vicious circle formed, poor feeding, unsatisfied infant, mother is tempted to feed it other than regular intervals and the rhythm of feeding is thoroughly upse Things are worse in the night and the whole household becomes disorga ized. The child begins to lose weight and go down hill, and eventually the mother seeks the advice of a doctor or nurse. Unless the private nurse can go into the house and take over the management and show the mother how to cope with the situation, it is best for the child to be taken to a hospital and separated from the mother for a time. A few trying days are to be gone through before the baby realizes that it is in different and more secure hands. The experienced nurse starts a routine for the baby and does not diverge from it, and gradually gets him into better habits.

In severe cases of nervous unrest certain nursing methods help to soothe the child's nervous system and give him sleep. Long periods of sleep will do him more good than anything else. The cubicle is kept fresh and cool. The baby must be dressed with great care and gentle movement seeing that tapes and garments are not too tight or irritating in any way. The slightest discomfort will irritate the child in its nervous state. Sometimes a cradle in the bed will ensure more comfortable sleep. Sometimes, for a very restless child a few months old, it is a good plan to roll him up tightly in a blanket with his arms to the side and pin the blanket with several large safety pins. He soon becomes comfortably warm, and drops asleep. Prolonged tepid baths, temperature 98° F. for half an hour at a time followed by a small, warm feed will often send this restless infant to sleep. The bath can be given three or four times a day in acute cases. Sedative drugs, e.g. chloral, are ordered to re-establish the rhythm of sleep. The feeds must be carefully planned to suit the child's age and weight. As the baby recovers and becomes normal in his sleep and feeding, the mother begins to realize that her management and attitude have been at fault. The doctor and the nurse will help her to reorganize her methods by drawing up a day's time table as it has been carried out in the hospital. The mother is strongly advised to attend a welfare clinic regularly with her child. It should give her confidence to feel there is someone who understands her case in every detail. At the clinic she will see the same nurse every week and the doctor also at regular intervals, as required.

Inanition or Marasmus. This condition may be a sequel to nervous unrest. The rhythm of feeding and sleeping becomes so disturbed that the digestive functions are seriously impaired. The baby refuses his feeds and vomits. Whatever food it is given is badly digested and to a large extent unabsorbed. The stools are either constipated or abnormally loose. The child loses weight and gradually becomes limp, pale and ill. The eyes are sunken, the skin of the face puckered and the fontanelle depressed owing to the general dehydration of the tissues.

Other causes of inanition in babies are congenital syphilis and the constant changing of feeds.

Treatment. It is difficult to lay down any specific rules for treatment. The infant needs expert nursing with regard to bathing, care of buttocks and warmth. The feeding, however, is the chief point. This is carefully graduated, beginning with milk and water in equal parts, gradually increasing the strength. If vomiting is troublesome, other feeds are tried. Lactic acid milk often gives good results in these difficult cases. Two-hourly feeds of two ounces are given at first if the vomiting appears to have become a habit, and it is a good plan to try equal quantities of lactic acid milk and ràther thick Benger's food. Mead's dextri-maltose should be used to sweeten the feeds of a marasmic baby. Difficult feeders are sometimes given a good start with Nestlé's condensed milk, made up in boiled water. Babies usually like it and begin to put on weight. After two or three weeks cow's milk should be added to the feed and the Nestlé's milk gradually decreased. It contains too much sugar and not enough protein to give lasting benefit.

It is usually unnecessary to worry about the bowel action of the child. As soon as his feeds begin to suit him, the stools will become more normal. The skin of the buttocks needs greatest care. The baby should be kept warmly wrapped up as the diet is not adequate to maintain the normal heat of the body.

One of the troubles in treating this type of baby in a hospital ward is his liability to contract infection due to his debilitated state.

To make lactic acid milk. The feed is made up in the required proportion of milk and boiled water. Lactic acid is beaten into the mixture with a fork, three minims to the ounce of milk, at a temperature below 80° F. This breaks up the milk into a very fine digestible curd which easily passes through a teat with a hole of reasonable size. When ready to give the feed, it should not be heated more than 98° F. or the curdling process goes too far.

Diarrhœa and Vomiting in Infants (Gastro-Enteritis). This disease, until recent years, has been responsible for the deaths of a large number of babies under a year old, in the late summer months. It is seldom seen in breast-fed infants. A combination of many factors seems to cause it:

1. Unsatisfactory milk supply. In hot weather in some neighbourhoods the milk is not kept cool and fresh.

2. Flies infecting milk, teats, and bottles.

3. Heat retention in the child. In slum conditions in hot weather, if the skin of the baby is not kept active by daily or twice daily baths, the pores become clogged with sweat and dirt. The temperature-regulating mechanism fails and the baby's temperature rises.

The natural reaction of any baby to pyrexia and infection is reflected in its alimentary tract. The digestive juices fail to function and the baby is sick. The mother imagines the feed does not suit the child and tries something different, usually a patent food which has been recommended to her. Just when the stomach is upset it is expected to deal with a food of a different nature. The baby continues to vomit and whatever food is taken erments in the stomach and intestines. Poisons are produced until the child is suffering from a dangerous degree of toxæmia.

Symptoms

1. The vomiting of feeds.
2. Frequent loose, green, offensive, frothy, acid stools.
3. Loss of weight.
4. Sore buttocks.
5. Rise in temperature; hot burning skin.
6. Ashen, grey look, with sunken eyes.
7. A dry mouth.
8. Sunken fontanelle.

Prevention. As soon as the baby vomits and has loose green stools he should be given nothing to drink except boiled water. This is only common sense—an adult who feels sick refuses to eat—and the baby becomes more sick if he is coaxed into taking feeds. The baby should be bathed and kept in a cool cot in a well-ventilated room. He should not be overdressed. If these precautions are taken at once, the baby will probably be better within twenty-four hours, and can resume its normal feeds, in a diluted form. The pantry and kitchen should be investigated to ensure that the milk is kept in a cool place and is used when fresh, and that flies are not infecting agents.

Treatment. The disease must be treated as infectious and all proper precautions taken. If it is not arrested immediately prompt measures are needed. The toilet of the baby must be attended to in every detail. If he is suffering from shock and is too ill to be taken out of his cot and put in a bath he must be sponged all over twice a day and kept cool. His mouth must be cleaned; the eyes swabbed with saline in severe cases; soft napkins should be used and changed very frequently. Each time he is changed the buttocks must be well washed with soap and water and a little olive oil rubbed in to prevent the acid stools causing irritation of the skin. The napkins must be put straight into a bucket containing a solution of formalin 1—500. After soaking they must be rinsed and re-rinsed before being mixed with the rest of the laundry. The temperature, pulse, and respiration are recorded four-hourly. Bed socks may be worn as the feet of these babies with a high temperature are often cold in spite of a hot, dry skin. Thirty minims of brandy in a teaspoonful of hot water is given four-hourly at the onset of treatment.

Feeding. Boiled water only is given, one ounce hourly. If this is vomited nothing should be given by mouth. Fluids are then given intravenously by the drip method, or into the peritoneum. Blood plasma is often found beneficial. As the baby recovers a little glucose is added to the boiled water feeds. The next advance is to give whey, after which lactic acid milk, followed by an ordinary milk and water feed may be given.

The nurse must wear a gown and mask and take careful precaution against spread of infection. She must wash her hands after attending to the baby, and each time after changing it before she does anything else. The baby must be kept quiet and cool and not overtreated. Rest and sleep will do it more good than anything. A record must be kept of the amount and character of the vomit and the number of stools passed.

Pyloric Stenosis. Pyloric stenosis is a congenital condition in young babies in which the pylorus becomes contracted so that food cannot pass into the intestine. It is generally found in boy babies and the symptoms develop at the age of two or three weeks. It is considered to be due to a lack of co-ordination in the neuro-muscular mechanism of the pyloric sphincter. The condition corrects itself as the child grows older and it is said that recovery is always complete before the sixteenth week. The difficulty is that in the meantime urgent symptoms arise which are due to starvation and cross-infection.

Symptoms

1. Sudden projectile vomiting of feeds.

2. Constipation, small orange-coloured stools, due to their being highly coloured by bile.

3. Loss of weight.

4. The child is very hungry, restless, unsatisfied.

5. Peristaltic waves are seen passing across the abdomen. The hard contracted pylorus can often be felt.

6. The temperature is normal, or may be subnormal due to malnutrition.

Treatment

1. *Medical.* A barium X-ray is given. Two drachms each of barium and lactose are mixed in a two-ounce feed of milk and water. An œsophageal tube is passed and the feed poured in through a small glass funnel. The child is X-rayed three times at hourly intervals and again later to see how much of the feed has passed through the pylorus into the intestine.

If the stenosis is not complete and the physician considers that the child can get sufficient food to keep him alive, medical treatment is advised. A stomach lavage is given to wash away the barium, and small two-hourly feeds of expressed breast milk or milk and water are administered (two ounces two-hourly).

A daily gastric lavage is often prescribed to wash away the remains of feeds which cannot be passed out of the stomach. Eumydrine $\mathfrak{m}$iii of a 6 per cent solution is given by mouth twenty minutes before each feed. This drug belongs to the atropine group (atropine methyl nitrate) and it relaxes the sphincter of the pylorus.

The baby must be well nursed and should not come into contact with infection while it is in its undernourished state. He is weighed daily and if the treatment is successful, although the weight may remain stationary or may only rise slowly for a week or two, a gradual gain is seen and eventually the child will pick up.

2. *Surgical treatment*. Although the use of the drug eumydrine has made medical treatment of pyloric stenosis much more successful, there are still severe cases which do not seem to respond to the drug and which need operative interference to save the baby's life. The muscles of the pylorus are incised (Rammstedt's operation).

Preparation for operation. No further skin preparation is required. The stomach is washed out half an hour before the operation and two ounces of normal saline may be left in after the lavage. The baby is well wrapped up, its legs and arms bandaged in warm wool, and a piece of wool is put on the chest and back, kept in position by a woollen jacket, fastening down the front. A woollen cap is put on the head. It is most important that heat should not be lost from the body surface. The operation is very quickly done and the wound is stitched up with salmon gut sutures.

Post-operative treatment. The baby is returned to a warm cot. He quickly recovers from the anæsthetic and is not likely to be sick; very light anæsthesia is given and the operation is usually done quickly. Carefully graduated feeds of saline, glucose and breast milk are given (see table below), and results are best if the increase in the feeds is made very slowly and gradually. It is unfortunate if for any reason breast feeding is not possible. In many hospitals it is possible to allow the mother to live in an annexe attached to the ward so that she is on the spot to supply the breast milk when necessary. The nurses also help her to look after her breasts and general health during this interruption of normal lactation. It is obviously a bad thing to have to change the baby on to artificial feeds at this time. If it has to be done, graduated milk and water feeds with glucose are given, or a lactic acid mixture or half cream Cow and Gate. By the fourth or fifth day the weight of the child begins to show a definite rise, and often a sensible mother may take the baby home on the fifth day and bring him to the hospital daily to be weighed and his dressing looked at if necessary. The stitches are removed on the seventh to eighth day. It is not necessary to treat the bowels as when normal feeding is resumed they should function normally.

Post-operative feeding in pyloric stenosis

Nothing by mouth for four hours, then:

Fourth and fifth hour half-normal saline with 6 per cent glucose ʒi.

Sixth and seventh hour half-normal saline with 6 per cent glucose with breast milk ʒ½.

Eighth and ninth hours breast milk ʒi½.

This gradually increases by ʒ½ and then by ʒi every two hours after twenty-four hours the infant is taking ʒi of breast milk two-h

By the third day, ℥ii should be taken two-hourly and then the amounts and intervals are increased until the feeds are ℥iii three-hourly.

Convulsions in Infancy. The cause of a fit is always irritation of the central nervous system. The nervous system of a child is unstable and uncontrolled, so a comparatively small cause may induce a fit. It is possible that some things which in an adult would cause a headache and pain will so upset the nervous system of a child that a convulsion ensues.

Some common causes are:

1. Infections, such as measles, pneumonia, gastro-enteritis, etc.
2. Constipation.
3. Meningitis.
4. Teething difficulties in rickety or debilitated children.
5. Digestive upsets.
6. Intra-cranial injuries at birth, especially after forceps delivery.

Treatment for a Severe Fit

1. Put the child in a mustard bath, half an ounce of mustard in a muslin bag, squeezed in a gallon of water, temperature 100° F. Sponge the head with cold water. The rigid muscles will relax and the colour of the skin and face will become pink as the child begins to breathe again. On recovery the baby should be put into a warm cot.

2. Medical advice is sought and the cause investigated. It may be necessary to reorganize the diet or to treat one of the diseases mentioned above. In most cases the doctor will order a sedative, such as haustus chloral infantum, one drachm four hourly.

3. A glycerine enema is often given.

Fits in children are not necessarily serious but medical advice is always required.

Jaundice in Infants. The newborn child has a larger number of red cells in the blood than it requires after birth. During the first few days of life numbers of cells are destroyed and pigments are released into the blood stream which may lead to a mild type of jaundice, called icterus neonatorum. The symptoms pass off within seven to ten days but during this time special nursing care is required. The baby is drowsy and difficult to feed. The production of heat by the liver is disorganized so that the temperature is often subnormal. The baby should not be bathed in case it catches cold. It should be rubbed with warm olive oil with the minimum of exposure. After the inunction the baby is dressed in warm woollen clothing with woollen socks and bonnet. It is often necessary to feed the baby two-hourly as in its drowsy state it is a feeble, lazy sucker and cannot ake at one feed sufficient to last much longer than two hours. The child ways recovers if the nursing care is adequate and he is kept warm.

Another cause of jaundice in infants is congenital syphilis. The jaundice develops after the first week and the diagnosis is confirmed by the Wassermann Reaction of the blood of baby and parents. Antisyphilitic treatment is given, very small doses of bismuth given intramuscularly, and a mercurial ointment is rubbed into the skin (see inunction).

Hare Lip and Cleft Palate. The operation for hare lip is done before the child is three months old. Before the repair the child has to be fed by spoon as it cannot suck. A small spoon should be used and the food put well to the back of the child's mouth leaving the spoon on the lips till the fluid is swallowed. If this is done carefully regurgitation should not occur to any great extent. Much patience is required to see that the baby gets an adequate diet and that he is in a good condition for the operation.

After the operation the lip is dressed with collodion. The child is fed with a small teaspoon, and after each feed the lip must be left clean and dry, first swabbing with saline and then drying with a little methylated spirit. A 'butterfly' dressing of strapping may be attached to the cheeks, to keep the incision from being stretched when the child cries. A Logan's bow is a small silver instrument which serves the same purpose. The child should be propped up in the cot and kept very warm, so that he does not catch cold after the anæsthetic. Mild sedatives are required at first, such as haustus chloral infantum, p.r.n.

Cleft Palate. This is not usually repaired until the child is over three. Up to this age feeding is difficult and regurgitation of food through the nose is likely to occur. Great care is required in nursing these children before and after operation. The child should be brought into hospital at least a week before the day of operation, as it is essential that he should not feel strange and should know his nurse and be in a happy and contented frame of mind. The feeding is important so that he is in as good a condition as possible for the operation. The operation must be postponed if he has a cough or a cold or if he is not in his normal good health in any way. His temperature, pulse, and respiration should be normal. No special preparation is required before the operation. The last meal should be taken four hours beforehand. Glucose can be given freely up to one hour before he goes to the theatre. An injection of atropine, grains 1/150 is given half an hour previously, and he is warmly wrapped up. The surgeon does a plastic operation on the palate, excising strips of mucous membrane from the sides and drawing them over the centre of the cleft. Very fine horse hair sutures are used.

Post-Operative Nursing Care. As soon as he has recovered from the anæsthetic, the child is propped up with pillows. The cot should be screened and out of draughts. On no account must the child catch cold or he may develop bronchitis or pneumonia. He can be given sips of boiled water in a sterile spoon as freely as required; he is usually very thirsty when he regains consciousness. The mouth is dry as a result of the atropine and plenty of water will do him good. Haustus chloral infantum is given as required. On no account must the child be allowed to cry and the success of the operation largely depends upon the nurse keeping the mouth very clean and the child contented, warm, and sleeping well. After the first day or two he is given nutritious and stimulating feeds, milky preparations, such as milky tea and cocoa, and soups. All utensils must be boiled and kept in a bowl of boiled water. A small spoon is best for feeding so that the child does not have to open the mouth wide. It should be put just to his lips with his head held well back, so that the food trickles into the mouth without any sucking effort. Glucose may be added to most feeds. Before and after feeds drinks of boiled water are given to wash the stitches. The nurse should not attempt to examine the palate and should never clean the mouth except by giving boiled water to drink. The stitches may be removed on the seventh day. To do this the child is placed with the head hanging well down. It is best done with him lying across the bed or table. He is rolled in a blanket and two people may be required to help, one to steady the head while the other holds the trunk. A very good light is needed to shine on the palate. Long fine, pointed forceps and scissors are required. Absorbable sutures of fine catgut are often used. An anæsthetic may be required for the removal of sutures.

Eczema. Infantile eczema is an allergic disease. It is caused by hypersensitiveness to certain substances, generally protein in nature. It is associated with other allergic diseases, hay fever and asthma, from which diseases very often other members of the family are found to suffer. In babies eczema is a particularly distressing complaint. The child is usually rather fat and well built. The eczema is usually worse on the face, head and buttocks and thighs, being widespread. The child scratches himself, rubs his head on the pillows, becomes very hot and sweats. His temperature rises, 100° to 101° F., and he is very fretful and miserable.

Treatment. The irritating protein is thought by some authorities to be the protein of cow's milk. The child is put on to feeds of soya milk or synthetic milk, such as Almata or Allergilac. Soap is not allowed on the skin, but the doctor may order saline baths in normal strength. These are cleansing, soothing and do not irritate the skin. Also, the baby enjoys the bath. He must be very carefully and gently dried by dabbing movements with a smooth towel. He should wear a cotton gown and the bed linen must be cool; a bed cradle is useful. The flexor surfaces of the elbows may be splinted with thick folds of paper; this is usually sufficient to prevent scratching, but if the child can still reach his legs, the wrists must be loosely tethered with wool and bandage to the sides of the cot, to limit his movements just sufficiently to prevent it. Local applications are used under the direction of the doctor: calamine lotion, calamine cream, olive oil. The parts should be kept covered. If the child scratches, the lesions are likely to become secondarily infected. Crusts and scabs are removed by the application of starch poultices or oil before the lotion is applied. The disease is very intractable and likely to last for years. It is not infectious but it is wise to keep the linen and towels of the child separate, from the point of view of cleanliness and hygiene. The napkins must be chosen of non-irritating material, muslin rather than turkish towelling.

Acidosis. Acidosis is a lowering of the alkaline reserve of the blood. It is recognized as a fairly common condition in a certain type of child (e.g. those who suffer from train-sickness), particularly between the ages of five to ten years. It is concerned with diet. The stores of sugar in the body are quickly used up by the nervous, over-active, and excitable child. It has been said that the emotional life of a growing child is lived on sugar. It is not the children of the poorer class who suffer from this condition. They usually get a high percentage of carbohydrate in their diet in the form of bread and jam and are more likely to be short of fats. The pampered and overfed child is more likely to be the sufferer, for example, one who is fed on an over-rich diet, containing milk and cream out of proportion to the other elements in the food. Fat is not satisfactorily metabolized without the proper proportion of carbohydrate. Acid poisons known as ketone bodies result and the condition is known as ketosis or acidosis. The same condition is found in diabetic subjects whose diet has not been properly planned and whose carbohydrates have been cut down to dangerous proportions. It is also found in conditions of starvation when the body begins to use up its stores of fat to maintain body heat. This fact should not be lost sight of, because children who are ill or who have had surgical operations soon slip into a condition of ketosis through prolonged starvation.

Symptoms. The symptoms of ketosis are:

1. Lethargy and drowsiness.
2. Pallor with dark rings round the eyes.
3. Emotionalism, in which periods of excitement are followed by vomiting (cyclical vomiting).
4. The smell of acetone in the breath and the presence of acetone in the urine.
5. Liability to other infections.

Treatment. Those who are in contact with growing children not only in hospital but in school and home should be quick to recognize the above symptoms. The treatment is to give more carbohydrate in the diet, plain cake, barley sugar, rather than rich foods and chocolate. For the child who is ill glucose is invaluable, it is pure carbohydrate in its most absorbable form.

Enuresis or Bed-Wetting. Enuresis is a problem with which all nurses have to deal sooner or later. The advice of school nurses is often sought, for these children are a burden to themselves and to everyone else. Each case should be carefully investigated and the parents interviewed. The doctor will examine to see if there is any organic disease to account for the condition. If a boy, he may need to be circumcised. The urine should be examined as it may be infected and irritating. A large proportion of the cases are considered to be in the nervous, over-anxious type of child, and during the evacuation period of the war when children were separated from their mothers and living under emotional stress the condition became one of the major difficulties with which householders receiving them had to deal.

Treatment. No line of treatment can be guaranteed to cure the condition but certain principles should be followed. The child should be dealt with sympathetically. It is wiser not to draw his attention each morning to the wet bed, otherwise he may become worried. If this happens he is likely to go to bed anticipating the worst which invariably occurs. Fluids can be withheld after five p.m. and if the child lies on a pad of sphagnum moss the urine passed will be absorbed by the pad so that the child is led to think he is overcoming his difficulties. Small doses of belladonna given at night inhibit the secretion of urine and the giving of this drug may be useful in re-establishing the child's confidence in himself. If there is any disease in the urinary tract it should, of course, be attended to. If the cause of the emotional stress can be removed, the condition often clears up.

Chorea (St. Vitus Dance). Chorea is a manifestation of rheumatism. It is due to toxins attacking the brain and is sometimes described as rheumatic encephalitis. The child is excitable, emotional and his movements are unco-ordinated. He grimaces, jerks and drops things. He twitches and fidgets all day and is only quiet during sleep. He is usually an overgrown child and, as with other forms of rheumatism, the danger is infection of the heart.

Treatment. The aim of the nursing treatment is to give rest to the heart. The child is nursed in a comfortable bed with one pillow. He should wear pyjamas of a non-irritating material such as Viyella or flannelette. He must be prevented in some way from falling out of bed, but restrainers of the normal type usually do more harm than good and make him more restless. In hospital 'side boards' can be fitted to the bed and these and the head of the bed are packed with soft pillows. The child should be in a quiet corner of the ward and screened. In some cases, however, if he is of an inquisitive nature, he is quieter if he can see what is going on around him. Toys should be chosen with care. Books and toys of a mechanical nature are bad; soft woolly ones are better. Other children should not be allowed to play with and excite the patient. The mother, if she is of the right type, can often have a calming effect on the child and may be allowed to visit and read to him. On the other hand, the mother might be the worst person to do this.

A blanket bath is given daily and every bony prominence should be inspected for signs of reddening. The child should not have a blanket next o him and the bedclothes should be firmly tucked in. The knees, heels, shoulder blades, elbows and occiput are given special attention as constant rubbing and fidgeting is very liable to cause sores to form. If signs of redness appear on the elbows, knees or heels they can be protected by wool pads and firmly bandaged. The mattress should not be lumpy, and care should be taken that the drawsheets are not patched, seamed or darned.

The temperature is taken rectally and the pulse recorded when the child is asleep. The patient must be fed. If he is allowed to do this for himself, the effort and the distress caused by spilling food, etc., damages the heart. He should never be allowed to feed himself until he is well on the way to recovery, which may be weeks or months. A spoon and thick china or enamelware should be used. The child's mouth may be damaged by forks or thin glass or china if his movements are unexpectedly jerky. All articles of food are allowed and the child should be encouraged to eat well. Sedative drugs are ordered, but are not of great value. Prolonged rest and convalescence is relied upon to cure the condition.

Cœliac Disease. Cœliac disease is sometimes met with in children's wards. It is due to inability to absorb fat. The cause is obscure, but it is thought that deficiency of vitamin B_2 has some damaging effect on the mucous membrane of the small intestine. The main features are wasting of the muscles, protuberance of the abdomen, 'pot belly'; and the passing of very large grey fatty offensive stools. The arms, legs, and buttocks show the muscle wasting very markedly and the child is anæmic and pale. The disease runs a chronic course up to the age of about seven years, when the child seems to grow out of it. In the meantime it is possible that death may occur, due to malnutrition and intercurrent infections.

Treatment. Treatment consists in building up the diet, giving one deficient in fat but rich in other constituents. It should contain soups, meat juices, bananas, tomatoes and other fruits, a sufficiency of good carbohydrates and skimmed milk. Marmite is given daily either on bread with just a scraping of butter, or it can be given as a drink if the child will take it. In some cases it is necessary to give it by stomach tube. Other proprietary preparations of vitamin B_2 are ordered and on a rigid diet the child generally improves, only to relapse if it is not strictly adhered to.

The child needs special nursing care as his health is delicate and he is particularly liable to contract other infections. It has been observed, however, by those who have looked after these children, that they are very tenacious of life and with care have a good chance of surviving.

Rickets. The early signs of rickets should be recognized by the nurse. They are not usually recognizable before the sixth to ninth month, and the first and most obvious sign is often sweating of the head. When the child is lifted out of its cot, the pillow is wet. The type of child is often characteristic, he is rather fat, flabby and pale, with a tendency to colds and digestive

disorders of a mild type. When one feels his arms and legs the muscles ar
not hard and firm as a normal child's; the ankles and wrists feel rathe
soft and swollen due to enlargement of the epiphyses as ossification doe
not take place at the same rate as growth. He may have an occasiona
green stool and vomiting attack. A severe case of rickets is sometime
complicated by convulsions. It is important to recognize that rickets is
nutritional disease with general symptoms in the early stages. The bon
symptoms make the disease obvious when the child begins to walk; bowe
legs, bowed arms, enlargement of the epiphyses, and a peculiar square hea
with late closure of the fontanelle. Dentition difficulties are common.

Treatment. The treatment is reorganization of the diet, giving plent
of animal fats, butter, eggs, fresh milk; with the addition of concentrate
vitamin D preparations—cod liver oil and halibut liver oil. The carbohy
drates in the diet should be cut down a little, but care must be taken no
to precipitate a condition of ketosis. Fresh air, sunshine, and ultra-viole
light are important factors. Vitamin D in all forms is necessary for th
proper metabolism of calcium, and calcium is required for the prope
growth of bone. It is also wise to add vitamin C to the diet. It is usuall
found that if there is a deficiency of one vitamin, others are also lacking

It used to be the practice to keep the child lying in bed with splints applie
to correct the deformities. This is not usually done now, however, wit
children in the early stages, say up to the age of three. They are allowed t
run about, especially out of doors, and as long as they are getting th
appropriate diet the deformities in these early stages will correct themselves
if the muscles are allowed to develop with normal exercise.

If the treatment is delayed too long, corrective treatment is necessary
Gross deformities as a result of rickets are becoming much less common
but in maternity departments cases of contracted and flattened pelvis are
still seen, and Cæsarean section often has to be performed if the shape o
the pelvis is not such as to allow the passage of the fœtal head.

Infantile Scurvy. Infantile scurvy is due to a deficiency of Vitamin C
It is often seen in conjunction with early rickets at the age of six to twelve
months and it is described as scurvy-rickets. The signs of scurvy in ar
infant are:

1. Sweating. 2. Pyrexia, 101° to 102° F.
3. Extreme fretfulness, due to tenderness of the long bones.
4. The lack of vitamin C damages the cells of blood vessels and hæmorrhages commonly occur under the periosteum. A swelling may be felt and
the child screams when it is lifted out of its cot or if the limb is touched,
or even when the nurse approaches. Sub-periosteal hæmorrhages in infantile scurvy may be misdiagnosed for fractures. X-ray evidence, however,
is conclusive.

Treatment. The child is kept comfortably in his cot and is not taken out for bathing. He is sponged all over with the minimum of movement and handling. A bed cradle is required. A diet is given containing fresh milk and the addition of vitamin C, orange juice, tomato juice, etc. If these are not available, ascorbic acid is given. Vitamin D should be given to counteract the tendency to rickets.

Operation for Inguinal Hernia on a Baby. No skin preparation is required. The last feed is given three hours before the operation and glucose and water may be given up to half an hour before. An injection of atropine, grains 1/150 is ordered. The baby is sent to the theatre well wrapped up as already described.

Post-operative care. The baby is arranged in bed with two pillows with an abdominal binder weighted with sandbags over his body. The dressing should be protected with a piece of jaconet in which a hole is cut for the penis, which may be put into the glass barrel of a syringe, secured round the waist by strapping or a bandage. The glass barrel drains into a small urinal between the baby's legs and the napkin is laid under the buttocks. Drinks of water are given as soon as the child recovers consciousness and some sedative drug, such as chloral, will be required. Diluted feeds with glucose are given after four hours at regular intervals. The dressing need not be touched for five days, if it remains dry. The baby must be kept warm to avoid chest complications. The stitches are taken out on the seventh day.

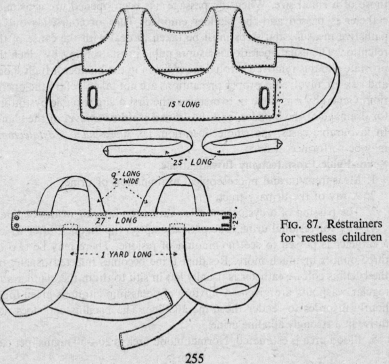

FIG. 87. Restrainers for restless children

Chapter Fifteen

THE NURSING OF GENITO-URINARY CASES

The anatomy of the male genito-urinary tract should be studied in connection with the nursing of these diseases. The conditions which call for the most detailed nursing care are those concerned with the prostate gland. This organ which is normally the size of a walnut, surrounds the neck of the bladder and the upper part of the urethra. In elderly men it often becomes enlarged and sometimes malignant. The outstanding symptom of an enlarged prostate is *acute retention*. The patient suffers great pain and distress through inability to pass urine.

Treatment. Hot fomentations over the bladder area, reapplied every few minutes, may help to relieve pain. The fomentations should be large pieces of flannel, wrung out in boiling water. If possible, the patient may sit in a hot bath. Tincture of hyoscyamus m.xl. is given in a mixture to relieve spasm. The urethral sphincter is dilated by bougies, beginning with those of a small size. When the passage has been opened up, a bicoudé catheter is passed and the bladder emptied. This, of course, is only a palliative measure and steps must be taken to deal with the cause of the retention. The usual operation is a supra pubic prostatectomy, by which the prostate gland is removed through an incision in the bladder. Much shock and risk are involved if proper precautions are not taken before the operation. Generally it is done in two stages, the first a supra-pubic cystotomy for drainage of the bladder, and the second for the removal of the gland. In favourable cases, the whole operation, i.e. *supra-pubic prostatectomy* may be performed at once.

Supra-Pubic Prostatectomy Investigations

1. Measurement and microscopical examination of urine.
2. X-ray of the urinary tract.
3. The passing of a cystoscope to examine the interior of the bladder.
4. Test for residual urine. The patient empties the bladder, after which a catheter is passed to see the amount of residue. There may be two or three ounces or much more. Residual urine becomes infected usually by the bacillus coli. A catheter is usually left in situ to drain the bladder and regular washouts are given. A mixture of potassium citrate is given four-hourly in order to render the urine alkaline. The bacillus coli does not thrive in a strongly alkaline urine.
5. Blood urea is estimated. Normal blood urea is 20—30 mgms. per c.c.

If it is higher than 40 mgms. the patient is considered unsuitable for operation until it has been reduced. This is done by giving the patient large quantities of fluid, at least six pints per day for some weeks if necessary.

6. Blood pressure is taken.

7. Urea concentration test is done. If the kidneys fail to concentrate 2 per cent of urea, they are not considered to be functioning properly. The estimation will not be accurate if there is residual urine in the bladder.

8. Chest examination.

9. Rectal examination is always done to ascertain the size and type of prostate.

10. The temperature, pulse, and respiration are recorded and the patient's temperament and mental condition assessed. The patient's age makes him apprehensive and fidgety and it is most important that he should be given confidence in the prospects of cure. In no case is it more important for the nurse to study the likes and dislikes of the patient or to make him feel that he can rely upon someone to look after him patiently in every detail. The thought of having to face such an operation is very distressing to an elderly man and most skilled and sympathetic treatment is required.

If the above investigations show that the patient's urinary tract is in a suitably healthy condition to stand a severe operation and if the patient himself is a suitable subject, the date of the operation is fixed.

Immediate preparation. The night before, the skin of the pubic area and abdomen is shaved and thoroughly washed; an enema saponis is given. The prepuce must be cleaned with eusol. The smegma bacilli thrive in the secretions round the urethral orifice, and are likely to cause irritation of the prepuce (balanitis) when catheters are left in the bladder. Fluids with glucose must be given freely all the time before operation. The patient is given a sleeping draught if required. No food should be given for five hours before the operation. The patient is prepared for the theatre in the usual way. Extra care must be taken to keep the patient warm, as the circulation of old people is not good. Long thick woollen stockings are always required. The dentures are removed.

If the operation is to be done under spinal anæsthesia, hyoscine gr. 1/100 and omnopon gr. ⅔ are given half an hour before the operation, and when the patient is drowsy, the eyes are bandaged. If a general anæsthetic is to be given atropine gr. 1/100 is given. The operation may be done under gas and oxygen after pentothal has been given intravenously; or stovaine may be given into the spinal canal. When the patient is anæsthetized a cystoscope is passed, and the bladder is washed out with a sterile saline or boracic lotion at a temperature of 100° F. Five ounces of lotion are left in the bladder to keep it distended. The surgeon then scrubs his hands again, changes his gloves and puts on a sterile gown. Fresh sterile towels

R

are arranged around the operation area and clipped in position. The table is tilted to the Trendelenburg position, so that the abdominal organs fall away from the pelvis. A vertical incision is made between the umbilicus and symphysis pubis, and the surgeon shells out the gland from the neck of the bladder with his right forefinger. Bleeding may be troublesome, and with special long suture holders, he ties off the bleeding vessels or plugs the prostatic bed with a gauze roll. Lighting must be perfect for this operation, as the surgeon is working deep down in the pelvis. The skin is sutured and a length of wide-bore rubber tubing with a large curved glass tube (Paul's) and a long piece of tubing attached, is fixed in before the dressing is put on. A catheter is often passed through the urethra into the bladder which is thus kept empty by two-way drainage. The catheter is spigotted, and the supra-pubic wound drains into a Winchester bottle at the side of the bed.

Post-operative care. The patient is put in a recumbent position, with one pillow at his head and if a spinal anæsthetic has been given 9-inch blocks to raise the foot of the bed are left in position for nine hours. After recovery from shock the patient may be raised into a semi-recumbent position with three or four pillows, an air ring, and a soft knee pillow. During the first twenty-four hours after operation hot blankets should be renewed frequently, and as soon as possible abundant fluids should be given.

Morphia gr. $\frac{1}{4}$ is given. The pulse should be recorded every fifteen minutes for at least twelve hours after the operation, and any marked increase during this time should be reported to the surgeon. Continuous bladder lavage is begun. Silver nitrate solution 1/15,000 at a temperature of 118° F. is used. It should be made up in distilled water; if made up with tap water, the silver is precipitated and causes irritation. A sterile tube is attached to the catheter and connected to a reservoir containing the lotion. The bladder is flushed through with the fluid at quarter-hourly intervals; a good deal of bright red blood and blood clot is washed out via the supra-pubic tube during the first few hours after the operation. As the bleeding decreases, the intervals between flushings increases and potassium permanganate 4 crystals to 1 quart of water or normal saline, is substituted for the silver nitrate. The temperature of the lotion is reduced gradually to 105° F. This method of bladder lavage is continued until all the hæmorrhage has quite ceased, usually for about three days. The supra-pubic drain is then removed and bladder lavage is continued t.d.s. by tube and funnel attached to the urethral catheter. In the interval between the washouts, the catheter drains into the Winchester bottle. Disinfectant should not be put into the bottle for the first twenty-four hours. The area of the penis around the catheter is dressed with a sponge soaked in glycerine and changed twice per day. The catheter is prevented from slipping out by affixing six narrow strips of tape on to the penis by means

f a circular band of strapping attached round the penis and the catheter.
During this time there is some leakage into the supra-pubic dressing
and the catheter is not removed until the dressing has been dry for at
least five days. The supra-pubic wound takes from sixteen to twenty-
nine days to heal in most cases, but it may be longer. While the urethral
catheter is in position, it need not be changed for ten days unless it
becomes blocked. Bladder washouts must be continued twice daily
whilst the catheter is in the bladder. All rubber tubing and glass connections are washed and boiled every day. When the urethral catheter is
finally removed, the patient is instructed to pass urine every hour for the
first twenty-four hours; every two hours for the second twenty-four hours
and after that time, every four hours. At least once a day for three days a
catheter is passed and the bladder emptied of residual urine, the amount
being measured each time; the patient is not considered fit for discharge
until the residual urine is less than 2 oz. If the vas on either side has been
ligatured, the small incisions should be dressed with powdered M. & B.
693. Through the whole course of the illness, the fluid intake must be
measured and it should not be less than 120 oz. in twenty-four hours. The
temperature should be taken every four hours, until it is normal. If it is
raised after forty-eight hours, a course of M. & B. 760 may be prescribed.
In addition to a very generous and appetizing diet, if the patient is used
to alcohol, a little may be given, and a bottle of stout or ale a day is often
ordered if the patient likes it.

The hygiene of the groins, scrotum and back needs special attention
when the patient is washed and at shorter intervals if the dressing is very
damp. It is usually best to keep the skin dry with powder, but sometimes
castor oil and zinc ointment helps to keep it waterproof if it becomes
irritated by the leakage of urine. The scrotum is supported by sandbags
or strapping to prevent infection of the testicle. Very often the vas deferens
on each side is ligatured to prevent infection reaching the testicles, but in
any case it is wise to give good support to the scrotum. When the bed is
made, care must be taken not to disarrange the tubes. Breathing exercises
should be given three times a day. An enema saponis is given on the third
morning before the supra-pubic tube is taken out. The bowels are kept
open by the judicious use of liquid paraffin or mild aperients. The post-
operative weeks are long and trying for the patient. It is very important that
the nurse should keep the patient in a hopeful and cheerful frame of mind,
encouraging and giving him confidence all the time. In this connection,
the importance of sleep is emphasized. In some cases a mild sedative is
required to ensure a really good night during the first week or two. Sedatives ordered may be: first night—morphia gr. $\frac{1}{4}$; second night—omnopon
gr. $\frac{1}{3}$; third night—nepenthe ℳ xxx s.o.s.

Mixtures containing acid sodium phosphate and hexamine are prescribed

THE NURSING OF GENITO-URINARY CASES

while the catheter is in the bladder, in order to reduce the risk of infection
Massage to legs may be started with advantage after five days. No surgical
patients need more persistent and skilful care than these. Visitors are
forbidden for the first few days, except the patient's wife who may visit
daily for about half an hour. After this time suitable friends are allowed
to visit, and the patient is encouraged to interest himself in every possible
way. The complications to be specially guarded against are: shock
hæmorrhage, uræmia and chest complications, but with thorough pre
liminary investigations and proper pre-operative care these can gener
ally be avoided. Although the operation is a serious one, in skilled hands
results are most satisfactory in spite of the age of the patient. For the first
few days the nurse should watch specially for the following symptoms
brown furred tongue, drowsiness, suppression of urine (signs of uræmia)

Nephrectomy is the removal of the kidney. It is generally performed for
unilateral tuberculosis, large calculi, hydronephrosis, or malignant growths

Preparation of patient. Thorough examination of the whole renal trac
must be done to make quite sure that the second kidney and bladder are
healthy and likely to be able to carry on their functions satisfactorily. The
investigations are almost the same as for supra-pubic prostatectomy but
include retrograde and intravenous pyelography and the examination of
specimens of urine from each kidney obtained by ureteric catheterization
Also in the case of tubercular kidney a guinea pig is injected with the urine
of the patient and the chest is X-rayed (see chapter on special tests).

The skin is prepared on the affected side from mid-line of the abdomen
to the spine behind. The patient is prepared as for an abdominal operation
An enema is given the night before.

The operation. The incision is made from behind. The muscles are
divided, the peritoneum pushed forward and the kidney is removed. By
approaching the kidney from behind, the peritoneal cavity is not entered
thus avoiding the risk of peritonitis. The wound is closed, probably with
Michel clips, and a corrugated rubber drain is inserted.

Post-operative care. The patient is nursed sitting up, but tilted over
towards the affected side. He must be very well supported with a pillow
in the back and a cleft is arranged so there is no pressure on the wound
A pillow is required between the knees. Deep breathing exercises are
given regularly after the first twenty-four hours in order to expand the
lungs fully and movement in bed is encouraged. The urine is measured
every twenty-four hours and the amount charted. The drain is not shortened
for forty-eight hours and then only if there is not an excessive amount of
drainage. Although it is ideal to remove the tube as soon as possible, this
must not be done until drainage has ceased. Fluids are given up to six pints
per day and a light generous diet. An enema is given on the third morning
after operation. An alkaline mixture containing potassium or sodium

citrate is given and all urine is measured. The dressing should be applied to the wound with firm strapping support to prevent incisional hernia. The toilet of the mouth must be attended to as in cases of prostatectomy. Symptoms of grave import are: brown furred tongue, drowsiness, and suppression of urine; all of which may indicate the onset of uræmia. Alternate clips are taken out on the fourth and sixth days, skin sutures on the eighth day, and deep tension stitches from the tenth to the twelfth day. The patient must stay in bed for at least three weeks and goes home after a four or five weeks' stay in hospital.

Nephrotomy is an opening into the kidney for the removal of calculi. The preparation and nursing is similar to that of a nephrectomy.

Operations on the bladder for: stones, papillomata. In all these cases thorough investigations of the renal tract are an important part of the preparation. An examination by a cystoscope diagnoses the condition and the procedure in the theatre is the same as in prostatectomy, i.e. (1) passing of a cystoscope; (2) bladder lavage; (3) the surgical treatment required in each case.

Stones are sometimes removed through a supra-pubic incision or are crushed. In the case of a small stone it is located by the use of a bladder sound. An instrument known as a lithotrite is then passed through the urethra. This is a crushing instrument between the blades of which the stone is gripped and crushed to small fragments. A catheter is fixed in the urethra and the grit is washed away by bladder lavage. A suction apparatus known as a bladder evacuator can be attached by means of tubing to the catheter. This empties the bladder more thoroughly.

Papillomata of the bladder are treated by diathermy.

Malignant growths in the early stages are excised by this method. In all cases after bladder operations the urinary output must be measured and at least 120 ounces of fluid given per day. Sedatives and alkaline mixtures are prescribed. A full diet may be given.

Phimosis or tightness of the prepuce. The operation for this condition is known as circumcision. An incision is made into the glans penis to loosen the prepuce. Several catgut sutures are inserted.

In the case of a child, a sterile vaseline gauze drain or gauze dipped in tincture of benzoin is wrapped round the penis. A large pad of wool is put to support the scrotum inside the napkin. This is most important if the child is to be kept comfortable. The incision should heal quickly if the child is kept clean and dry.

In the case of circumcision in the adult potassium bromide is given for two or three days before and for two or three days after the operation. The patient is not allowed to have visitors and is kept quiet in bed. A roll of gauze dressing is anchored in position round the end of the penis by being fastened by an extra knot in each catgut stitch. As the stitches absorb the dressing falls off. If the penis looks at all inflamed and sore the patient may sit in a warm bath of boracic lotion two or three times a day In case of hæmorrhage after adult circumcision, a piece of wool and a light piece of rubber tubing may be clipped round the penis to act as a tourni quet, until medical help can be obtained.

Plastic Operations. These are usually performed for the following con genital malformations:

Hypospadias in which the opening of the urethra is on the underside of the surface of the penis.

Epispadias in which the opening of the urethra is on the upper surface of the penis.

Ectopion vesicae in which the anterior wall of the bladder has failed to unite. These errors in development cause the patient to be incontinent of urine. Repair operations are done upon the child during the first year of its life.

The post-operative care involves keeping the dressing as dry as possible to encourage healing. This is not easy, as the bladder generally leaks all the time. The area becomes sodden and sepsis ensues. The child is fretful and ill and needs great care. The dressing is changed as frequently as required. The skin is treated with castor oil and zinc ointment or if this is too strong with lanoline. Scrupulous cleanliness and good feeding contri bute more than anything to recovery, and it is customary for the repair to be done in several stages at intervals. In some cases ureters are transplanted into the rectum.

Hydrocele. A collection of fluid in the tunica vaginalis, which is the serous covering of the testicles. It is treated by tapping.

Varicocele is a varicose condition of the vessels of the spermatic cord. After the operation for this condition the drain in the scrotum is shortened after twenty-four hours and removed after forty-eight hours. The scrotum needs firm support by a suspensory bandage of some kind. A firm T bandage serves the purpose well or a piece of elastoplast attached as a sling to the thighs. Salmon-gut stitches are removed on the seventh day and the patient is allowed to get up at the end of a week.

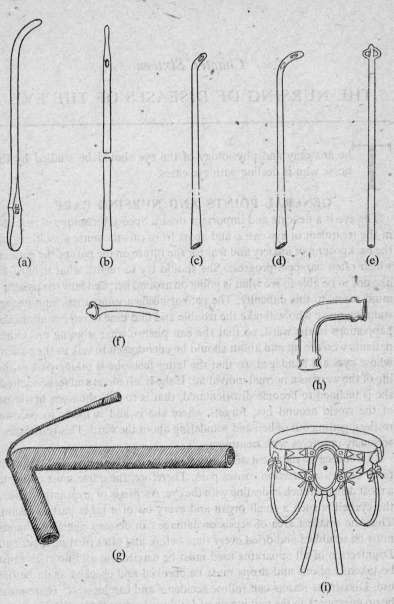

FIG. 88. (a) Bladder sound. (b) Olive-headed catheter. (c) Coudé catheter. (d) Bicoudé catheter. (e) Malecot's self-retaining catheter. (f) de Pezzer's self-retaining catheter. (g) Supra-pubic drainage tube with catheter attached for irrigation. (h) Glass supra-pubic drainage tube (Paul's). (i) Hamilton Irving's drainage apparatus with celluloid box

Chapter Sixteen

THE NURSING OF DISEASES OF THE EYE

The anatomy and physiology of the eye should be studied by the nurse who is dealing with eye cases.

GENERAL POINTS AND NURSING CARE

The eye is a delicate and important organ. Special technique is required in the treatment of eye cases, and apart from this the nurse should realize the background of anxiety and fear for the future on the part of the patient, which often hampers progress. She should try to realize what it must be like not to be able to see what is going on around her, and how the patient's mind reacts to this difficulty. The patient needs a sympathetic and understanding nurse who will take the trouble and find time to tell her about the happenings in the ward, so that she can picture what is going on. Other patients who are up and about should be encouraged to talk to the patient whose eyes are bandaged, so that the latter feels she is taking part in the life of the ward as a normal individual. If she is left alone and feels isolated, she is inclined to become disorientated, that is to say, she loses her sense of the world around her, forgets where she is and is likely to become restless, getting out of bed and wandering about the ward. This restlessness seriously interferes with treatment.

The cornea is the most sensitive structure in the body. The slightest piece of dirt or infection causes pain. Therefore, the nurse must cultivate a most delicate touch in dealing with the eye. Asepsis is of great importance; the eyeball is such a small organ and every bit of it takes part in vision. Thus the smallest area of sepsis or damage can destroy sight. The hands must be scrubbed and dried every time before and after treating a patient. Disinfection of all apparatus used must be carried out and no risks must be taken. Lotions and drops must be checked and checked again before use. Disastrous results can follow accidents and carelessness. There must be no guesswork in the making up of lotions or when testing the temperature. For dressings and bandages the lightest materials must be used. In many conditions, an eye shield is worn, either Buller's shield or one of the Cartella pattern. Eye pads are not used if there is much discharge. Headache results if these appliances are not expertly put on, with the minimum of pressure and weight.

EYE TREATMENTS

Bathing. The best simple method of bathing the eye is to cover the bowl of a wooden spoon with wool, fixing it firmly with cotton. The patient is given a bowl of very hot boracic lotion—equal parts of saturated solution of boracic and water. The patient then steams the eye by holding the bowl of the spoon near the lids. Thus it is possible to use the solution very hot, and it is not contaminated by the fingers. This is very useful treatment, often ordered for styes and other inflammatory conditions of the lids. The eyes may also be 'steamed' by opening and closing them over a bowl of very hot boracic lotion.

Compresses. Ice compresses are ordered after certain painful eye treatments; e.g. after the squeezing out of granulations under the lids in cases of trachoma and after the application of caustics to the conjunctiva. Woollen eye pads or swabs are squeezed in ice-cold water. The patient lies on her back and the compress is put on her lids, and changed very frequently.

Irrigation

Requirements
1. Mackintosh and towel.
2. Irrigating dish (shallow kidney pattern or triangular).
3. Jug of lotion.
4. Undine.
5. Lotion thermometer in distilled water or saline.
6. Dry wool or lint swabs, receiver.

Method. The patient sits up in a chair with the head well back; if in bed, the pillow is removed, the patient is moved down the bed and lies with the head as far as possible to the side of the bed, so that the nurse can stand well behind. The mackintosh and towel are tucked round her

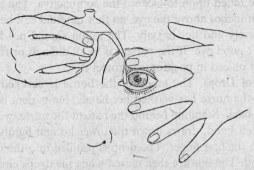

FIG. 89. Irrigation of the eye

265

neck, and the patient holds the dish, which she presses firmly against the cheek. The nurse scrubs her hands thoroughly, dries them on a clean towel and returns to the patient. The temperature of the lotion in the jug is tested, it should be 95° F. It is poured into the undine. The nurse then runs a little over the back of her hand to test the temperature again. The lower lid is pulled well down. The lotion is allowed to run over the cheek into the eye and the patient is asked to move the eyeball up, down, in and out, so that the fluid circulates in the conjunctival sac.

Irrigation Dish

When the irrigation is finished, the eye should be swabbed from within outwards, using one swab only once. The cheek is dried and the mackintosh and towel removed. If skilfully done, no fluid should have trickled down the neck, nor should the collar be wet.

In infected cases, five to ten ounces of lotion should be used for the irrigation. It is not possible to use lotions strong enough to kill germs

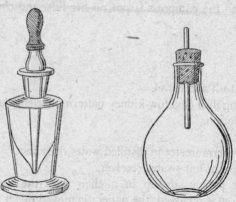

FIG. 90. Two types of drop bottle

without damaging the delicate structure of the eye; therefore the thoroughness with which the treatment is done, rather than the strength of the solutions, must be relied upon to cleanse the conjunctiva. The undine is held one and a half inches above the eye, so that the fluid can be directed into the sac accurately and not heavily. The lotion should not be allowed to splash into the good eye. If the patient is at all difficult or restless, an eye pad should be placed in position to protect it.

Instillation of Drops. The label on the bottle is checked by a second person. After the nurse has washed her hands, the patient is told to hold her head well back. Standing behind the patient the nurse, with the second finger of the left hand, draws down the lower lid and lightly controls the upper lid with the first finger. The drop is instilled into the outer canthus of the lower lid. The lids are then closed while the drops circulate around the conjunctival sac.

The Application of Ointment. An eye rod, sterilized by boiling, is used. After washing the hands, the nurse takes the ointment on one end of the rod, draws down the lower lid as for instillation of drops and places the rod on the inside of the lower lid. She asks the patient to close the eye, and gently withdraws the rod in an outward direction, thus smearing both lids with the ointment. If the second eye has to be treated similarly, the other end of the rod is used, so that infection is not carried from one eye to the other. The rod is washed and boiled immediately after treatment. If the right eye is to be treated, the nurse generally stands behind the patient; if the left eye, it is easier to stand in front of the patient.

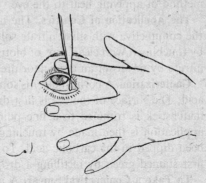

FIG. 91. Instillation of drops into the outer canthus

Eversion of the Lids. It is quite easy to treat the conjunctiva of the lower lid. The nurse, however, should practise eversion of the upper lid on one of her friends until she can do it neatly. This lid contains a rigid structure of cartilage called the *tarsus*. Standing behind the patient, a glass rod, or matchstick which has been trimmed and smoothed, is laid on the lid. Gripping the eyelashes with the thumb and first finger of the right hand, the eyelid is turned back over the rod. With practice it is quite easy to do this, without the help of either rod or stick, and the lid stays everted

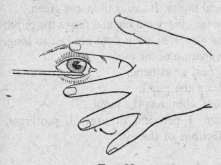

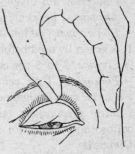

FIG. 92.
Application of ointment to the lids

FIG. 93.
Eversion of upper lid

for some length of time without much discomfort. This is not so easy to do if the lid is inflamed.

Application of an Electric Coil. Heat can conveniently be applied to the eye by means of an electric coil. It is bandaged in position over a woollen eye pad, and the current is gradually adjusted to a comfortable heat. The nurse should be at hand while this treatment is in progress, so that she can readjust the current if required. Hot fomentations are a very unsatisfactory method of applying heat to the eye.

The Application of Caustics. The nurse is sometimes required to paint the conjunctiva with silver nitrate solution. She first dries the conjunctiva by touching it with clean slips of blotting paper, and then applies the silver nitrate by means of an applicator dressed with wool.

Cauterization. A corneal ulcer is sometimes cauterized with pure carbolic acid. The surface of the eye is first dried with strips of blotting paper. A matchstick is trimmed to a fine point with a penknife and boiled. The application is then made by touching the ulcer with the point which has been dipped in the carbolic acid. To identify the spot, the ulcer may be first stained green by instilling a drop of fluorescine into the eye.

To Take a Conjunctival Smear. A platinum loop is used. It is sterilized by holding it in a spirit lamp until it is red hot. When it is cool, it is smeared along the inner surface of the lower lid, as the lid is drawn down. The loop is then immediately smeared on the surface of the culture medium. This is usually gelatine broth in a petrie dish.

Lotions used for irrigation

1. Boracic lotion, equal parts of saturated solution and boiled water.
2. Normal saline.
3. Perchloride of mercury, 1 in 10,000 to 1 in 12,000.
4. Oxycyanide of mercury, 1 in 10,000 to 1 in 12,000. (Less irritating than the perchloride, but it must be made up fresh.)

Eye drops

Zinc sulphate, 1 grain to the ounce, for inflammatory conditions.

Fluorescine for diagnosing corneal ulcers. It stains the ulcer green.

Atropine, 1 per cent, to paralyse the ciliary muscle and dilate the pupil.

Homatropine, action the same as atropine, but it does not last so long. It is generally used before an examination of the eye.

Cocaine, 2 to 5 per cent, as a local anæsthetic.

Pilocarpine, 1 per cent, to contract the pupil.

Eserine (physostigmine) $\frac{1}{2}$ per cent, contracts the pupil.

Silver preparations (silver nitrate, 1 per cent or argyrol, protargol, collosol argentum), for severe infections of the eye.

Ointments

Golden ointment (ung. hydrarg ox. flav. 1%).

Atropine ointment $\frac{1}{2}$—1%, a convenient way of instilling atropine into the eyes of young children and infants.

All lotions used for eye treatments are made up in distilled water with full aseptic precautions. When carrying out eye treatments, the nurse's hands must be scrupulously clean, and after operation or where there is an open wound, strict surgical technique is required.

Requirements for examination of the eye
1. Ophthalmoscope.
2. Mydriatics, atropine 1 per cent, homatropine.
3. Letter cards.

THE NURSING OF SOME EYE CASES

Conjunctivitis. (a) *Simple.* There is mild inflammation of the conjunctiva which may be due to irritation by grit or dirt or sun. It may also be caused by a variety of organisms, staphylococci, Koch Weeks bacillus, Morax Axenfeld, etc.

The symptoms are: (1) A watery and blood-shot eye. (2) Smarting pain. (3) Photophobia. (4) A feeling of grittiness.

Treatment. If caused by an infection, care must be taken to keep all utensils, mackintoshes, towels, etc., separate. These mild infections can spread rapidly, if proper care is not taken. The eye is usually irrigated with boracic lotion or normal saline. Zinc sulphate drops may be instilled, and a perforated eye

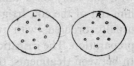

FIG. 94.
Cartella eye shields made of perforated cardboard

FIG. 95.
Buller's adhesive eye shield with glass centre

shield is used to protect the eye from light. The patient must be warned against rubbing the eye. If a child, the arms should be splinted. The sound eye can become infected by carrying the discharge from one to the other, therefore great care must be taken.

(b) *Purulent conjunctivitis.* This is a much more serious condition caused by streptococcal or gonococcal infection. The gonococcal type is seen in new-born babies whose eyes have been contaminated during their passage through the vagina by gonococcal discharge (ophthalmia neonatorum). Ophthalmia neonatorum, however, is by no means always caused by the gonococcus. The official definition of the disease is 'any inflammation occurring in the eyes of a baby within the first twenty-one days of birth'.

Ophthalmia Neonatorum. Symptoms appear on the second or third day after birth. The affected eye or eyes are sticky and when the baby wakes from sleep the eyelids are stuck together. The lids are swollen and inflamed and before long pus wells out between them. It becomes difficult to separate the lids.

Treatment. Medical advice must be sought at once, at the first sign of a sticky eye. The case must be notified on the appropriate form to the Medical Officer of Health of the district. Full barrier precautions are instituted as the discharge is highly infectious. If only one eye is affected, the baby is nursed on the side of the bad eye, being put in its cot very carefully so that although it is turned on to its side, it cannot roll over on to the face. The arms are not put in the sleeves of the gown, thus preventing the child from putting its hands to its face. The good eye may have a pad and bandage applied to prevent it becoming infected. The bad eye is not covered up. The pillow should be covered with a jaconet case and pieces of old linen should be laid under the baby's head, to catch discharge. These pieces should be burnt at once when soiled. The eyes are treated every two hours or more often, and the services of a special nurse are required. If she is single-handed, she can roll the child up in a blanket and mackintosh and hold him between her knees while she irrigates the eye over a pan. If she has someone to hold the child, she can carry out treatments with the baby on a table. It is not practicable to do it without taking him out of the cot. Irrigation with perchloride of mercury, 1 in 12,000 is usually ordered, with twice daily instillation of drops of some silver preparation. The irrigation must be very thorough, to wash away the pus. In between treatments, the discharge should be wiped away with a damp swab as soon as it appears. Once a day the cornea should be examined for signs of ulceration. The doctor may do this on his daily visit, but if not, the nurse must do so.

Some authorities recommend painting the conjunctiva once a day with silver nitrate. Eye rectractors are used to expose the under surface of the lids, and it is said that the results from this less frequent but more drastic treatment are very much better. The severity of the conjunctivitis can be gauged by the amount of swelling of the lids and if they are very swollen it is almost impossible to separate them sufficiently to irrigate thoroughly.

It is important that breast feeding should be continued during treatment for ophthalmia neonatorum. The few hospitals which specialize in the treatment of this disease have accommodation for lying-in mothers.

Owing to the more thorough examination of women at ante-natal clinics, and because preventive measures are taken at birth, cases of ophthalmia neonatorum in this country are few and far between. The preventive measures at birth consist in swabbing the eyelids with perchloride of mercury before the eyes are opened, and the instillation of silver nitrate drops, 1 per cent. For the first fortnight, the face of the baby is washed with wool swabs and water in a separate bowl, so that the eyes are not contaminated by the bath water. There should be a separate towel for drying the face.

Ophthalmia neonatorum is the commonest cause of blindness in children. If it is not dealt with quickly and thoroughly, the cornea ulcerates, and pus penetrates into the anterior chamber, causing irreparable damage to the internal structures of the eyeball.

Cataract. Cataract is an opacity of the crystalline lens. The four commonest types are:

THE NURSING OF SOME EYE CASES

1. Senile.
2. Diabetic.
3. Traumatic.
4. Congenital.

The opacity may start in the middle of the lens and spread outwards, or it may begin on the circumference and spread inwards. The senile and diabetic cataracts develop slowly and when the cataract is 'ripe' and hard, the treatment is extraction of the lens.

Preparation for operation. The patient is generally an old subject between the ages of seventy and eighty years. The routine before and after operation must be clearly and carefully explained to him in every detail, as the operation cannot be a success without the full co-operation of the patient. The following points are included in the preparation:

1. Examination of the chest by the house surgeon. The operation is postponed if the patient has a cold or cough, as violent movements of the head and chest, as in coughing and sneezing, are very damaging to the eye after operation.

2. The patient should have time to become well acquainted with his day and night nurses, and to become familiar with the other people coming and going in the ward. He should feel a friendly and comfortable atmosphere, and should be able to recognize the different voices and footsteps, so that he is not likely to be startled or worried by unaccustomed sounds. Anything which startles the patient suddenly when his eyes are bound up makes him flinch and screw up his eyes and this squeezing action of the muscles can do a good deal of harm.

3. The patient must become accustomed to the use of the bedpan before the operation. There must be no argument about getting in and out of bed afterwards. The difficulty must be overcome beforehand.

4. A mild sedative such as potassium bromide is given twice daily.

5. A mild aperient is also given beforehand regularly to ensure a daily normal action of the bowels, without strain.

6. The eyes are irrigated daily with saline, to accustom the patient to the procedure.

7. A conjunctival swab is taken to make sure that no infection is present which will complicate recovery.

Preparation on the day of operation. The patient has an ordinary breakfast. If the operation is at 2 p.m. he has fish, potato, and milk pudding for early dinner. If the surgeon wishes, the lashes are cut; the nurse smears the blades of a pair of sharp scissors with vaseline and carefully trims them. The instillation of cocaine drops, 4 per cent, into both eyes is begun twenty minutes before the patient goes to the theatre. They are instilled at 1.45, 1.50 and 1.55 p.m. and again by the surgeon before he begins the operation.

THE NURSING OF DISEASES OF THE EYE

In the theatre. The patient is put flat on the table and his head is bound up in a sterile towel. When he is ready, the surgeon separates the lids with retractors and irrigates the conjunctival sac with sterile normal saline. The operation is very quickly done, taking only two or three minutes. A curved incision is made in the upper circumference of the cornea and a small one into the iris. The lens is then delivered by pressing it out from below, and the structures are smoothed back into place by an iris repositor; no sutures are required. The lids are carefully shut, some surgeons put in a stitch to keep them closed. Pads and a double eye bandage, sterile, are applied. Special cambric eye bandages, tied with tapes are an advantage, in order to avoid moving the patient's head when treatments are carried out. The surgeon, before he begins the operation, reassures the patient and gains his co-operation. It is, of course, essential that he should keep absolutely still for this short, but delicate operation. The results are usually very good.

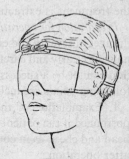

Fig. 96.
Moorfields eye bandage

When the patient is lifted on to the stretcher to be conveyed back to bed, it must be one nurse's special care to hold the head still. The lifting must be carefully done and the trolley wheeled slowly back to the ward.

Post-operative Care. A great deal of this has been suggested in the treatment preparatory to operation. As no sutures have been put in the cornea or iris, complete rest for the eye is essential for the first few days. Any squeezing movement may cause *prolapse of the iris* before it is healed. The patient lies on his back with two or three pillows, the number does not matter very much, as long as the patient is comfortable and quiet. He should not turn on his side. Bromide mixtures are continued, also liquid paraffin or whatever aperient the patient has been having. The diet consists of soft foods which require no chewing movement, e.g. milk, jelly, soups, bread and milk, fish, mashed potatoes, stewed fruits, custards, milk puddings, crustless bread and butter, soft boiled eggs, etc. If the patient becomes restless and mentally confused, the nurse must realize that it is only because he has lost the sense of his surroundings. If he cannot be reassured and quietened, it is best to uncover the good eye, and if at night, to put a shaded light on the bed table, so that the patient is allowed to see for a time where he is. This usually calms him and he will settle down again.

If, in spite of the pre-operative preparations, the patient refuses the bedpan afterwards, it is sometimes safer to allow him to get up and sit on a chair or commode, rather than have him upset and resisting the nurse's efforts.

When she goes to the bed to attend to the patient, if he appears to be asleep, the nurse should speak quietly to him, and if necessary, wake him by taking hold of his hand. This is the best way to avoid startling him.

If nursing a private patient in a separate room, the nurse should not tread too noiselessly, so that the patient may have warning of her approach.

The local treatment is usually somewhat as follows: all treatments are done with aseptic precautions.

First day after operation. Irrigation over the lids with normal saline. Instillation of atropine drops, 1 per cent into the affected eye.

Second day. The patient may open his own lids while the irrigation is being done. Atropine drops repeated.

Third day. The nurse draws down the lower lid and irrigates more thoroughly.

The local treatment is continued for about five days.

The good eye is uncovered on the second or third day; the patient gets up, and the other eye is uncovered, on the seventh to tenth day. He goes home wearing dark glasses on the tenth to fourteenth day. He sees the surgeon after an interval of six to eight weeks and bi-convex glasses are prescribed. Until the patient has spectacles he can only distinguish light from dark.

The two complications to be feared are:

1. Prolapse of the iris, against which all precautions have been taken.

2. Sepsis. All treatments are done with full aseptic precautions after the operation.

Congenital cataract in babies is treated by needling. The child's eye is anæsthetized by cocaine drops and a little general anæsthetic is also given. The capsule of the lens is torn with a needle, to allow the opaque, milky fluid to escape. In young babies this is replaced by a clear lymphoid substance, and, if the operation is done several times at intervals, the lens may clear and develop normally. It is only necessary to keep the child in hospital twenty-four to forty-eight hours.

Glaucoma. Glaucoma is an increase in intra-ocular tension, usually due to eye strain in elderly people. In acute cases, the patients suffer very violent headache and vomiting and coloured haloes may be seen round lights. Eserine drops are instilled to contract the pupil and to open up the ducts from the canals of Schlemn from which drainage of the aqueous fluid normally takes place. A trephining operation is sometimes done, a hole being made at the margin of the cornea to allow fluid to escape. Iridectomy may also be performed. Pre-operative treatment and nursing care of the cataract case is applied in a modified form, according to the type of operation which has been done. Leeches may be applied to relieve pain and congestion.

Strabismus or Squint. Strabismus or squint is due to unequal action of the extrinsic muscles which move the eyeball. In young children orthoptic exercises are taught to strengthen the weak muscle and thus correct the squint. The child may have the good eye bandaged so that he is obliged to use the weaker one. If this treatment is not successful, the tendon of the muscles affected may be cut and the eyeball 'advanced'.

Pre-operative and post-operative care is again similar to that of a cataract operation.

Corneal Ulcers. These may be caused by foreign bodies penetrating the eyeball abrading the cornea. They are also seen in elderly and debilitated people and they are sometimes of syphilitic origin. The treatment is rest in bed, the application of heat by electric coils, irrigation with normal saline, instillation of atropine drops and cauterization of the ulcer with pure carbolic. The eye is kept covered. The ulcer is seen as a white spot on the cornea and can be shown up green by staining with fluorescine.

Iritis. The iris becomes muddy and loses its clear colour. It is usually accompanied with some degree of conjunctivitis, the conjunctiva being injected or bloodshot in a radiating fashion. The disease is due to a blood stream infection from a septic focus or syphilis. The treatment is rest in bed, heat, warm irrigations and atropine drops. It is most important that the pupil should be kept dilated so that inflammatory adhesions do not form between the iris and the cornea. The eye is kept covered.

Sty (hordeolum). A sty is a staphylococcal infection of a lash follicle. It appears as a small boil at the root of an eyelash. The treatment is by steaming the eye and the application of golden ointment to the lids to prevent other follicles becoming infected. If the lash falls out, pus discharges, but epilation should not be done.

Perforation of the Eyeball by Foreign Bodies. Many war injuries are complicated by perforated wounds of the eye. An electro-magnet may be used for the removal of pieces of metal. A serious danger which the surgeon has to consider is sympathetic ophthalmia of the good eye. The injured eye is called the 'exciting eye' and the other the 'sympathetic eye'. The surgeon has a difficult decision to make, as to whether he must remove the 'exciting' eye before it can affect the other, or whether there is a possibility of saving it. If he leaves the decision too long, both may be lost.

THE EYE THEATRE

The aseptic rather than the antiseptic method is used, because antiseptics strong enough to kill organisms would also damage the delicate tissues of the eye. All instruments, including sharp ones, are boiled for three minutes. They are fixed into metal racks placed in a sterilizer containing soda bicarbonate, to prevent blunting. The surgeon tests each sharp instrument before he decides to use it, on a small drum, covered with thin white kid. The point of the knife should cut it by its own weight, as it is gently dropped

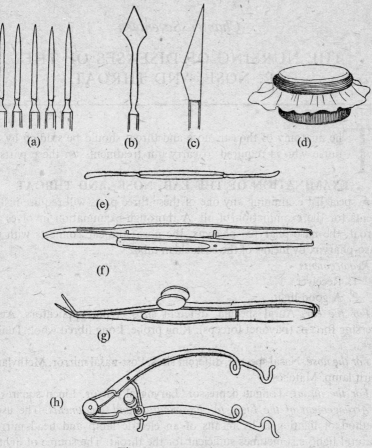

Fig. 97. Eye Instruments

(a) Graefe's knife.
(b) Keratome or iridectomy knife.
(c) Beer's cataract knife.
(d) Kid drum for testing sharp instruments.

(e) Iris repositor.
(f) Iris forceps.
(g) de Wecker's iris scissors.
(h) Eye retractor.

on the taut kid surface. The instruments are dished up on small trays covered with small sterile towels. They are kept covered until the moment the surgeon is ready to use them. Drops are prepared in sterilized form at the dispensary or by the manufacturers. Lotions are made with distilled water. Undines are put in cold water and brought to the boil. Pipettes are boiled in the same way. The surgeon scrubs his hands thoroughly with soap and water for several minutes and rinses them in disinfectant and then under running distilled water. He dries them on a sterile towel and does not wear gloves.

Chapter Seventeen

THE NURSING OF DISEASES OF THE EAR, NOSE, AND THROAT

The anatomy of the ear, nose and throat should be studied by the nurse who is required to carry out treatments on these parts.

EXAMINATION OF THE EAR, NOSE, AND THROAT

A specialist examining any one of these three parts will require instruments for the examination of all. A thorough examination involves the throat, the naso-pharynx, pharynx, the nose; the ear connects with the naso-pharynx by means of the eustachian tube.

Requirements
1. Receiver.
2. A good light.

For the ear. Aural specula, different sizes. Wool applicators. Aural dressing forceps (bayonet forceps). Ring probe. Long fibred wool. Tuning fork.

For the nose. Nasal specula, different sizes. Post-nasal mirror. Methylated spirit lamp. Matches.

For the throat. Tongue depressor. Laryngeal mirror. Linen squares.

Arrangement of the Light for Examination and Treatments. The usual method of lighting is by means of an electric lamp and head mirror. Natural light is sometimes sufficient for the throat. The source of light is put behind the patient's head; the head mirror is fastened to the forehead of the doctor or nurse and adjusted so that the light is directed on to the mirror and reflected into the ear or throat. For examination of the ear, an auroscope is often used. This is an instrument which has a small electric light attached to the aural speculum. For use in operations, the surgeon wears an electric lamp fixed to a band on his forehead. The flex of the lamp goes behind the head to a battery on his back, or electric current may be taken from the main supply, through a resistance box, which cuts down its strength to the requirements of the bulb.

NURSING TREATMENTS

Mopping an Ear. The amount and character of the discharge should be noted. From a meatal boil the pus may be thick, and in small quantity. From the middle ear it is usually thinner, copious and may be bloodstained

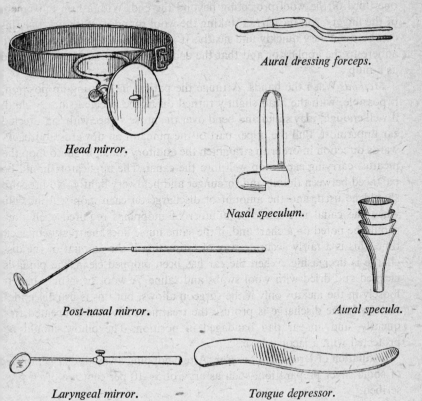

Aural dressing forceps.

Head mirror.

Nasal speculum.

Post-nasal mirror.

Aural specula.

Laryngeal mirror.

Tongue depressor.

FIG. 98. Instruments used for examination of the ear, nose, and throat

or mixed with mucus. If the skull is fractured in this region, cerebrospinal fluid and blood may escape in a watery discharge. Chronic aural discharges are usually offensive and this fact should be reported.

Requirements

1. Mackintosh and receiver.
2. A good light.
3. Number of wool applicators.
4. Sterile normal saline.
5. Gallipot.
6. Wool swabs.
7. Drops if ordered (standing in warm water).
8. Pipette.

FIG. 99. Wooden applicator dressed with wool for mopping the ear

To prepare the applicator, take between the first finger and thumb of the left hand a finely shredded piece of long fibred wool (a special variety can be obtained for this purpose), about one inch square. Take the stick (or metal wool carrier) in the right hand and lay the end of it on the wool, leaving one-third of the wool projecting beyond the end. With a firm movement of the fingers, roll the carrier, taking the wool round it. With practice this can be done very quickly and neatly. It is essential that the wool should adhere to the applicator and that the end of it should be free, to be used as a mop.

Method. Wash the hands. Arrange the patient in a sitting-up position, if possible, with the head slightly turned on to the affected side. A child, if well enough, may stand and bend over the nurse's knee with the affected ear uppermost. Pull the upper part of the pinna in an upwards and backwards direction in order to straighten the auditory canal, begin to mop the meatus, carrying each mop well into the canal. The applicator should be balanced between thumb and forefinger and held very lightly. No pressure should be used, and the amount of discharge on each mop will indicate when the canal is clean. The number of moppings required each time should be noted on a chart and, if the same nurse does the treatment each time, this is a fairly accurate way of estimating if the amount of the discharge is decreasing. When the ear has been mopped clean, the pinna is cleaned and dried with wool swabs and saline. A wool swab may be left loosely in the meatus only if the surgeon allows, but this is usually undesirable. If the discharge is profuse the treatment should be repeated frequently, and an ear pad bandaged in position. The pillow should be protected with a jaconet case.

Instillation of Drops into the Ear. After mopping away discharge, drops of some silver preparation, such as argyrol 5—10 per cent are often prescribed.

A pipette should be boiled and the bottle containing the drops stood in warm water. The head is turned to the opposite side while two or three drops are instilled: the head should be maintained in this position for a minute or two.

Other drops ordered are peroxide of hydrogen, ten volumes, or olive oil, to soften wax before syringing. A mixture of carbolic lotion and glycerine is used in cases of earache and meatal boils. Aluminium acetate on a gauze wick is good treatment for boils. Two or three drops are put on the end of the wick four-hourly and the wick is changed every twenty-four hours. Gentian violet 1 per cent solution, or ung. hydrarg. ox. flav. may be smeared on the pinna if it becomes sore.

Syringing an Ear. This treatment is only done if ordered by a doctor. It is usually prescribed to remove wax and is seldom or never ordered for a discharging ear. A doctor may syringe an ear in order to remove a foreign body.

Requirements
1. Mackintosh and receiver.
2. A good light.

3. Bowl.
4. Aural syringe.
5. A pint of lotion, normal saline or soda bicarbonate, Ʒi to water Oi, lotion thermometer.
6. Wool swabs.
7. Towel.

Method. Sit the patient up, arrange the mackintosh and towel round the shoulders, tucking them well in over the clothing. Ask the patient to hold the bowl—a kidney-shaped dish is good for this purpose. Draw the lotion, temperature 100° F., into

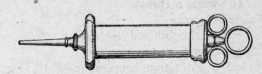

FIG. 100. Aural syringe

the syringe several times till the syringe is warm. With the left hand draw the pinna in an upward and backward direction and direct the point of the nozzle to the posterior wall of the meatus. The fluid will then circulate up to, and in front of, the drum, and return and be able to escape. In a case of wax, the lotion thus gets behind the concretion and will dislodge and sweep it out. When syringing an ear for the first time, the nurse should be shown exactly how to hold the syringe. It is important that the temperature of the solution should be tested. If it is not at blood heat, the patient may feel giddy owing to disturbance in the semicircular canals. Dry the meatus carefully after treatment.

Application of Heat. For earache and meatal boils, a rubber hot water bottle with a cover gives comfort and relief. An electric pad may be covered with a piece of lint or wool and bandaged in position and applied four-hourly, for ten to twenty minutes. Fomentations are not very satisfactory, as they do not hold the heat long enough, but if no electric pad is available a fomentation and a hot water bottle is a good method of applying heat.

Nasal Douche. A patient can give herself a nasal douche of warm normal saline by sniffing it up the nostrils from a bowl and the fluid will run out of the mouth. This is quite a good method of cleansing and clearing the nose.

Douching may be done with a syphon douche or a Higginson's syringe.

Requirements
1. Mackintosh and receiver.
2. Towel.
3. Syphon douche apparatus or Higginson's syringe with a nasal bulb.
4. Jug of saline solution or soda bicarbonate Ʒi to water Oi, temperature 99° F.

Method. Drape the mackintosh in front of the patient and cover it with the towel, tucking both well in round the neck. Sit the patient up and give her a large bowl to hold. Fill the douche or syringe and test it to exclude air. Tell the patient to hold the head downwards over the bowl keeping the mouth open and panting as she breathes. Put the bulb of the douche into one nostril and start the flow of lotion; if using the Higginson's syringe, use as little force as possible. The fluid returns through the other nostril and mouth.

To Syringe a Throat

Requirements

1. Mackintosh and receiver.
2. Towel.
3. Jug of lotion, temperature 99° F., lotion thermometer.
4. Higginson's syringe with a long-pointed nozzle.

Method. Sit the patient up, placing the mackintosh and towel in position. She holds the bowl and is asked to hold her head over it with her mouth wide open. The flow of fluid, generally normal saline, is directed on to the tonsil bed. Some surgeons order this to be done to remove sloughs after tonsillectomy.

To Paint a Throat

Requirements

1. Mackintosh.
2. A good light.
3. Receiver.
4. Tongue depressor.
5. Painting solution and gallipot.
6. Camel hair brush.

Method. Sit the patient up with the head well back, a good light is essential. Dip the brush in the solution and when quite ready to apply it depress the tongue with the spatula held in the left hand, and quickly paint one tonsil. With a fresh supply of paint treat the other tonsil in the same way. Mandl's paint (iodine $1\frac{1}{4}$ per cent with glycerine, potassium iodide and oil of peppermint) is generally used.

To Take a Throat Swab.
This should be done before the throat receives any treatment. Early morning is the best time.

Requirements

1. Culture outfit, consisting of a sterile swab stick dressed with wool in a small tube; a second sterile tube containing culture broth.
2. Throat spatula, matches, a good light.

Method. The patient's head should be held well back. Remove the wool plug from the tube with the little finger of the right hand. Withdraw the swab stick, holding it with the thumb and forefinger. Replace the wool plug and put the tube down. Depress the tongue with the spatula held in the left hand, and smear the areas of both tonsils with the dressed end of

he stick, taking care not to touch the tongue or cheeks. Smear the swab
over the surface of the gelatine slope and replace the swab stick in its own
ube, being careful not to touch the sides of the tubes in either case. Flame
he wool plugs with a match and replace firmly in the tubes. Send at once
o the laboratory with the form which will have been filled in beforehand.
The swab may be sent to the laboratory without being planted on a culture
medium when it is certain that it will reach the laboratory within a few
hours.

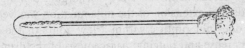

Fig. 101. Sterile throat swab stick

THE NURSING OF SOME DISEASES OF THE EAR

1. **Meatal Boils.** These are very painful though they do not involve
essential internal structures. The patient complains of severe earache which
should be investigated by a doctor in all cases.

Treatment. The treatment is to keep the patient warm in bed and to
apply heat to the ear by means of an electric coil or by fomentations and a
hot water bottle or short wave diathermy. Drops of warm glycerine and
carbolic or aluminium acetate 10 per cent are instilled, and aspirin or
veganin tablets are prescribed to relieve pain until the boil comes to a head
and discharges.

Otitis Media. Otitis media is inflammation of the middle ear. This tiny
cavity in the temporal bone is lined with mucous membrane continuous
with the lining of the eustachian tube, which leads from the naso-pharynx.
Hence any infection extending from the nose or throat via the tube may
cause otitis media. It is a common complication of the common cold,
influenza, measles, and scarlet fever.

Symptoms. In the acute stage, earache, rise in temperature, and in all
cases, some degree of deafness.

Nursing Treatment. Earache is always serious, and the ear should be
examined by a doctor. The tympanic membrane is seen to be inflamed and
bulging, owing to the pressure in the middle ear. As soon as tension causes
rupture of the drum and discharge begins, the pain is relieved. The patient
must be kept in bed and heat is applied and drops of warm carbolic and
glycerine or argyrol 10 per cent are instilled. The temperature, pulse, and
respiration are recorded four hourly and the patient given plenty of fluids.
Aspirin or veganin tablets are prescribed for the relief of pain. When the
ear begins to discharge, ear moppings are begun, and drops, as ordered, are
instilled. The lobe of the ear must be kept clean and the discharge wiped
away frequently. It is a good plan to put a little yellow oxide of mercury

ointment (ung. H.O.F.) on the skin if the discharge is irritating. The patient rests in bed in the semi-recumbent position, inclined towards the affected side.

To encourage drainage from the middle ear, through the eustachian tube, some surgeons like the patient to chew and use the throat muscles thoroughly. The act of swallowing is a movement of the muscles of the pharynx, and this opens the eustachian tubes.

The use of the sulphonamide drugs clears up many cases of otitis media in a few days, whereas in the past the discharging condition might take weeks to subside and extension of the inflammation was very common.

If the drum does not rupture within a few hours of the onset of pain and if it appears tense and bulging, paracentesis of the drum is performed (myringotomy). Under a general anæsthetic, a curved incision through the drum is made with a myringotome to allow the pus to escape.

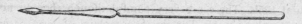

FIG. 102. Myringotome

Requirements for myringotomy
1. Mackintosh and receiver.
2. Good light—electric auroscope or head mirror.
3. Aural specula.
4. Lifting forceps.
5. Sterile towel.
6. Sterile applicators with sterile long-fibred wool.
7. Sterile aural dressing forceps, myringotome, pipette.
8. Ear drops standing in warm water (e.g. glycerine and carbolic).
9. Ear pad and bandage.

This small operation is often performed in the ward. The ear is thoroughly cleaned by mopping, and the patient is given a short anæsthetic such as pentothal or ethylchloride. The mackintosh and sterile towel are arranged in position, after which the incision is made. The ear is mopped, the drops instilled and the pad and bandage are applied. The patient is encouraged to lie on the affected side.

In satisfactory cases the incision usually heals within a few days, and the hearing is not affected, but in others the discharge may continue and the infection is likely to spread to other parts of the ear. To understand the complications to which otitis media may lead, it is necessary to understand the anatomical relations of the middle ear. For the purpose of simplicity, the cavity can be likened to a box with six sides.

The cavity is bounded by:
1. The tympanic membrane, externally.

2. The internal ear internally.
3. The meninges and brain above.
4. The lateral sinus below and behind.
5. The aditus and mastoid antrum behind.
6. The facial nerve, in close relationship with the medial wall.

The cavity is lined with mucous membrane which continues into the aditus and antrum, and into the hollow cells of the mastoid process. Therefore the commonest complication is mastoiditis, and the other complications may follow from this.

Mastoiditis

Symptoms

1. Continuing purulent discharge from the middle ear.
2. Rise in temperature, pulse, and respiration.
3. Tenderness over the mastoid process behind the ear.
4. Projection of the pinna forward (often very marked in young children), due to œdema of the soft tissues behind the ear.
5. Headache and malaise.
6. Sickness.

In cases where the discharge has been present for weeks or months, there may be no rise in temperature, very little swelling, and the pain may not be acute.

Treatment. The treatment of mastoiditis is operative. Several operations are performed of which three may be mentioned :

1. *The Schwartz operation* in acute cases. The incision is made over the mastoid process, and all the infected cellular bone is removed. The cavity thus produced is drained.

2. *Radical mastoidectomy* in chronic cases where the bone disease is involving the middle ear. Again the incision is behind the ear, and any infected bone in the mastoid process is removed. The aditus is opened, and the whole excavation made continuous with the meatus and middle ear, by the removal of the posterior wall of the meatus. The ossicles, usually diseased, are removed. Hearing is impaired by this operation. The post-aural incision is sewn up, and a packing, often of rubber, is left in the bony cavity, the end of the packing protruding from the meatus.

3. *Conservative operations*. These are various. The aim of the surgeon is to remove the structures which are infected, but he tries to avoid the radical operation by conserving as much as possible of the parts which are essential for hearing.

Preparation for Operation.

In addition to the usual preparation for the theatre, as described in the chapter on surgical nursing, the preparation of the operation area must be very carefully done. The area of the scalp surrounding the ear is shaved, the size depending upon the wishes of the individual surgeon, but it is usually about two inches square round the ear. The shave must be very close, no stray hairs must be left, as hair is always heavily infected with organisms. The remaining hair must be brushed well over to the other side of the head and secured by plaiting or ribbon or bandage. In cases of short hair, it is sometimes necessary to make several small plaits to keep the hair out of the way. The pinna and meatus are thoroughly cleaned by mopping every crevice and corner with hydrogen peroxide, or saline. It is then dried and again mopped with methylated spirit. The skin behind the ear after shaving is cleaned with saline and a sterile 'compress' applied. Some surgeons prescribe a wet compress of saline or soda bicarbonate solution, but others prefer the 'compress' of methylated spirit. Some surgeons only require the area to be cleaned and shaved.

Post-Operative Care. The patient is put to bed turned on to the unaffected side, until she is sufficiently recovered from the anæsthetic. This is to avoid vomit contaminating the dressing. Within a very short time, however, she is given one or two pillows, and turned on to the affected side to secure good drainage. The pulse is taken frequently and the patient is given copious fluids up to six pints daily.

For the first few days she should be kept very quiet. Sedative drugs are given for the relief of pain. The dressing is not touched as a rule for twenty-four to forty-eight hours, according to whether the simple or radical operation was done. The surgeon may do the first dressing himself, or he may instruct the sister to do it. Special packets of sterilized dressings are prepared for ear cases. Each one contains a wool ear pad, wool swabs, small gauze sponges, and dressed wool applicators. These are wrapped and sterilized in a square of linen or lint. When doing the dressing, the nurse

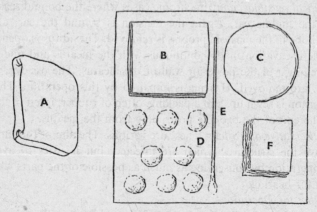

Fig. 103. Aural dressing packet

(a) Contents wrapped in square of lint.
(b) Gauze sponges.
(c) Wool ear pad.
(d) Wool swabs.
(e) Dressed wool applicator.
(f) Long-fibred wool.

hould note particularly the amount of discharge. The edges of the wound hould be moist. Each time the dressing is done, the drain is removed, the rea cleaned with saline and a fresh drain reinserted. The pinna is cleaned nd the external meatus mopped every time, the progress of healing in the middle ear being indicated by the lessening of discharge in the meatus. The urgeon may like the bandage arranged so that some turns are behind the pinna and some in front. Thus the pinna is left free and the meatus can be mopped at frequent intervals without disturbing the mastoid dressing. This is usually the case after a Schwartz operation when the middle ear has not been opened up.

After the radical operation, the dressing is changed after forty-eight hours. On the fourth day any packing on the meatus is removed, and the meatus mopped clean and the mastoid cavity insufflated with sulphonamide powder via the meatus.

Sutures are removed on the fifth or sixth day, and from the seventh day onwards the meatus and cavity beyond are gently irrigated with warm sterile saline, using a tube and funnel. When clean, the cavity is insufflated with sulphonamide powder. This is repeated each day. Eventually the cavity becomes lined first with healthy granulation tissue, and subsequently with epithelium which spreads over the surface of the cavity from the torn edges of the meatal skin. This end result will probably take many weeks to complete.

On the day after a mastoid operation, the patient is given an aperient. A generous diet is prescribed as soon as she is able to take it, and the temperature, pulse, and respiration are taken four-hourly, until the patient's condition is satisfactory. The patient sits up in a few days, and, in the simple cases, may get up on the fifth day if there is no headache. The more extensive the operation, the longer the patient stays in bed afterwards.

Unfavourable Symptoms to be Observed by the Nurse. They are arranged in groups relating to the structures which are involved:

1. *The Brain.* Pyrexia, headache, drowsiness and delirium; vomiting; slowing of the pulse (extra-dural abscess; meningitis; cerebral abscess).

2. *Lateral Sinus.* High swinging temperature and rigors (lateral sinus thrombosis).

3. *Internal Ear.* Vertigo and tinnitus (labyrinthitis).

4. *Facial Nerve.* Sagging of the muscles of the cheek; dribbling from the corner of the mouth; inability to smile or whistle (facial paralysis due to damage to or inflammation of the facial nerve).

THE NURSING OF DISEASES OF THE NOSE

The Common Cold. The symptoms are too common to need description. Nurses working in a general ward should remember how very infectious a cold is, and where it may be of little importance in ordinary healthy people apart from the inconvenience, catching a cold can be a serious matter in a patient suffering from some other illness. In children's wards, particularly, the nurse who goes about with a streaming cold without taking precautions is a menace. The most infectious stage is the first forty-eight hours. It is wise, if possible, to isolate oneself in bed for twenty-four hours, to have a hot bath, to keep warm and to take an abundance of hot drinks, especially fruit juices. Unfortunately, however, it is not practicable for workers to treat the condition so seriously. They are usually obliged to mix with their fellow workers. But they should keep at a distance, as far as possible, from other people, and be taught that the spread is by droplet infection. Handkerchiefs are particularly infectious, and, if possible, paper ones should be used and burnt. If nurses are obliged to be on duty with a cold, as is often the case, masks should be worn whilst attending to patients, and, if it can be avoided, they should not be required to nurse sick infants. Inhalants containing camphor, menthol, eucalyptus, etc., are useful. There are many such preparations on the market. Gargles also help to prevent the spread of a cold to the lower respiratory passages. It should be remembered that influenza and measles often simulate a streaming cold. If the temperature is raised with what appears to be an ordinary cold, the patient should certainly be isolated. If patients in a ward have a cold, they must stay in bed.

Submucous Resection of the Septum

Preparation for operation. No enema is required if the bowels have been opened satisfactorily. The nasal cavity is packed with gauze drains soaked in liquor adrenalin hydrochloride, 1 in 1,000 and cocaine 2 per cent, though the surgeon may prefer to do this in the theatre.

At the operation, after the mucous membrane has been dissected from the cartilage and bone of the septum, the deviated part of the septum is removed. The mucous membrane flaps are carefully put together again and will become sealed by blood clot. Sterile nasal plugs are put in each nostril to keep the mucosal flaps in apposition. They consist of two fingers of a rubber glove, each containing a gauze drain—lubricated with sterile vaseline and kept in position by a piece of strapping fixed across the anterior nares.

Post-operative care. If there is any bleeding, ice poultices are applied across the bridge of the nose. The patient sits up. The plugs are removed after twenty-four hours, the gauze drains being taken out first, but if they should come out before this time, the nurse reports the fact but should never try to reinsert them. An inhalation of friar's balsam may be given to relieve the soreness of the throat resulting from the enforced mouth breathing.

An aperient is given the day after the operation as blood may have een swallowed during the operation. As the septum heals the patient lust be encouraged to breathe through the nose and to do deep breathing xercises. For the first few days the patient should not blow the nose. Ialf a teaspoonful of warm liquid paraffin is poured into each nostril daily) soften any dry blood clot which may be left in the nasal cavity. This is one during the first week. The results of the operation will not be good if ood habits of breathing are not established. The patient usually goes ome in four to seven days' time, but she should not go into crowded places or a few more days, owing to the risk of inhaling germs before the mucous nembrane is healed, and able to resist infection. She must be told to wrap erself up well and not catch cold.

For other operations on the nose, for example turbinectomy, removal f nasal polypi, the preparation and after treatment is similar to the above, xcept that any gauze packing is removed as the patient recovers con-ciousness.

Infection of the Nasal Sinuses. Infection of the nasal sinuses is a com-non complication of colds and catarrhal conditions. The cavity of the ose is connected with air spaces in the bones which surround it. These re lined with mucous membrane similar to that of the nose, and infections om the nose and naso-pharynx often extend to the sinuses, causing sinu-tis. The sinuses are:

1. The two frontal sinuses in the frontal bones.
2. The two maxillary sinuses in the upper maxillæ (antra of Highmore).
3. The two sphenoidal sinuses (seldom infected).
4. The hollow cells in the ethmoid bones.

nfection of the Frontal Sinus

ymptoms

1. Intense frontal headache aggravated by stooping or coughing and is specially severe in the middle of the day.
2. Slight swelling over the sinus, and of the upper eyelid.
3. Tenderness.
4. Pyrexia and malaise.

Treatment. The patient should sit up in bed in a warm room, at a emperature of 65° F. Draughts should be avoided. Inhalations of steam rom a large bowl containing 1 drachm of tinct. benzoin co. to the pint of oiling water, are ordered. Prior to the inhalation the nose is often sprayed vith a solution of adrenalin hydrochloride 1 in 3,000. Aspirin relieves the ain. Fluids should be given very freely to encourage drainage. Small lectric cradles may be used as a method of applying heat. If the condition ecomes chronic, osteomyelitis of the frontal bone may develop. Surgical nterference and drainage is required. The condition is a dangerous one, as

the sinuses are only separated from the meninges by a thin plate of bone
Short-wave therapy may be prescribed in mild cases.

Infection of the Maxillary Sinus (antrum). The pain and tenderness ar
felt over the cheek bone on the affected side, and there may be toothach
in some of the upper teeth.

Treatment. If natural drainage is not established quickly, the antrum
may be emptied of its accum-
ulated secretion by puncturing its nasal wall with a
trocar and cannula, and
applying suction with a glass
syringe. This operation is
usually carried out under
local anæsthesia. In chronic
cases an operation to permit
permanent drainage of the

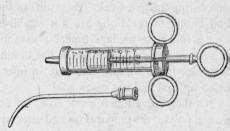

FIG. 104. Antral cannula and syringe

antrum is required. (Caldwell-Luc operation.)

Ethmoiditis. Ethmoiditis frequently accompanies infection of the fronta
or maxillary sinus and is treated in the same way. For chronic cases it may
be dealt with by an intranasal or external (facial) operation. A rubber tube
drain is often left in the nose, extending from the region of the opened
sinuses to the nostril, both in operations on the ethmoidal cells and on th
frontal sinus. It must never be removed until the surgeon gives instructions
either intranasally or externally.

The nurse's part in connection with these infections is to recognize them
as common complications of nasal infection and to realize that if the patien
is not kept warm and well nursed the conditions can become very chronic
and highly dangerous, whereas if inhalations and fluids and good nursing
treatment are instituted as soon as the first symptoms appear, the condition
generally clears up. The surgeon is loath to interfere unless medical meas
ures have failed. When the temperature is normal and the patient is other
wise fit, a sinusitis which has failed to clear completely will often be
stimulated to recover by judicious fresh air treatment, but care must be
taken that the patient is not too suddenly exposed if the winds are cold

THE NURSING OF THROAT CONDITIONS

Tonsillitis. Infection of the tonsils can be due to a variety of organisms
by far the commonest are the streptococci. Other diseases with which a
sore throat is associated are diphtheria, Vincent's angina, and secondary
syphilis.

Acute follicular tonsillitis. The tonsils are swollen and red and the ton
sillar crypts become full of pus which exudes and gives a patchy, yellow
appearance. The cervical glands are swollen and tender. The patient feel

ill, is unable to swallow and has a rise in temperature, 100° F. to 103° F.

Nursing Treatment. The case should be regarded as infectious. A mask should be worn by the nurse. Eating and drinking utensils should be kept separate. Coughing and sneezing are likely to spread the infection. A swab may be taken to identify the organism. The patient is kept warm in bed and is persuaded to drink as much fluid as she can take. Glucose or cane sugar should be added to all drinks. It is important to see that the patient takes sufficient nourishment and sometimes soft foods such as bread and milk or oatmeal gruel are swallowed more easily than fluids. Nourishing meat and wine jellies and ice cream may be given. Inhalations of steam and friar's balsam are given. Antiseptic gargles of glycothymoline or carbolic, 1 in 100, as hot as can be borne, are given frequently, at least every two hours. Gargles of potassium chlorate and iron (mist. pot. chlor. and ferri) are given and swallowed. Aspirin and veganin are prescribed for the relief of pain. Five grains of aspirin crushed in an ounce of hot water and used as a gargle before meals helps the patient to swallow, or insufflation of the tonsillar area with powdered aspirin may be ordered. Linseed or antiphlogistine poultices applied to the swollen glands of the neck give great relief. Sulphonamide drugs may be ordered in streptococcal infections. The bowels are kept open by saline aperients.

The inflammation subsides within a few days and the patient is allowed up in some cases after the temperature has been normal for two days. At least a week's holiday in the fresh air is necessary after an attack of tonsillitis. In some cases more than this is required, as a severe sore throat can make the patient feel very ill and exhausted.

Quinsy (peri-tonsillar abscess). This condition generally begins as a sore throat and the abscess may develop beneath the tonsil; in some cases the condition may be bilateral. It is extremely painful, and swallowing, even of saliva, becomes almost impossible. The abscess may burst spontaneously. When this does not occur and pain is severe the surgeon will open the abscess. This is done without a general anæsthetic in order to avoid any sudden respiratory obstruction which might occur during the induction of the anæsthetic, and secondly, to safeguard against the inhalation of blood or pus by an unconscious patient.

Requirements for opening a quinsy
1. Mackintosh and receiver.
2. A good light and head mirror or head lamp.
3. A hot mouthwash.
4. Tongue depressor.
5. Cocaine 10 per cent and spray.
6. A pair of long dressing forceps.
7. Wool.
8. Guarded scalpel and a pair of long fine sinus forceps.

T   289

Method. The nurse arranges the patient sitting up in bed, or preferably in a chair. The surgeon depresses the tongue, paints or sprays the tonsil with cocaine, and then makes a small stab incision into the swelling, or opens it with the points of the sinus forceps. Plenty of hot mouthwashes are given and the patient gargles very thoroughly to get rid of the discharge. Relief is so great after the

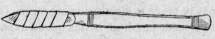

Fig. 105. Scalpel guarded with strapping exposing the point only

quinsy has been opened, that there is no difficulty in encouraging the patient to do this.

Frequent attacks of sore throats and quinsy may necessitate removal of the tonsils especially if the lymphatic glands become inflamed and remain swollen.

Tonsillectomy

Preparation. If the patient is an adult, little preparation is necessary, apart from seeing that the bowels have been well opened, and that the teeth and mouth are clean. The patient is prepared for the theatre in the usual way and is given a dose of atropine, gr. 1/100 hypodermically. No food is given for five hours before the operation. The operation is postponed if the patient has a cold or herpes or any respiratory infection or gives a history of having had such an illness in the previous few weeks. If the patient is a child, some basal anæsthetic such as nembutal may be given. The tonsils may be dissected out or removed by the guillotine.

Post-operative care. In the case of an adult, the post-operative discomfort is worse than in children. On returning from the theatre, the patient is nursed in the lateral position with a pillow in the back. In some cases the tonsils are removed under local anæsthesia. These patients are sat up in bed or in a chair straight away after the operation. After a general anæsthetic, most careful watch must be kept. The nurse must watch for any signs of excessive bleeding. This may be seen as blood trickling from the mouth, if the patient is lying properly on her side, otherwise by frequent movements of swallowing. A quarter-hourly pulse chart must be kept. The airway is removed when the patient shows signs of not tolerating it, and the face is sponged with cold water. The gown is changed if necessary, and the patient is sat up. Sometimes there is a slow hæmorrhage from the tonsil bed. If this is the case, the patient must remain sitting up, ice may be given to suck, and the surgeon should be informed. He may then find it necessary to remove a clot of blood which has formed in the tonsil bed and which is a big factor in maintaining the slow hæmorrhage. This procedure is often sufficient to stop the bleeding. In other cases he may apply pressure to the tonsil bed by means of a swab held in forceps. If this does

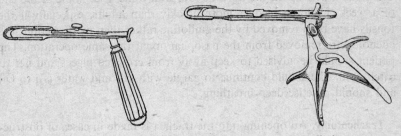

Tonsillectomy guillotines. (a) *Mackenzie's pattern.* (b) *O'Malley's pattern.*

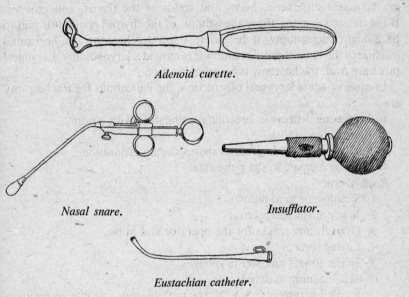

Adenoid curette.

Nasal snare.

Insufflator.

Eustachian catheter.

Fig. 106

not arrest hæmorrhage the patient must go back to the theatre for ligature of the bleeding point under an anæsthetic. In many cases, however, there is no hæmorrhage at all after tonsillectomy, and in the large majority of cases it is slight and stops after a few hours.

On the second day the patient is given aspirin gr. x in an ounce of warm water to gargle and swallow before meals. Syringing is sometimes ordered. As soon as possible the patient should be given plenty to drink, avoiding milky fluids which tend to coat the mucous membranes. Ice cream and jellies are appreciated. After the first twenty-four hours, the more the patient is encouraged to eat the better. She should even be given toast on the second day. An aperient should be given after twenty-four hours to get rid of any swallowed blood. The patient may complain of earache. This is usually a referred pain and is not serious but it must be reported.

The patient gets up on the third or fourth day and goes home at the end of a week. Children recover more quickly than adults, especially if the tonsils have been removed by the guillotine rather than by dissection; the adenoids are removed from the nasopharynx at the same operation. The patient should be advised to keep away from crowded places and not to catch cold. She should continue to gargle with salt and water ($\mathfrak{Z}$i to Oj) and should practise deep breathing.

Tracheotomy. An opening into the trachea is made in cases of obstruction of the upper respiratory passages. Common causes of obstruction are laryngeal diphtheria, burns and scalds of the throat, and growths. If the incision is made above the isthmus of the thyroid gland, it is said to be a high tracheotomy, if below it, a low tracheotomy. A horizontal incision in the crico-thyroid membrane is termed a laryngotomy. Laryngeal tubes are oval, tracheotomy tubes round in section.

In cases of acute laryngeal obstruction, the indications for tracheotomy are:

1. Increasing distress in breathing, sometimes with stridor.
2. Increasing cyanosis.
3. Sucking in of the intercostal spaces during inspiration.
4. Marked increase in the pulse rate.

Requirements

1. Sandbag or hard pillow.
2. Mackintosh and receiver.
3. Overalls and masks for the operator and nurse.
4. Lifting forceps.
5. Sterile towels and sterile sponges.
6. Skin-cleaning materials.
7. Sterile instruments: Scalpel, tracheal dilators, one pair rectractors, one sharp hook, tracheotomy tubes (inner and outer) of various sizes, complete with pilots and fitted tapes.
8. A 'keyhole' dressing of lint; cyanide gauze.
9. The following may be required: small artery forceps, needles and salmon gut sutures; local anæsthetic. In cases of diphtheritic laryngitis, spectacles should be provided for doctor and nurse.

Method. In an emergency case the patient is wrapped tightly in a blanket with the arms at the side and covered with a mackintosh and towel. The sandbag is placed under the shoulder blades so that the head falls well back. One assistant then holds the head firmly keeping it absolutely in line with the neck and body. The skin is cleaned with methylated spirit and the incision made and the dilators introduced into the tracheal opening. At this point the emergency should be over and the patient begin to breathe more easily and become a better colour. The tube is inserted with the lint

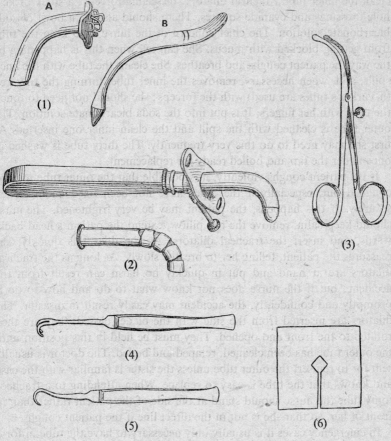

FIG. 107. Tracheotomy instruments

(1) Parker's tube. (a) Outer and
    inner tube. (b) Pilot.
(2) Durham's tube with pilot and
    inner tube.
(3) Tracheal dilators.
(4) Tracheal retractor.
(5) Tracheal sharp hook.
(6) Keyhole dressing.

dressing between the flange and the skin. A little ointment on the dressing prevents the skin from becoming sore. A piece of cyanide gauze is put over the tube to filter the air as it enters the trachea.

The patient is sat up in bed. A steam tent is very helpful in preventing chest complications through the inhalation of air which is neither moistened nor warmed in its passage through the upper respiratory passages. The patient should be reassured and given a pencil and writing block. She is encouraged to drink fluids almost at once.

A trolley or tray is kept at the bedside, and on it should be a clean inner tube of correct size in a covered dish of saline; a receiver, linen spills to clean the inner tube; tracheal dilators; dissecting forceps; a stock of key-hole dressings and cyanide squares. There should also be a bowl of soda bicarbonate solution. The chief concern of the nurse is to keep the tube from getting blocked with mucus. She can tell when this is happening by the way the patient coughs and breathes. She cleans the tube with the linen spills, and, when necessary, removes the inner tube, turning the tiny key (if Parker's tubes are used) with the forceps; she should not need to touch the tube with her fingers. It is put into the soda bicarbonate solution. The outer tube is cleaned with the spill and the clean inner one inserted. At first she may need to do this very frequently. The dirty tube is washed at once under the tap and boiled ready for replacement.

If the patient coughs violently, it is possible that the outer tube may be coughed out, especially if the tapes have not been fixed and fastened securely. If this happens, the patient may be very frightened. The nurse should keep calm, remove the top pillow, extend the patient's head backwards, and insert the tracheal dilators. As she does this quickly, she reassures the patient, telling her to breathe slowly. As long as the tracheal dilators are at hand and put in quickly no harm can result from the accident; but if the nurse does not know what to do and how to do it promptly and confidently, the accident may easily result in disaster. The dilators are inserted from the side with the blades closed, they are then rotated to the front and opened. They must be held in this position until the outer tube has been cleaned, retaped and boiled. The doctor is usually sent for to reinsert the outer tube unless the sister is familiar with the case and knows that the tube is easy to replace. When attending to a tracheotomy tube the nurse should stand at the side of the patient rather than in front of her, so that she is not in the direct line if the patient coughs.

In emergency cases it is usually only necessary to have the tube in for a few days. In the case of children, it is important that it should not be left in longer than necessary as they become used to it and are frightened when it is removed. If the cause of the obstruction is a growth, the opening may be permanent. The patient is supplied with suitable rubber tubes and she is taught to change them herself.

Inexperienced nurses are often frightened by tracheotomy cases. They should be reassured that no harm can come to the patient if the dilators are always at hand and if the nurse knows how to use them.

It is most important to keep the patient warm and out of draughts. If a steam tent is not ordered, screens should be used. The cold unfiltered air entering the trachea directly is liable to cause bronchitis or pneumonia. Soft nourishing foods are given at first. It is important that the general health and morale of the patient should be maintained during this trying illness. As she gets better she should be encouraged to mix with the other patients and take part in the general life of the ward.

Intubation. An alternative to tracheotomy is the insertion of an intubation tube through the mouth between the vocal cords. This keeps open the respiratory passage without making an incision. The tube is difficult to insert. It is an impracticable method unless a doctor is available at a moment's notice to replace the tube if it comes out.

Chapter Eighteen

THE NURSING OF INFECTIOUS DISEASES

NOTIFIABLE DISEASES

Acute influenzal pneumonia; acute polioencephalitis; acute polio-myelitis; acute primary pneumonia; anthrax; cerebro-spinal fever; cerebro-spinal meningitis; cholera; continued fever; diphtheria; dysentery; encephalitis lethargica; enteric fever; epidemic cerebro-spinal meningitis; meningococcal meningitis; erysipelas; membranous croup; ophthalmia neonatorum; puerperal fever; relapsing fever; scarlatina; scarlet fever; smallpox; trench fever; tuberculosis in any part of the body; typhoid fever; typhus fever.

Cases of anthrax, arsenical, lead, mercurial and phosphorous poisoning; toxic jaundice, ephitheliomatous ulceration, or chronic ulceration, contracted in a factory or workshop, must be notified immediately to the Chief Inspector of Factories, The Home Office, London, S.W.

All cases of food poisoning must be notified to the Medical Officer of Health of the district in which the patient resides. Cholera is notifiable to the Port Sanitary Authority.

Patients suffering from any of the above diseases are treated as infectious. The case must be notified to the local medical officer of health by the doctor in charge of the case. The patient must not be transported in a public vehicle of any kind.

THE GENERAL COURSE OF AN INFECTION

The organism spreads by the following methods:

1. Droplet infection.
2. Fomites—clothing, books, bed linen, etc.
3. Food—commonly water or milk.
4. Animals, insects and parasites.
5. By direct inoculation.

Having gained entrance to the body, the organisms multiply in the blood (incubation period) until the infection is sufficiently generalized to cause symptoms. In response to the infection, the blood and tissue fluids produce substances (antibodies and antitoxins) which combat the germ and the toxins produced. By the liberation of these protective substances the infection is gradually overcome in a more or less definite period of time, and immunity is gained. The patient recovers and is usually protected by immune substances in the blood from a second attack of the disease. Resistance or immunity is specific, that is to say, an attack of measles will protect the patient from a further attack of measles, but will not render her immune to other infections.

Incubation period is the period which elapses between the time of infection and the onset of the first symptoms.

Prodromal period is the time which elapses between the onset of the first symptom and the appearance of the rash.

Defervescence—the days during which the symptoms are abating.

Quarantine—the period of isolation for all those who have been in contact with the disease.

The general trained nurse who has not made a special study of infectious diseases in a fever hospital must have some knowledge of them in order to protect her patients and herself, and to prevent the spread of infection amongst others.

1. She must be able to recognize the earliest symptoms and know what to do. If in hospital, she must seek medical advice at once; the case must be notified to the proper authorities; the ward sister supplies the appropriate forms for the notification. She must get in touch with the relatives and warn them that the patient may be moved and that they must be prepared to answer inquiries as to how the disease may have been contracted.

2. She must know how to isolate the patient satisfactorily in a general ward and give the nursing care required during the interim period before the patient is moved to an isolation ward or special hospital.

3. If she has to nurse the patient during the illness, as very often happens in spite of her not having had a special training, she must know sufficient about the disease to follow its course. She must be able to discriminate between the normal and the abnormal features of the illness. The large majority of patients suffering from an infectious illness recover when the disease has taken its usual definite course.

4. Apart from the general nursing and the relief of symptoms, it is most important that the onset of complications should be recognized as soon as they appear. It is always the complications which make these diseases so serious, and if they can be avoided the outlook is good.

5. Apart from the general precautions against the spread of infection as described below, the nurse should make quite sure that she knows in every case how the infection spreads, what part of the body the organism is attacking, and what excretions are particularly dangerous. Thus she adapts her general rules of isolation to the requirements of the case, and by application of her knowledge protects herself and others from contracting the disease. For instance, in the cases of those diseases which spread by droplet infection, masks must be worn. In the typhoid group of diseases, where

the infection is in the intestine, it is the care and disposal of the excreta and precautions with the bedpan and bed linen that are particularly important Where direct inoculation is the danger, as in primary and secondary syphilis, gloves must be worn and the greatest care taken to protect the hands from abrasions. Further details of 'Barrier Isolation' are given at the end of this chapter.

GENERAL PRINCIPLES FOR THE NURSING OF INFECTIOUS CASES

The hygiene and comfort of the patient is of first importance. A daily blanket bath is given and detailed nursing care of the mouth and pressure points. The room or ward must be kept fresh with the windows open as much as possible. When the severe symptoms have abated the diet should be increased and well planned. At all stages fluids, especially fruit juices and glucose, are valuable. Sedatives are prescribed to ensure good periods of sleep, and aperients are likely to be required. If there is an irritating rash, frequent sponging with warm water containing soda bicarbonate is done. Calamine lotion can be used, and blankets should not be put next to the patient. Irritation is usually worse when the patient is hot, and sometimes the use of a bed cradle keeps her cooler and more comfortable. If serum has been given, the rash, which is part of the reaction, can be very troublesome. It is usually of an urticarial type and, apart from local treatment, injections of liquor adrenalin hydrochloride, ℳ v—x are useful. Sponging the areas with carbolic lotion 1 in 40 or with soda bicarbonate solution may help to allay irritation. When the temperature is very high the patient is often restless and delirious. Frequent sponging of the whole body should be done and the bed cradle used.

In all cases of infectious illness, however slight the attack, the patient must be confined to bed and kept warm. Too much emphasis cannot be laid on the fact that it is the complications which are likely to make the illness a dangerous one, and if the patient catches cold while resistance is lowered, bronchitis and pneumonia may develop.

The urine must be tested for albumen in cases where there is high fever. Where swabs are required for diagnostic purposes they should, if possible, be taken first thing in the morning, before a mouthwash is given. Swelling of the glands, pain in the joints, albumen in the urine and the presence of a cough, are all symptoms which should be reported to the doctor. During convalescence, when the temperature has subsided, particular attention should be paid to the pulse, especially when the patient begins to get up. It should be recorded just before the patient leaves bed and after she has been up for half an hour. A raised pulse which persists in these cases may be an indication of some damage to the heart. When the patient is ready to be discharged, a disinfectant bath, e.g. lysol, 1 in 500, is given. The hair

s washed and the patient is given clean clothes. Everything she has used
s disinfected, including bedding and mattress.

In up-to-date fever hospitals, the method of bed isolation has been
brought to a fine art, that is, different infectious diseases are nursed in the
same ward by the same nurses, with precautions which prevent cross
nfection. Cubicle nursing is a modification of this method. Both these
need careful studying as they can only be practised by staff specially trained
n these methods of nursing infections.

THE RECOGNITION AND NURSING OF CERTAIN INFECTIONS

1. **Measles** (morbilli). Incubation period, 10 to 14 days. Spread by
droplet infection.

Symptoms
1. Heavy cold; cough.
2. Running eyes.
3. Quick rise in temperature, 101° to 103° F.
4. Severe malaise, headache, and photophobia.

Second day. Koplik's spots on the mucous membrane of the cheek,
opposite the molar teeth.

Fourth day. Blotchy crescentic rash appears behind the ears and on the
chest; later it becomes generalized. The temperature may rise to a higher
level as the rash appears.

Seventh day. The temperature falls to normal and the rash fades.

On the tenth day the patient gets up, and on the fourteenth day is ready
for discharge.

Complications. Bronchitis, broncho-pneumonia; conjunctivitis; ble-
pharitis; keratitis; otitis media; mastoiditis. The patient is particularly
susceptible to other infections when the resistance is lowered (e.g. whooping
cough, tuberculosis). Measles is specially serious under the age of five.

Nursing Points
1. Warmth in bed: two or three pillows; bed jacket and chest blanket.
2. Lights shaded to avoid eyestrain; the bed should not be facing the
window; no reading is allowed.
3. Mouthwashes and gargles.
4. Eyes are irrigated if necessary.
5. Cough medicine; the chest may be rubbed with camphorated oil.
6. Blood serum from a convalescent patient is useful to make the attack
less severe.

N.B. Report specially, *cough, pain in the chest, earache* and *sore eyes*.

2. **Scarlet Fever.** Incubation period, 1 to 6 days (often 3 days); spread

by droplet infection. The cause is a streptococcus which attacks the tonsils. There is a very thin dividing line between an acute streptococcal throat and scarlet fever. If the attack is severe with the appearance of a rash, it is generally termed scarlet fever. 'Barrier' nursing is required, but the patient is not necessarily removed from a general ward.

Symptoms
1. Sore throat—the tonsils are enlarged and inflamed.
2. Rising temperature, from 102° to 104° F. The face is flushed and the pupils are dilated.
3. Headache and vomiting.
4. Swollen glands in the neck.

Second day
1. Scarlet rash all over the body with a paler area round the mouth (circum-oral pallor).
2. Strawberry tongue (red and rather swollen).
3. Restlessness and delirium.

Fifth to seventh day
The temperature falls and the skin begins to desquamate.

The period of isolation varies. Some authorities discharge the patient after two weeks, others insist upon six weeks' isolation. The quarantine period is eight days.

Complications
1. Otitis media.
2. Mastoiditis.
3. Cervical abscess.
4. Nephritis.
5. Rheumatism.
6. Damage to the heart (endocarditis and pericarditis).

Nursing Points
1. Gargles.
2. Throat swabs taken to identify the organism.
3. Sponging for hyperpyrexia.
4. Fluid diet.
5. Poultices to the neck for painful glands.
6. Administration of sulphonamide drugs.
7. Testing of the urine for albumen and blood.
8. Anti-streptococcal serum.

N.B. Report earache; joint pains; albuminuria; persistently rapid or irregular pulse; lethargy and pallor during convalescence.

Dick test is a skin test for susceptibility to scarlet fever. An intradermal injection of scarlet fever toxin produces a red area (erythema) at the site of injection after twelve hours in susceptible persons (Dick positives).

3. Diphtheria. Incubation period, 2 to 7 days. Spread by droplet infection. Infecting organism, Klebs-Loeffler bacillus. It commonly attacks the mucous membrane of the throat, nose or larynx. Occasionally it is seen growing on the conjunctiva or even on a wound. The characteristic lesion is a greyish membrane which is seen on the affected part. When detached, it leaves a bleeding area, and on examination is found to consist of necrotic tissue, showing a heavy growth of bacilli. The germs do not spread into the blood stream, and the serious effects are due to the severe toxæmia which results from the rapid absorption of toxins (exotoxins) from the focus of infection. Cases vary from those of a mild type to very severe and dangerous attacks.

Symptoms—Faucial (average severity)

1. A sore throat, not necessarily very severe.
2. Malaise and a feeling of exhaustion and faintness.
3. Temperature raised, 99° to 100° F. Pulse 90 to 100, usually of poor volume.
4. Pallor.

Complications

1. Heart failure, due to toxins attacking the heart muscle. There may be less severe heart symptoms, denoting less grave damage.
2. Albuminuria.
3. Paralysis especially of the soft palate and eye muscles. In this case, the toxins attack the nervous system and the symptoms usually last for about six weeks after which the patient recovers. Paralysis involving the heart muscle or muscles of respiration may be fatal.

Laryngeal diphtheria. This is usually seen in young children. An additional complication arises, i.e. laryngeal obstruction due to œdema of the glottis. Tracheotomy may be necessary.

Nursing Points

1. Complete rest. The patient is nursed quite flat with one small pillow. In some cases even one pillow is not allowed.
2. The patient must be washed, fed and kept perfectly still. He is not allowed to turn himself in bed nor to reach for anything from his locker. This is especially important in the early stages, as the toxins circulate so rapidly, and attack the heart.
3. *Anti-diphtheritic* serum, 5,000—10,000 units, at the earliest possible moment, even before a positive throat swab has been obtained.
4. Frequent throat swabs for diagnostic purposes, and to show the progress of the disease.
5. The toilet of the mouth and nose is important. The nurse must cleanse them frequently. The patient must not exert himself by gargling.
6. Fluid diet.
7. Testing of the urine for albumen.

8. Rest in bed for two or three weeks, or much longer. Isolation until three consecutive negative swabs have been obtained.

N.B. Report abnormalities of the pulse; fainting attacks; breathlessness; pain in the region of the heart; albumen in the urine; weakness of the legs or arms; regurgitation of fluids through the nose (paralysis of the soft palate). Sudden death may occur due to paralysis of the heart muscles or the diaphragm.

The Schick test. Intradermal injection of a minute dose of diphtheria toxin into the arm with a 'control' injection into the other arm. If the person is 'Schick positive', i.e. susceptible to diphtheria, an area of redness will be seen at the site of injection of the toxin. This increases for about a week and then fades and desquamates. A 'Schick positive' person should be immunized with modified diphtheria toxin. The results, as regards prevention, are very satisfactory.

4. Whooping Cough (pertussis). Incubation period 7 to 14 days. Spread by droplet infection. Infecting organism—bacillus pertussis.

Symptoms

1. Slight rise in temperature.

2. Cough which develops sooner or later—any time within three weeks —into a typical whoop, that is, a series of coughs on expiration followed by a long inspiration. The patient, usually a child, expectorates a quantity of tough, white, ropy mucus. The coughing may make the child sick and exhausted.

Complications

1. Bronchitis and broncho-pneumonia; bronchiectasis; tuberculosis.

2. Sometimes the violence of the coughing causes blood vessels to rupture in the conjunctiva and nose. Rectal prolapse or hernia occasionally result.

Nursing Points. The child should be confined to one room which is kept fresh, well ventilated and at a constant warm temperature, 65° to 68° F., or in suitable weather the bed may be taken on to a sunny balcony. He should not be allowed to go into draughty passages, but need not necessarily be kept in bed all day. He should be allowed to amuse himself quietly. After a fortnight, if the weather is warm, he may go out in the sunshine. The diet should be generous; vitamin D in the form of cod liver oil or halibut liver oil is particularly beneficial and helps to prevent chest complications. Artificial sunlight is prescribed. A meal should not be given immediately before an attack of coughing, and, as these attacks often occur at definite regular intervals, the nurse should try to time the meal carefully otherwise the food may be vomited. The individual should be studied in this respect.

Unless thorough nursing with warmth and good food can be obtained, he child is likely to be left with a chronic cough which lowers the resistance and renders him susceptible to other respiratory infections.

The period of isolation varies from three to five weeks, according to the instructions of the doctor. Sometimes the 'whoop' lasts longer than this, but is not necessarily infectious. The quarantine period is fifteen days.

5. **Chicken Pox** (varicella). Incubation period, 14 to 21 days. Spread by direct contact or infected articles.

Symptoms. Apart from the rash, the symptoms are not usually very severe.

1. Some cases develop a moderately high temperature.

2. The rash appears during the first three days and consists of raised red spots, developing into vesicles. They are distributed most thickly on the trunk and less thickly on the limbs. They begin to dry up and fade after the fourth or fifth day.

The patient is infectious until every scab has fallen off, and particularly for the first five days of the illness. He is usually isolated for three weeks.

Nursing Points. The chief point is to see that the vesicles do not get rubbed or infected with pus-forming organisms—staphylococci. The skin should be powdered with boracic or calamine powder. In ordinary cases there are no complications, nor is there any scarring.

6. **German Measles** (rubella). Incubation period, 7 to 21 days. Spread by droplet infection.

Symptoms

1. Swollen glands in the neck, particularly at the back and in the nape of the neck. Supra-clavicular glands are often swollen also.

2. A red rash appears on the second day; it may be generalized.

3. The temperature is slightly raised, 99° F. and, in a few cases, the symptoms may be much more severe with a pyrexia up to 101° or 102° F. and moderate malaise.

4. Catarrh.

5. Slight conjunctivitis.

Complications. Usually none.

Nursing Points. In slight cases no nursing is required, nor is the patient isolated or kept from school or work. If, however, the temperature is raised to any degree, or the patient feels ill, a day or two in bed is advisable. Poultices may be applied to the neck and the eyes may need irrigation.

7. **Mumps** (infective parotitis). Incubation period 12 to 26 days. The disease is spread by droplet infection.

Symptoms

1. Swelling of the parotid glands in front of the ear.

2. Rise in temperature, 100° to 101° F.

3. Dysphagia.

4. Swelling of lymphatic glands in the neck.

5. Malaise.

Complications. Enlargement of other glands in the body, especiall, orchitis in male patients. These complications are not very common no, are they usually serious.

Nursing Points. 1. Fluid diet; if the patient is a child, it is importan to see that he gets sufficient to drink, with the addition of glucose, ever though swallowing is painful. It is possible for a young child to suffe from acidosis due to lack of carbohydrate. It is recognized by drowsines and a smell of acetone in the breath.

2 Poultices are applied to the painful glands, linseed, antiphlogistine etc.

3. Gargles and mouthwashes.

4. If there is pain in the scrotum it should be supported on a sandba, or by means of a suspensory bandage. Applications of lead and opiun lotion give relief, or hot fomentations.

The isolation period is three weeks; the disease is very infectious. I, every case the patient should be isolated for at least a week after th, swelling subsides. The quarantine period is twenty-eight days.

8. **Smallpox** (variola). Incubation period usually 12 days. This disease should be recognized, although it is so seldom seen in this country. If ar outbreak does occur, it is usually in a mild form, known as *varioloi, smallpox* in persons who have been vaccinated. Vaccination against small pox consists of scarifying the skin and inoculating the incision with glycerinated calf lymph from an animal suffering from cowpox. This gives the subject a mild attack of the disease, which protects him against the disease in its severer forms.

Symptoms

1. A sudden rise in temperature, 102° to 104° F.

2. Malaise and rigors.

3. Pain in the back; headache.

4. The rash appears on the third day in the form of red papules. On the sixth day they change to vesicles; on the ninth day to pustules. By the tenth to twelfth day scabs form and begin to drop off. The lesions appear in groups and are most thickly distributed on the face and limbs. In the varioloid type of disease, the symptoms are much less pronounced and there may be only a few pocks.

Complications. The patient may rapidly die from toxæmia, pneumonia or collapse. The eyes may suffer severe damage.

Nursing Points. If, in a general ward, a patient is suspected to be suffering rom smallpox, certain measures must be taken promptly. The local Medical Officer of Health will be notified and his advice sought. A special-st who has had experience of the disease will probably come to see the patient. The ward is put into strict quarantine; all the patients and nursing staff may be re-vaccinated if more than seven years have elapsed since their last inoculation.

The patient will be removed to an isolation room or to a fever hospital. Thorough investigations will be made into the patient's family and place of work, etc., and all contacts will be carefully traced and watched. New patients will not be admitted to the ward for sixteen days, nor will the patients in the ward be discharged. Strictest precautions are necessary to prevent those in contact with the patient from contracting the disease. Skilled nursing is required, especially with regard to the hygiene and toilet of the patient. A well-ventilated room is essential. There is usually an offensive odour, and eau-de-Cologne may be added to the washing water and plenty of talcum powder should be used. Sponging all over at least twice a day should be done. Bright lights should be avoided and the eyes irrigated with boracic lotion. The toilet of the mouth should be thorough. An air bed is an advantage, as the skin becomes septic in the third stage of the rash. The discharge from the vesicles and pustules is very infectious. The diet should be as generous as the patient can take, in order to maintain his general condition, and plenty of fluids and glucose should be given. Two or three pillows are required and the patient should be moved about the bed as much as possible to avoid chest complications. The rash may be treated with carbolic lotion, 1 in 60; this keeps the skin clean and stops the irritation. If delirium is present, sedative drugs are required.

9. **Anterior Poliomyelitis.** This disease is due to a virus which attacks the central nervous system, causing paralysis of different groups of muscles. The virus is present in discharges from the mucous membrane of the naso-pharynx, hence it is spread by droplet infection. Its infectivity is low, but it occurs in small epidemics, especially when living and sleeping quarters are overcrowded and ill-ventilated. The infection settles in the anterior horns of the spinal cord from which the motor fibres of the spinal nerves to the skeletal muscles and the diaphragm arise. The inflammation in the cells prevents the impulses from reaching the muscles.

Symptoms

1. A cold, accompanied by a rise in temperature (100° to 101° F.), and pain in back and limbs resembling the onset of influenza.

2. Sudden loss of function of one or more groups of muscles. It is not uncommon for the paralysis to supervene without any other symptoms of importance being noticed. The paralysed muscles are cold and blue and sensitive to touch, as the sensory nerve roots in the cord are not affected.

Tingling pains are complained of. If the diaphragm or intercostal muscles are paralysed, respiration fails and the patient may die.

Complications

1. Permanent deformities.
2. Death from respiratory failure.
3. Encephalitis or meningitis occurs in a few cases.

Nursing Points. 1. The patient is nursed in a general ward with modified barrier precautions. Masks and gowns should be used, as the catarrhal symptoms spread the infection. If the patient is a child, the nurse should not get in too close contact with his breath as she lifts him out of his cot. The nurse herself should use a gargle regularly. All discharges should be received into paper handkerchiefs or swabs which can be burned. Any discharge from the ears is likely to be infectious. All crockery should be boiled after use.

2. The position of the limbs or limb is important. Splints or light plasters are applied as soon as possible to give support to the extensor muscles. Until this can be done, the nurse should wrap the limb in warm wool and arrange it as carefully and correctly as she can in a good position, because it is important to prevent the sagging of muscles at this early stage.

3. Lumbar puncture is often done for the relief of pain and aspirin or veganin is prescribed. Sometimes poultices or fomentation may soothe an aching back. Active massage or electrical treatment is not given for about two months, until the inflammation of the nerve structures has subsided. Antiseptic gargles should be given. In favourable cases the paralysis recovers within a few weeks, although it is unusual for complete recovery to take place, and the damage to one or more groups of muscles is likely to be permanent. The patient is considered infectious for at least a month and is not usually transferred to an orthopædic clinic or hospital until this time has elapsed. The rehabilitation period lasts anything up to two or three years in the hope of restoring the function of the muscles, and during this time the patient should be in charge of a trained masseuse. Operative treatment is often required later, and a walking iron or other supporting apparatus may be required permanently in many cases.

Serum from convalescent patients has been found useful as a prophylactic measure, and in recent years lives have been saved by the use of an 'Iron Lung' for cases of respiratory failure.

10. **Cerebrospinal Meningitis** (spotted fever). Incubation period, 1 to 5 days. Infecting organism, the meningococcus. Sometimes the disease is called 'meningococcal meningitis'. The focus of infection is the mucous membrane of the naso-pharynx, and from here the germ is circulated in the blood and lymph stream to the meninges. Thus the spread is again by droplet infection. The disease occurs in small epidemics, generally due to overcrowding of sleeping quarters.

MENINGITIS

Symptoms

1. Severe headache with pain in the neck and back.
2. Rise in temperature, 101° to 103° F.
3. Arching of the back and head retraction (opisthotonus).
4. Vomiting.
5. Drowsiness, deepening into coma.
6. In children convulsions occur and squint (strabismus) is not uncommon.
7. In some cases there is a rash, consisting of small hæmorrhages under the skin.

Nursing Points. 1. The patient is nursed in a general ward with barrier precautions. Masks must be worn and special care taken with discharges from the nose, throat and ears. The crockery must be boiled after use.

2 The patient is nursed flat, the eyes are shielded from the light and the patient is kept very quiet.

3. The daily toilet is attended to with care; the mouth and nose must be kept very clean.

4. Headaches can be relieved by the application of cold compresses or by an ice bag. Sedative drugs are required if the patient is delirious.

5. Lumbar puncture is performed for diagnostic purposes and for the relief of headache. It may be done daily, towards evening.

6. The diet should be light and nourishing and given in frequent small feeds.

7. A small enema can be given on alternate days, if necessary.

The outlook and treatment of this disease has been completely changed during the last three or four years by the use of M. & B. 693 which is given in full dosage, up to nine days. The results are remarkable: the patient practically always recovers quickly, and the only complication which has been observed to follow is a slight deafness. This is in contrast to the outlook before the introduction of sulphonamide drugs. In those days the patient relapsed into coma and gradually died in an emaciated, exhausted, and collapsed condition. Nasal feeding was always necessary during the last days of the patient's life. Those patients who recovered were generally left with some nerve lesion, more or less severe. Anti-meningococcal serum was given intrathecally and was considered helpful, but nowadays it is not thought necessary to give it if M. & B. 693 is given.

11. **Typhoid** (enteric fever). Incubation period, 5 to 23 days; infecting organism, *bacillus typhosus* which is ingested through contaminated water or milk. It attacks Peyer's patches of lymphoid tissue in the ileum, causing inflammation and ulceration.

The disease generally lasts from five to six weeks and can conveniently be divided into three stages, according to the pathology and symptoms which develop. The nurse cannot nurse the patient intelligently unless she understands the condition of the intestine and unless she can interpret the symptoms accordingly.

Symptoms

First stage (first and second weeks). The Peyer's patches are inflamed. The onset is insidious and misleading.

1. Gradual rise in temperature in the staircase fashion, 100° to 104° F. The pulse rate increases, but not always in proportion to the temperature, 90 to 110.

2. Abdominal discomfort, diarrhœa or constipation; the abdomen feels soft or 'doughy'.

3. Persistent headache.

4. Rose-red spots on the abdomen are seen after the seventh day. They appear in groups and may be few or numerous.

5. The patient's condition deteriorates and after seven to ten days she is gravely ill. The Widal test which shows the presence of antibodies (agglutinins) in the blood serum may be positive on about the tenth day.

Second stage (second and third weeks). The patches are ulcerated and, in a severe case, the patient lapses into the 'typhoid state'; pyrexia is persistent; the appearance is pale and toxæmic; there is loss of flesh; incontinence of urine and fæces; diarrhœa with 'pea-soup' stools; swollen, red tongue; foul breath; relaxation of the muscles and muttering delirium; liability to bed sores.

Third stage (third to fifth week). Sloughs from the surface of the ulcers loosen and are discharged in the fæces. The ulcers begin to heal. The symptoms gradually abate and the temperature falls by lysis. The patient's condition improves generally.

Nursing. The patient can be nursed in a general ward if careful precautions are taken. The organism is found in the fæces and urine. Overalls are worn. The contents of bedpans are covered with two or three pints of carbolic lotion, 1 in 20, for two hours before disposal. The bedpan is disinfected and kept for the one patient only. Bed linen is soaked in formalin, 1 in 500, for eight hours before being sent to the laundry. A separate bed brush and duster must be kept for bed-making and all the patient's washing and eating utensils are kept separate.

Toilet of the patient. The washing of the patient must be done with great thoroughness, remembering that any excreta not removed is a potential source of infection. A full blanket bath is given in the morning and the patient is sponged down again in the evening. Every time the patient defæcates the buttocks and perineal area must be washed with soap and water to remove all traces of fæcal matter. The back and pressure points require four-hourly attention as the patient becomes so thin and ill that bed sores easily develop. Use should be made of air rings, heel rings, and water beds. The patient's position should be changed two-hourly in the acute stage. She can have two or three pillows and should be turned and propped on her side, both to avoid pressure sores and to encourage deeper respiration. The patient must be given mouthwashes frequently and she must be helped to clean her teeth. It is often necessary for the nurse to clean the patient's mouth four-hourly in the second stage of the disease. Rusks, raw pineapple, and chewing gum can be given to the patient to chew and stimulate the flow of saliva thus helping to keep the mouth clean. As the toxæmia causes relaxation of the muscles, the patient often lies with the knees flexed and turned to one side. She is often more comfortable with a small soft knee pillow, and the nurse must arrange the legs if necessary, and pad them to prevent rubbing. There is often a tendency to foot drop, and a small cradle is helpful in preventing the weight of the bedclothes resting on the feet. Every detail of the patient's toilet must be carefully attended to by the nurse.

Diet. Nothing is allowed which will irritate the ulcers. The doctor prescribes the diet and it should be as generous and sustaining as possible, in order to keep up the patient's strength during this long and exhausting illness. (For further details, see page 76.) Fluids are always important in a condition of such grave toxæmia.

The headache is relieved by ice or vinegar compresses and veganin or aspirin tablets, if prescribed. It is often not necessary to give sedative drugs in quantity, as in the 'typhoid state' the patient is quietly delirious and likely to doze and sleep the greater part of the day and night.

The bowels. Aperients are seldom ordered apart from regular doses of liquid paraffin. If the patient becomes constipated, an enema saponis, ten ounces, can be given on alternate mornings. If diarrhœa is troublesome a starch and opium enema may be given every day, if necessary, or tincture opii, 5 minims, t.d.s. by mouth may be prescribed.

The urine should be measured and tested for albumen.

There is no disease in which the patient is more dependent upon consistently good and detailed nursing and observation, and the nurse has her reward when she sees the patient gradually taking an interest in her surroundings and feeling ready to enjoy some food. The diet, however, must be very carefully increased as errors in feeding cause the ulcers to break down and the patient suffers a relapse.

Complications. The most critical stage of the illness is during the third week when the sloughs are separating. If the ulcers are deep, the separation may cause a hæmorrhage. Blood may be seen in large quantities in the stools and the symptoms are those of internal hæmorrhage.

Perforation of the intestine, due to separation of the sloughs, is a complication almost invariably fatal. The patient complains of abdominal pain, the pulse rises, the abdomen becomes rigid and the patient's condition is one of collapse. Operation, although it is the only hope, is almost always unsuccessful for two reasons. After three weeks of severe toxæmia the patient is in no condition to stand an abdominal operation; and secondly, the intestine in its unhealthy, ulcerated state has little chance of healing, even though large portions of the gut are removed. It is most important that the nurse should be alive to the dangers of perforation and hæmorrhage, and that from the second to the fourth week she should handle the patient with the greatest of care. When washing the abdomen there should be no unnecessary manipulation. If hæmorrhage occurs, opium preparations are prescribed. The patient must not be lifted or rolled more than is necessary. Pads of wool are put under the rectum, to avoid lifting her on and off the bedpan. A kidney dish can be put in position when the patient micturates. If it is necessary to change the drawsheet, the clean one can be pinned to the soiled one with six safety pins, and, with the minimum of lifting, the soiled one is drawn out and the clean one slipped into position.

Another cause of death in typhoid fever is pneumonia and all nursing measures must be taken to prevent this. Typhoid abscesses in bone sometimes occur late in the disease.

Inoculation against typhoid is a preventive measure. The injection given is T.A.B. vaccine. This emulsion contains dead typhoid bacilli and bacilli A and B of paratyphoid. The paratyphoid diseases are due to organisms of the same group, but they are much less virulent. The condition of the patient is similar, but not nearly so serious.

VENEREAL DISEASES

It is a well-known fact that the incidence of syphilis and gonorrhœa increases in time of war. Both diseases are commonly spread when the national moral standard is lowered and sexual behaviour becomes promiscuous; but it should also be remembered that many innocent people contract these diseases. In any case, the nurse is there to nurse the victims and not to pass judgment upon them. In most cases one might say it is due to ignorance. The nurse is likely to do much more good by handling her patients sympathetically. If she learns to inquire tactfully about the home life and surroundings of her patient she can put in little words of advice and teaching, while she is doing her treatment, which would never be tolerated unless she were on really friendly terms with her patients. The nursing of these cases gives an unrivalled opportunity for teaching on health and social problems. Most nurses who take up this work find it increasingly interesting.

It is important that the nurse should recognize the symptoms of these diseases, so that they can be treated in the early stages, and also that she may understand how to protect herself and others from infection at the various stages.

Syphilis. Syphilis is due to infection by the spirochœta pallida and occurs in three stages.

Primary syphilis. A sore occurs at the site of infection, usually on the lip, vulva, or nipple. The germ cannot puncture healthy skin, but it can penetrate a crack or abrasion. Thus a sore on the lip can be contracted through a patient drinking from a cup infected by discharge from another person. The nurse can contract a sore on her finger through getting a cut or abrasion infected, when examining or treating a patient with an infectious discharge. The sore or chancre develops about three weeks after infection, and is seen as a hard swelling under the skin or mucous membrane. It breaks down and ulcerates and the discharge is very infectious. The infection travels by the lymph stream to the nearest group of lymphatic glands which begin to swell.

Secondary syphilis. The symptoms develop three weeks to three months after the primary sore is seen. By this time the infection has reached the blood stream giving rise to the following symptoms:

1. Rise of temperature (in some cases).

2. Sore throat.

3. A white exudate is seen on the fauces and uvula. This is called a 'snail track'.

4. The hair falls out and the patient suffers from occipital headache; various eye troubles develop (iritis and keratitis).

5. A rash is commonly seen and takes many forms, e.g. red papules or vesicles. The rash of syphilis is said to imitate that of many other diseases, but observers have noticed that it never irritates and when it fades it often leaves a permanent brown stain on the skin.

6. Lymphatic glands all over the body show enlargement.

Tertiary syphilis. After the acute stages of the disease it becomes latent for anything from two to twenty years when fresh symptoms begin to appear. These are due to hard, painless swellings in the bones and various organs of the body. These swellings are called 'gummata'; they break down and destroy tissue wherever they occur. They are seen as gummatous ulcers of the skin, and the results are seen in the broken down nasal bones, giving the typical 'saddle nose'. They may form in the liver, stomach and larynx.

Neuro-syphilis occurs in the tertiary stage, that is, syphilis which attacks the nervous system. It is very serious and results in tabes dorsalis or general paralysis of the insane, according to whether the syphilitic lesion is in the spinal cord or the brain. Mental deterioration of all types of severity is commonly seen and mental hospitals and homes accommodate numbers of these patients in the later stages.

Treatment. The disease in its first and second stage is highly infectious. Full details as to the precautions to be taken in nursing both syphilis and gonorrhœa are given as an appendix to this chapter. The disease in the tertiary stage is not infectious.

The primary sore is treated by various mercurial preparations as ordered by the doctor. The discharge contains the organisms. Wassermann reaction and Kahn tests are performed on specimens of blood taken from a vein and on cerebro-spinal fluid taken by lumbar puncture. If they are negative, the disease is in its very early stages, but if positive the blood stream is obviously already infected.

The disease in the second stage can be very acute, and the patient must be confined to bed. The throat condition and the rash are particularly infectious, especially if the eruption is vesicular, exuding fluid. Rubber gloves should be worn and the utmost care taken with crockery, etc. The patient is given a non-stimulating diet with plenty of fluids. Condiments and rich foods increase the local symptoms. If the mouth is affected the temperature should be taken in the axilla. In many cases, unfortunately, the second stage symptoms are very vague and not sufficiently severe to cause the patient to seek a doctor's advice; mild sore throat and a feeling of malaise, with perhaps a transitory rash which is missed. Hence it is common for the disease not to be recognized until third stage symptoms develop.

General anti-syphilitic treatment is given in all stages and must be continued until blood and cerebro-spinal fluid tests are negative. It may be necessary to continue treatment for two or three years. The drugs used are preparations of arsenic, bismuth, mercury, and, in the third stage, potassium iodide is found to be valuable. Bismuth is given intramuscularly, mercury by inunction and arsenic intravenously. The teeth of the patient must be attended to before any prolonged treatment is given by these drugs. Special precautions are required in the case of arsenic. It is given as a proprietary preparation in the form of N.A.B. (novarsenobenzol), kharsivan, salvarsan, etc. It is a very dangerous drug and these preparations contain poisonous doses in a non-toxic form. It is usually given in weekly doses for two months and after an interval another course is given which often has to be again repeated if tests are still positive.

Preparation for arsenic injection

1. The patient is told to take a good aperient the night before, and to report if the bowels have not been opened.

2. A meal should not be taken for four hours before the injection.

3. The urine is tested for albumen.

4. The patient is weighed each week.

5. Plenty of sugar or glucose should be taken to counteract the poisonous effect of the drug upon the liver.

After the injection the patient is kept under observation for fifteen to thirty minutes. Collapse, due to a sudden fall in blood pressure caused by the arsenic, has occurred where patients have not been properly prepared. This will happen within ten to fifteen minutes of the injection, and the proper antidote is to give a hypodermic injection of adrenalin hydrochloride, 10 minims. The other signs of arsenic or mercurial poisoning must be looked for in patients being treated by these drugs.

Congenital Syphilis. The child born of syphilitic parents does not exhibit the primary sore. The disease is already in the secondary or tertiary stage of blood stream infection. If in the second stage, it is recognized when the child is about three or four weeks old. His health begins to deteriorate and in a severe case the child becomes marasmic. A rash is a common symptom; the skin peels off the hands and feet, and large areas of the body may be raw. There is a harsh croaking cry and a characteristic nasal discharge accompanies the 'snuffles'. The skin is described as 'café au lait' in colour in the parts where the rash does not develop. Many infants die of these symptoms. On the other hand, many children only have one or more of them in mild degree.

The rash and all discharges are very infectious.

Treatment. The treatment is the same as in an adult case, the child being given small doses of anti-syphilitic drugs by injection. The rash is treated with some mercurial preparation such as lotio nigra. The parents should be under observation and treated at the same time.

If second stage symptoms are not seen in the infant, tertiary developments may appear at puberty. Mental defects of various kinds become obvious, sight and hearing are defective, and juvenile tabes may develop. Later on in the female the syphilitic toxins damage the uterus; many cases of sterility and abortion are due to syphilis.

In whatever sphere the nurse is working, she should recognize the variety of symptoms presented during the different stages of syphilis and do all she can to teach the public how widespread and disastrous are the results on the health of the nation. She should urge them to seek medical advice at the earliest possible moment, in order to prevent the disease from being transmitted to future generations.

Gonorrhœa. Gonorrhœa is a venereal disease caused by the gonococcus. The organism is found in the discharge from the affected part. The gonococcus is delicate and grows only on mucous membrane, and hence the most commonly attacked parts are the vagina in the female. From there it may spread upwards causing cervicitis, endometritis, and salpingitis. The urethra may be infected and the small ducts at the entrance to the urethra, Skene's ducts. Bartholin's glands, just inside the vagina, are frequently a focus of infection. The rectum may become infected. Ophthalmia neonatorum, or conjunctivitis of the newly born, is contracted during the passage of the head through the infected vagina.

The disease is spread by sexual intercourse, but may be spread also by discharge from soiled lavatory seats, towels, bed linen and infected fingers. The essential points to be remembered are that a purulent discharge from the genital tract is often gonococcal; that the discharge is infectious and that mucous membranes only are the site of disease.

Symptoms. The symptoms may be acute or chronic, and again it is the chronic cases which are more likely to spread infection through their not being recognized and treated. An acute case of gonorrhœa in the female causes swelling and inflammation of the vulva, burning pain on micturition, and a greyish milky discharge. The temperature may rise, 100° to 101° F., and the patient feels ill, as with any other acute infection. The mouth is furred and the appetite fails. The patient is usually very worried and often tries to hide the symptoms.

In a chronic case there may be no symptoms apart from a more or less continuous discharge. There is so little inconvenience to the patient from this that it can go untreated for months and be a source of danger to others. If the Bartholin's glands are infected, the labia swell and a painful abscess forms.

Treatment. Proper precautions are taken to prevent the spread of infection. Smears are taken on glass slides from the urethra, cervix, vagina, Bartholin's glands, Skene's ducts and the rectum, so that it may be ascertained exactly which parts are infected. An acute case should be taken into hospital and nursed in bed. Local treatment is now largely unnecessary since the introduction of the sulphonamide drugs. Treatment with M. & B. 693 and 760 gives very good results. In heavily infected cases the gonococcus is found to be absent from all discharges after a five days' course of the drug. Some specialists give continuous treatment for seven days and many of them prescribe plain water douches to cleanse the vagina and also to emphasize to the patient the unpleasant nature of the disease; otherwise a certain type of patient is liable to think the disease is too easily cured. A good deal of health teaching should accompany treatment otherwise the patient cannot realize that infection of the tubes leads to sterility through blocking with scar tissue; nor are they likely to understand that blindness may result from ophthalmia neonatorum in infants, if the mother has an infected birth canal. The treatment of this condition has been dealt with in the chapter on eye conditions.

In chronic cases the infection may spread to the blood stream causing damage to the heart and joints. Arthritis usually attacks one of the larger joints such as the hip or shoulder or wrist. It is a very painful condition. The joints are not as a rule immobilized, although a light splint is often applied at night so that the patient can rest free from pain. Applications f glycerine and ichthyol are often made, and heat, massage and exercises ordered. The condition is likely to be seen less frequently now the disease can be treated successfully with sulphonamide drugs.

PRECAUTIONS AGAINST THE SPREAD OF INFECTION IN A WARD FOR VENEREAL DISEASES

Each patient has her own:

Thermometer. Crockery. Washing bowls and tooth mugs. Sitz bath. Bedpan and bedpan cloth. Pad bowl. (All are numbered to correspond with her bed number.)

Crockery. Different colour of beatl ware for each patient.

Cutlery. Marked with cotton of corresponding colour: each set is kept in a separate locker, and has a separate teacloth for drying.

Each patient has:

A face towel, face flannel and soap.

A back towel, back flannel and soap, the latter being kept separately in a numbered jar over each bed. The back towel has a distinguishing mark and is kept on a separate towel rail on the patient's locker.

Patients are instructed to mop out the bath with lysol 2 per cent before and after use, the bath being cleaned thoroughly once daily by the nurses. Acute cases do not use the bath; they have a blanket bath in bed.

Lavatories. No patient is allowed to sit directly on the lavatory seat; she must take her own bedpan into the lavatory and use it on the seat, afterwards emptying it, mopping it with lysol 2 per cent, and drying it with her own bedpan cover. Pads are put aside in individual bowls for inspection by the sister, and are burnt later.

Blankets, dressing-gown, hot-water bottle covers, etc., are kept for each patient's separate use. They are afterwards sent for fumigation.

After each treatment the treatment table, which is covered with mackintosh, is mopped down with lysol 2 per cent and a fresh paper towel put on. All instruments used are soaked in lysol 2 per cent until they can be thoroughly washed and boiled. All swabs and soiled dressings are deposited in a covered bucket.

Gloves are soaked between treatments in biniodide of mercury (1 in 2,000 concentration), and are dried on a towel kept for that purpose only. They are boiled when finally finished with for the day. Hands are soaked in biniodide of mercury (1 in 4,000 concentration) and dried on a special towel.

Overalls and screens. Separate overalls and screens are kept for syphilitic and gonorrhœal cases, and they are kept in separate places. Nurses wear overalls and gloves for bedmaking and wash between each case.

All soiled bed linen, personal linen, towels, etc., are soaked overnight in formalin (1 in 250 concentration) before going to the laundry. Blankets and other woollens which do not need to be so frequently washed are sent to be fumigated.

Children wear knickers night and day. Pads are only worn when there is a profuse discharge, as the rubbing caused by them is apt to set up an irritation.

Toys. These are kept separate and must be destroyed when finished with if they cannot be fumigated or soaked in disinfectant.

Books. Acute cases are given magazines, etc., which can be destroyed.

Patients' clothes. These are sent home if possible, being fumigated first if necessary. If the patient has no relatives the clothes are fumigated and stored in a parcel.

Hairbrushes and combs, toothbrushes, etc. Patients may bring in their own, or are supplied with individual ones. On discharge, brushes and comb are soaked in disinfectant and then washed. Toothbrushes are destroyed.

No patient is allowed to handle the babies in the ward.

On discharge of patient. All crockery—beatl ware and therefore non boilable—and enamelled ware are soaked in formalin 1 in 250 for twelve hours. Spoons and forks are boiled.

All blankets and mattresses are sent for fumigation. Linen is soaked in formalin (1 in 250 concentration).

INSTRUCTIONS TO PATIENTS SUFFERING FROM SYPHILIS

The Patient

1. Syphilis is a *dangerous* disease; and if not treated promptly, or if wrong treatment is given, disablement or death may result. It can be cured if promptly and systematically treated.

2. Treatment by quacks, herbalists, druggists or persons advertising so-called cures is likely to lead to disastrous results.

3. The disappearance of outward evidence of disease after treatment has begun is not certain evidence that the disease is cured. *Neglect of treatment under these circumstances may be highly dangerous. Treatment should not be stopped until the doctor says that this is safe,* the doctor's instructions should be carefully followed.

4. Treatment need not as a rule interfere with work or necessitate stay in hospital.

5. During treatment the teeth should be cleaned night and morning. If the mouth is not kept clean, treatment may have to be stopped.

The patient should dress warmly, live simply, and avoid wine, beer or spirits. Indulgence in stimulants may seriously interfere with treatment.

6. If for any reason a change of doctor becomes necessary, a note showing what treatment has previously been given should be obtained by the patient from the first doctor and given to the new doctor.

7. If, after treatment has been stopped, rashes on the skin, sore throat, or any other evidence of ill health appears, a doctor should at once be consulted and informed of the previous treatment. *This is extremely important.*

8. After recovery a doctor should be consulted every three months, even though there are no symptoms of a return of the disease.

Risks to Others

9. Syphilis is a contagious disease, and if untreated, or if the right treatment is neglected, may last several years; and during this time the disease may be conveyed to others by sexual intercourse, by kissing, or by using the same eating and drinking utensils, tobacco pipes, etc.

10. The patient's habits should be regulated so as to avoid these dangers. Cleanliness of the hands is essential.

11. Sexual intercourse must be avoided. No one who has or has had syphilis should marry unless a doctor, after going fully into the facts, states that this is safe; otherwise the disease will probably be given to wife or husband and any future children.

INSTRUCTIONS TO PATIENTS SUFFERING FROM GONORRHŒA

The Patient

1. Gonorrhœa is a *dangerous* disease; and if not treated promptly and systematically may lead to serious disablement and may be attended by grave consequences.

2. Treatment by quacks, herbalists, druggists and persons advertising so-called cures is likely to lead to disastrous results.

3. Treatment should be continued until the doctor is satisfied that the disease is cured, and that there is no fear of return of discharge.

4. Treatment need not as a rule interfere with work or necessitate stay in hospital.

5. During treatment condiments must be avoided, and large quantities of simple fluids should be drunk. Indulgence in alcoholic drinks (wine, beer or spirits) seriously interferes with the efficiency of treatment, and often brings back the disease after apparent recovery.

6. Extreme cleanliness is necessary. Care must be taken not to convey any discharge to the eyes by hands or by towels. If this precaution is neglected, acute eye inflammation and blindness may result.

7. The doctor's orders as to the avoidance of chill and as to the amount of exercise allowable in the various stages of the disease must be followed carefully. Horse-riding, cycling, or motor-cycling will hinder recovery.

Risks to Others

8. Gonorrhœa is a *contagious* disease. So long as there is any discharge,

however slight in amount, no matter how long it has lasted, the patient is liable to convey the disease to others.

9. The patient's habits should be regulated to avoid this risk. Cleanliness of the hands is essential. The use of towels, etc., shared by others should be avoided, especially by children.

10. Infection is especially liable to be conveyed by sexual intercourse, and this must therefore be avoided. Under the conditions mentioned in paragraph 8, a man may infect his wife, causing her protracted ill health and suffering. She may become a chronic invalid, and unable to bear children.

REGULATIONS FOR BED OR 'BARRIER' ISOLATION IN CASES OF INFECTIOUS DISEASE IN THE WARDS

(A)—The following regulations apply to any case in which an infectious fever is suspected, but not yet diagnosed; to any infectious disease when diagnosed; and to any other case in which the member of the medical or surgical staff under whom the patient is admitted requires it.

1. In the event of a cot occupying the position next to the bed of a barrier case, the cot should be removed to another part of the ward.

2. Next adjacent to the 'barrier' bed a table should be provided, which is used for the nursing of this case and for no other purpose.

3. On this table there shall be placed:

a. Jug and basin.

b. Soap dish with soap.

c. Bowl of lysol or other prescribed lotion, with scrubbing brush.

d. A towel with a number of other towels folded within it or a number of paper towels.

e. A bowl containing pieces of wool or lint wrung out in mild antiseptic solution.

f. A second bowl, in which these can be thrown when used.

g. A clinical thermometer in a vessel of disinfectant.

4. An empty bucket shall be placed under the table, also a bucket for the reception and disinfection of soiled bed linen.

5. Hanging on the screen shall be two gowns, one for the nurse attending the patient, the other for the doctor or student who needs to examine or dress the patient. In the event of the patient needing two nurses or two doctors, a second gown of each kind must be provided.

6. A special and conspicuous label shall be fixed to the bed, indicating that it is a barrier case.

7. Any person who has occasion to touch the patient or the bed shall, before doing so, put on the gown provided, taking care that the clothes and the forearms are protected by it. When finished he/she shall, after washing, remove the gown and return it to its proper place; then again wash the

ands in the basin on the special table and, finally, deposit the towel in he bucket under the table. When removing the gown, the tapes are first ntied. The arms are shaken free, and the gown folded with the infected ide inside.

8. The end of any stethoscope or other instrument which has touched he patient must be disinfected in the bowl of antiseptic provided.

9. In the event of there being any nasal, aural, oral or vaginal discharge, a piece of the wool or lint mentioned in paragraph 3 must be used for wiping the discharging orifice and be then placed in the empty receiver.

10. The equipment on and under the table mentioned in paragraphs 3 and 4 should be moved or replaced *only* by the nurse in charge of the case, who must wear her gown whilst doing so and must ask someone else to open for her any door through which she may have to pass.

11. All soiled bed linen, towels, etc., must be placed at once in the pail with lid at the bedside, and carried directly from the ward, and not mixed with the rest of the ward linen.

12. Excreta (fæces and urine) from cases of typhoid, paratyphoid, dysentery, cholera and plague must be thoroughly disinfected by appropriate methods, as directed by the physician or surgeon in charge of the case.

13. The nurse must wash, scrub and disinfect her hands after handling utensils for excreta or soiled linen, paying particular attention to the nails.

14. On the discharge or death of a barrier case, soiled bed linen should be disinfected in the ordinary way and all other bedclothes and the mattress should be disinfected by steam or formalin.

15. Food and toilet utensils shall be dealt with in accordance with the instructions under the heading *D*1.

16. In the event of a case needing any surgical dressing, none of the utensils, etc., on or under the special table (paragraph 3) must be used. Everything that is necessary for the dressing must be brought to the bedside in the ordinary way.

17. Rigid surgical technique (aseptic and antiseptic) shall be applied in the dressing of all infected wounds, including cases of erysipelas, whether dressed by a student or a nurse.

18. All those engaged in dressing infected wounds must, for their own protection, be particularly careful of cuts, cracks or other abrasions of their fingers or hands, and it is imperative that gloves should be worn during such dressings.

(*B*)—1. For the prevention of the infection of the members of the medical, surgical, and nursing staff, in attendance on an infectious patient these regulations are, except in a very few cases, amply sufficient, but extra precautions are needed in the following conditions:

Diphtheria. All those attending cases of *diphtheria* are advised to submit

319

to the 'Schick' test, and if necessary receive a prophylactic dose of diphtheria antitoxin or an immunizing dose of toxin plus antitoxin mixture.

Typhoid or paratyphoid or food poisoning. All those liable for the duty
of attending cases of *typhoid* or *paratyphoid* or *food poisoning* are advised
to seek protection by T.A.B. vaccination, repeated every two years.

(*C*)—These regulations shall similarly be applied to the following named
diseases :

1. *Glanders and Plague.* In the event of a patient admitted to one of the
wards being found to be suffering from one of these diseases, 'bed isolation'
shall be instituted forthwith and an application at once be made to the
medical superintendent for a room to be prepared to which the patient can
be moved.

2. *Acute syphilis.* 'Bed isolation' shall be applied to any cases of acute
syphilis which may happen to be admitted to the general wards. (Bed
isolation is unnecessary for cases suffering from late results of syphilis
such as are usually admitted.)

3. *Vulvo-vaginitis in childhood.*

4. *Dysentery, cholera, and zymotic diarrhœa.*

5. *Cerebro-Spinal (spotted) fever.*

6. *Encephalitis lethargica acuta.*

(*D*)—1. In cases of *pneumonia, tuberculosis of the respiratory tract* and
open cancer a separate set of utensils for feeding and washing shall be
provided for each case; all mugs and crockery shall be marked in a dis-
tinctive way. These various articles, together with separate glass cloths for
the use of the patient are kept, when not in use, in a separate cupboard
or on a separate table. Immediately any of the utensils have been used by
the patient it/they shall be transferred to the patient's own disinfecting
bowl, where it/they shall be immersed in 2 per cent lysol for, say, fifteen
minutes before being washed in very hot water and dried with the patient's
own glass cloth. If a special sterilizer is available it is simpler to boil
crockery after each meal.

2. Cases of *rectal cancer* shall be provided each with its own bedpan
marked and treated in a precisely similar fashion to that indicated under *D*1

(*E*)—Bed isolation is unnecessary in the following diseases :

a. Typhus. Immediately on admission the patient must be freed from
lice by shaving and washing.

b. Anthrax. In the ordinary surgical cases the precautions under paragraphs 17 and 18 of Bed Isolation Regulations.

If, and when, the patient becomes septic the case comes under the
category of *C*2.

c. Leprosy. It should be possible to admit a case into any ward, subject
to the precautions mentioned in paragraphs 17 and 18 of the Bed Isolation
Regulations.

Chapter Nineteen

AN APPROACH TO PSYCHIATRIC NURSING

Psychology is the study of mental life. It is the science which investigates how the mind functions. A good nurse studies the mental reactions of her patients and adapts her management and treatment accordingly. This 'applied psychology' as it is called, is largely common sense and sympathy. All of us use psychology unconsciously in dealing with other people, but a study of the science helps us to understand more thoroughly the working of the mind and therefore adds to our inborn psychological gifts.

Medical psychology or psychiatry is the study of *mental disorders*. These fall into two main groups:

1. The Neuroses

Physical illness can be caused, aggravated and prolonged by psychological factors. Every observant nurse will find that the same type of illness has often a different appearance in different patients. Examples:

(a) Two patients may suffer from the same form of cardiac failure; the one works in spite of it until the last minute, while the other comes to hospital in a much earlier stage of the illness, having stopped work before he broke down. This may be due to differences in what is called 'personality make-up', the latter patient being more sensitive and less robust than the former. The robust patient recovers quickly, whilst the more sensitive one lingers on and has difficulty in returning to normal life.

(b) Two patients have the same kind of head injury. One returns to work after a fortnight whilst the other is still an invalid and complains of headaches and giddiness months later. Here again the difference may be explained by differences in psychological and social factors. On closer inquiry it may be found that the latter has an unhappy married life and dreads returning to it, or that he is unemployed and hopes for compensation money, or that he has other social or economic troubles.

Psychological factors of this kind are easily understood and it is obvious that a nurse who thinks of them can do a great deal in helping to discover and overcome them.

When a person is spoken of as neurotic the untrained nurse is inclined to assume that whatever the symptoms complained of, the person is 'putting it on' and all that is required is that he should 'pull himself together' and exert his will in an effort to forget himself and get on with

x   321

his work. But to the specialist in mental illness a neurosis means much more than this.

First and foremost, there is no question of the patient consciously complaining of symptoms which do not exist. If he says he has a pain, the pain is there; if he says he cannot see, or that his legs are paralysed, it is a fact that these organs are not functioning at all or that their function is impaired.

If the organ concerned is examined clinically, however, it is found to be normal; no disease process, such as inflammation or ulcer or pressure from tumour, can be detected. The condition thus resolves itself into a *functional* disorder; that is to say, that although the organ itself is normal, the patient has lost the idea of its function, as in the case of blindness or paralysis. These two symptoms are not commonly met as neuroses. It is much more usual for a patient to complain of more ordinary symptoms, i.e. headache, palpitation, indigestion, irritation of the skin. The same explanation holds good; the heart is examined and found to be sound, no ulcer or gastritis can be detected, nor are the common causes of skin irritation found to be responsible.

The relationship between the mind and the body is so close that fear or worry can upset the function of any organ in the body, and it cannot be too strongly emphasized that it is not that the patient only imagines the function is upset, it actually is upset, e.g. fear can derange gastric secretions, upset cardiac rhythm, cause diarrhœa, frequency of micturition, and innumerable other symptoms. Fear can cause such symptoms in normal individuals. *In the neurotic some mental conflict is prolonging them.*

The symptoms of other neuroses, are themselves psychological, i.e. attacks of fear and anxiety, loss of memory, inability to concentrate, mental depression, or certain ideas and impulses. Many of these symptoms are present in mild degree in healthy people and are insignificant as long as they do not disturb normal work and a happy life. Only if they become so severe that the patient and his environment suffer as a result of his abnormalities does one speak of a 'neurosis'. Then he may be said to have a mental breakdown and the problem of the psychiatrist is to discover the cause.

It is not always necessary for the patient to have hospital treatment, but the more severe forms of neurosis benefit by change of environment and intensive and sympathetic treatment. The shrewd observant nurse can be of great help to the psychiatrist in his task of assisting the patient in his readjustment and the tackling of his difficulties.

The *neuroses* are commonly divided into four groups.

(a) Anxiety states (exhibiting themselves in such symptoms as palpitation, diarrhœa, pallor, sweating, extreme nervousness, frequency of micturition).

(b) Hysteria (exhibited in such symptoms as loss of voice, vomiting, muscular twitchings, paralysis).

(c) Obsessions (phobias and fears).

(d) Psychoneurotic depression.

The *methods of psycho-therapy* in use are:

1. *Persuasion and suggestion.* A detailed history of the patient's life is obtained by the psychiatrist. Any phase of it which might appear to throw light on the symptoms is discussed fully. The patient thus may be brought to realize his own state of mind and by gaining a clear insight into his symptoms and their origin may rid himself of his complaints.

2. *Psycho-analysis.* This is the name given to the form of psycho-therapy devised by Freud and his followers and is a deep method of analysis which may take months or years to accomplish. It is not usually a hospital treatment. The method of 'free association' is used, i.e. the patient expresses freely whatever thoughts follow each other in his mind. Much use is also made of the interpretation of the patient's dreams.

3. *Hypnosis.* This is carried out for certain cases of hysteria. The patient is put into a trance, that is, his conscious mind is put to sleep, and he submits to the stronger will of the psychiatrist. The subconscious mind of the patient is then contacted and exposed to the influence of the therapist who can, by the force of suggestion, influence the patient's symptoms.

4. *Narco-hypnosis.* This is induced by the injection of a hypnotic drug, e.g. pentothal. The technique of influencing the subconscious mind is the same.

By one of these methods the patient is made to understand the conflict in his own mind and its results in his daily life. As soon as this is done he is on the way to recovery. Needless to say, the patient must be co-operative and anxious to recover.

An understanding of these conditions by the nurse will show her at once the importance of a sympathetic attitude, combined with a measure of firm reasonableness, which may influence the patient's general morale. Also, as these patients are often of the introspective type (and indeed their treatment often necessitates their being so) the general routine of their life should be so organized as to counteract this tendency. It is essential that the general health should be maintained by a regular and full diet, that all minor disorders, e.g. constipation, septic teeth, etc., should be corrected and that the patients should be kept active and interested by occupational therapy, games, intellectual discussions and lectures, etc. No small part of the nurse's work is to keep her patients healthily occupied so that they feel their days are full and worth while.

2. The Psychoses

There is no hard and fast line between the neuroses and the psychoses, but on the whole the psychoses are mental illnesses of a more severe type. In the early stages symptoms often appear similar to those of the neuroses and are therefore not diagnosed, and so the case progresses until it is too late for effective treatment. The patient's mind becomes confused and his personality changes. For example, he may become suspicious, violent, melancholic or extravagant. The *psychoses* may be divided into the following:

1. *Manic-Depressive Psychosis.* This includes:

(a) *Mania.* A condition in which the patient is over-active, excitable, and over-talkative. His ideas follow each other in a rapid flight and he may become extremely restless and difficult to control. He frequently has delusions of grandeur and an aggressive manner.

(b) *Melancholia.* A condition in which the patient is depressed, slow in thought and action (i.e. retarded), and frequently has delusions of unworthiness, self-reproach, etc. These patients are often suicidal. These two illnesses frequently alternate in the same patient during his lifetime, hence the term 'manic-depressive psychosis'. The prognosis is good, but for the marked tendency to relapse.

2. *Schizophrenia.* This is the most frequent form of psychosis. It is a severe form of mental illness usually occurring in the younger age group of patients. It may come on gradually or quite suddenly and the symptoms are too numerous and varied to be described here. It must be sufficient to say that the word itself means a 'splitting of the mind' and in extreme cases the patient lives in a world of his own, having withdrawn himself from the world of reality until his fantasies have become more real to him than his own surroundings. This may result in such gross symptoms as delusions, hallucinations, and disorientation.

3. *Changes in personality* due to organic disease of the brain, e.g. tumours, general paralysis of the insane, alcoholic degeneration resulting in delirium tremens, and senile arterio-sclerotic conditions.

Mental deficiency. This is not a psychosis in that it is not an acquired condition. It is due to a failure of cerebral development before or soon after birth as a result of disease, injury or hereditary defect. Mental deficiency has many degrees from mere dullness to complete idiocy. Only those who are stranded in life through their intellectual defect need medical care. These patients are treated in special institutions.

Treatment of the Psychoses. It can easily be understood that the management of psychotic patients is the most important part in the nursing care. Tact, patience, and a great measure of understanding is required. The last can only be gained by living amongst the patients and observing them carefully. No text-book can teach it.

Occupational and recreational therapies are probably the most generally useful forms of treatment for the psychoses as well as for the neuroses, and modern mental hospitals have specially trained exponents of these treatments. The re-adaptation and rehabilitation of the patient should be the main concern of the nursing staff. The regular administration of sedative drugs may be required in the early stages, e.g. bromide, chloral and the various barbiturates, especially in cases where sleepnessness is a prominent symptom. Special methods of treatment may be given in certain cases, e.g.:

(a) *Continuous Narcosis*. The object of this treatment is to keep the patient asleep for 20—22 hours out of 24 for a period of 10—14 days. The technique varies, but the usual procedure is to give 2 c.c.s of somnifaine twice or three times daily, and in addition two drachms of paraldehyde four hourly s.o.s. The patient is able to be roused sufficiently for feeding and nursing treatment. Great care is required in the nursing of these patients and special attention must be paid to the diet and temperature and to the bowels and urine.

(b) *Convulsive treatment*. This consists of the production of epileptic fits, which may be induced either by intravenous injections of a convulsant drug, e.g. cardiazol, or by electrical stimulation of the brain. This latter method is most generally used as it is the least unpleasant for the patient. In certain cases it may be given to out-patients. The number of fits given varies according to the patient's condition, but anything between six and twelve is an average number and they are usually given two or three times weekly.

(c) *Insulin treatment*. The patient is given a sufficient dose of insulin to induce a hypoglycæmic coma which lasts for 1—2 hours. After this time he is brought round by glucose given intranasally or in some cases intravenously. When the treatment is over there should be no undesirable after affects. The patient gets up, dresses, has his meal and joins in the day's routine and activities. It is particularly important that he should eat his full meals during the rest of the day to avoid the possibility of uncontrolled hypoglycæmia. This treatment is given six days a week for three months, the ultimate number of comas induced in one patient being approximately sixty.

(d) *Leucotomy*. This operation aims at cutting the white matter of the frontal lobes of the brain in such a way as to divide the frontal thalamic association fibres.

The nursing of acute psychotic patients is not easy. The staffing of the ward presents special problems to ensure that there are sufficient nursing attendants, not only to control the patients, but to observe them in every detail. The patient must be safeguarded from hurting himself by the removal of furniture and any breakable or harmful articles. The windows should be shuttered and the lights well out of reach. It may be necessary to fit bed boards to the sides of the bed, or more often to put the mattress on the floor. Sheets of specially strong material are required so that the patient cannot tear them. It is obvious that a patient in such a restless condition cannot be nursed in a general ward but must be in a private room. Restraint is usually inadvisable and makes the patient worse. It must not be applied without medical instruction. The nurses and attendants must be very alert and inquire into the meaning of any unusual noise or happening in the ward. Many a disaster may be saved by the alertness of the nursing staff especially when patients have suicidal tendencies.

It is essential that a suicidal patient should never be left, even for an instant, for any cause whatever. The nurse should not leave the patient to attend to any visitor or member of the staff entering the ward; nor must she allow her attention to be distracted by any other happenings in the ward. If there are two patients of this type being cared for by one nurse, there *must* be a second nurse within call. The sister in charge of the ward must be quite certain that every member of the staff is aware that the patient has suicidal tendencies. In mental hospitals, it is customary for each nurse and attendant to sign his or her name on a special form issued and signed by the medical officer stating that the patient has suicidal tendencies.

Every observation of the behaviour of the patient is worth note and the experienced observer learns to know which are the reactions to be expected in the different types of case and which are new developments. The shrewd and careful nurse is an important member of the team of workers who are trying to improve the mental state of these patients.

The ordinary daily nursing care of psychotic patients who are confined to bed depends upon their condition. For instance, the patient should be bathed when he is in an amenable and docile frame of mind. The routine of meals must be kept as far as possible in order to maintain the patient's strength, but in intervals of extreme restlessness it is often unwise to attempt feeding and a meal must be specially prepared when the time is more opportune. It is an invariable rule that the temperature must be taken in the axilla and there must be no departure from this, even in apparently normal cases. If hypodermic injections have to be given a fairly strong needle should be used to avoid it being broken. An injection should never be given without adequate assistance in controlling the patient. The same applies to any treatment which the patient is likely to resist, e.g. giving of medicines, enemas, etc. Tube feeding is often necessary for difficult patients. It is usually done by the doctor, or by an experienced sister, again having adequate assistance. The safeguarding of keys is of great importance to avoid the patient gaining access to drugs or other articles, e.g. instruments, by which he might do himself harm.

The nurse has a special responsibility in looking after the patient's personal possessions, not only taking away from him sharp and harmful objects, but also in looking after his more valuable property, e.g. money, watch, fountain pen, cigarette case, etc., until he is in a fit state to look after them himself. Explanations and answers to inquiries from the patient's relatives are never given by the nursing staff, except after explicit directions from the doctor. The nurse must be very careful not to commit herself by any vague or hazardous comment on the patient's condition. If she is in doubt should always refer the relatives to the doctor himself. Finally, not only must the nurse dealing with cases of mental illness he able to cope with the patient himself, but in a general ward particularly, she must be able to control the talk and gossip of the other patients. Thus she will try to avoid an atmosphere which would do further harm to the patient's condition.

Psychiatric treatment and nursing are but at the beginning of their development and the keenest and best type of nurse is undoubtedly needed.

Chapter Twenty

RADIO THERAPEUTICS

RADIUM

Radium was first discovered by Monsieur and Madame Curie in 1895, who, after many months of research, extracted it from a uranium ore called pitchblende, which is largely found in the Belgian Congo and a little in South America and Cornwall. About 150 tons of pitchblende produces half an ounce of radium. It is because of the great difficulty of extraction that it is so extremely expensive. Before the present world conflict the price was about £12,000 to £15,000 per gramme (30 grammes=1 ounce). In 1901, M. Henri Becquerel, whilst carrying out experiments on radio-active substances, accidentally discovered that radium produced an inflammatory reaction on the skin. He had been carrying a specimen in his waistcoat pocket and found that an area of skin, exactly corresponding to the pocket in which he carried the uranium, became inflamed and eventually ulcerated. The ulcer took several weeks to heal.

Radium is described as being a radio-active substance, spontaneously, without any known chemical change, giving off rays, and, at the same time, it undergoes a process of atomic disintegration, so that eventually, after 3,380 years, it becomes a non-active substance, i.e. lead. The half value period is 1,690 years. It is an extraordinary fact that the product of the first process of disintegration is a radio-active gas, or emanation, called Radon, and this may be collected and used for treating certain conditions.

Radium gives off three definite groups of rays which differ in nature, wavelength, and penetrating power. The second group is about one hundred times more penetrating than the first, and the third one hundred times more penetrating than the second.

These groups are called the alpha (α), beta (β), and gamma (γ) rays, respectively.

The alpha rays have very little penetrating power; in fact, they are absorbed by a sheet of paper or a few centimetres of air and are therefore of no use therapeutically.

The beta rays are more penetrating than the alpha, but are absorbed or stopped by 1 mm. of aluminium. They are of very little use therapeutically. Ninety-nine per cent of beta rays are stopped by the use of filters placed between the radium and the part being treated.

METHODS OF APPLICATION OF RADIUM

The gamma rays. These form the most important group of radiations from radium. They are very similar to X-rays but are of a much shorter wavelength and therefore of greater penetrating power than any X-rays which have yet been produced. Six inches of lead are needed to stop or absorb the gamma rays. When gamma rays strike metal substances a secondary radiation is given off from the substance. This radiation is of less penetrating power than the gamma radiation and may, in consequence, be harmful to the skin. On this account it is extremely important not to place any metal, for example, safety pins, between or near the radium and the part being treated. Also for this reason metallic ointments and lotions are never used in association with treatment by radium.

METHODS OF APPLICATION OF RADIUM

For therapeutic purposes the salt, radium sulphate, is used. It is insoluble in water, and in appearance resembles a white powder rather like bismuth. It is measured in milligrammes or grammes. There are three universal types of container used—needles, tubes, and plaques—and the amount and intensity of the radium radiations depends on the amount of radium in the container, the amount of time of application (length of exposure) and the amount of filtration provided by the walls of the container and the distance between the radium and the part being treated. The actual dose is measured in milligramme hours: e.g. 200 milligrammes of radium applied for 12 hours equals a dose of 2,400 milligramme hours.

Needles. These are small containers, usually made of platinum iridium, with walls usually 0.3 to 3 m.m. thick. They consist of a central hollow chamber for the reception of the salt, at one end of which is an eyelet and at the other a point which is soldered to the chamber with gold. Gold is used because of its high melting point. This is the weakest point of the needle. Needles contain from 8 to 25 milligrammes of radium sulphate. Each needle is marked with a registration number and a number denoting the amount of radium in the needle.

Methods of use. Needles may be used for either interstitial or surface application. The interstitial or implantation method consists of first sterilizing the needle by boiling, and then actually introducing the needles into the tissues by means of a specially constructed introducer. Before

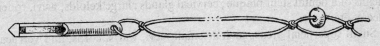

Fig. 108. Radium needle with thread and bead attached

sterilization, a thread is placed in the eyelet of the needle with the free ends tied to a coloured bead. Different coloured beads are used for different strength needles. The ends of the threads with the beads attache are always left outside the dressing. Thus an accurate check on the numbe of needles and the amount of radium used may be made frequently durin the treatment, without disturbing the dressing.

The actual amount of radium used and the length of time of applicatio are prescribed by the medical officer in charge of the case. The sister i charge of the radium department then prepares and sterilizes the needle in accordance with his prescription. She is always present in the operatin theatre when radium is implanted.

Cases treated by the interstitial method are carcinoma mammæ, car cinoma of the mouth; carcinoma of the cervix and rodent ulcer.

Surface application of needles. In this method special substances ar used which can be moulded to the shape of the area being treated, afte which the needles are placed in the mould or plaque. The two chief sub stances used are columbia wax and dental stent. Columbia wax consists o beeswax, paraffin, and sawdust. Before use it is hard, but it may be softened by manipulation in warm water and then moulded to the shape required Different thicknesses of wax or dental stent may be obtained so that the intensity of radiation may be varied by this means. The needles are secured to the wax by first heating them in a bunsen flame and then placing them on the surface of the wax. They are then covered by a thin layer of melted wax. Finally, after all the needles have been placed in their required positions, the whole plaque is covered by rubber adhesive strapping, which prevents loss of needles during treatment. The finished plaque may be fixed to the patient by tapes and a firm bandage.

The patient must remain in bed during treatment. The great advantage of this method of application is that at intervals the plaque may be removed and the patient allowed up. A strict account of time and the number of hours when the plaque is actually in position must be kept. When the plaque is removed it is very important that it should be replaced in exactly the same position so that the area thus obtains its final full amount of radiation. To facilitate this, the area of skin may be marked with an indelible pencil or gentian violet.

Cases treated by this method are carcinoma mammæ, post-operatively, as a prophylactic treatment to the affected area, including the axillary and supraclavicular and subclavicular glands; carcinoma of the mouth, by means of a dental stent plaque; cervical glands; large keloids, nævi, rodent ulcers, etc.

Small superficial areas, such as small nævi, warts, corns, and verrucas, may be treated by attaching needles to the adhesive side of rubber strapping and placing the strapping on the area. Filtration of the rays may be made by means of layers of lint or wool or gutta-percha tissue, placed between the radium and the skin. Such treatment may be carried out in an out-patient department because each application lasts usually only up to two hours.

Tubes. These are similar to needles, except that they have no points. They may be put into specially shaped containers designed for treating carcinoma of cervix and uterus; carcinoma of the rectum and œsophagus.

Plaques. Special small containers made of platinum, gold or silver are used for surface application. These universal types contain full strength, 10 milligrammes of radium sulphate; half strength 5 milligrammes; double strength 20 milligrammes. They may be round, square or oblong. They are usually about an inch in diameter and on one side there is a screw for manipulation of the plaque with forceps.

Radium Bomb Therapy. Five to eight grammes of radium sulphate are sometimes enclosed in a special applicator called a 'radium bomb' which is kept in a special department to which the patients go for treatment.

Precautions to be taken to Guard against Loss of Radium

1. The beds of radium patients need very careful placing and spacing, so that they are not too near others; usually a corner bed in the ward is chosen.

2. Patients must be kept in bed all the time during treatment.

3. While the radium is in position the bed linen must be kept separately, dressings are not thrown away, but put in a special bucket kept for the purpose, until the radium is taken out, checked and returned to the department. The ward sweepings are kept in a special bin in the same way.

4. If a radium needle or applicator should come out of its position during treatment, it is at once placed in a special lead-lined box kept for the purpose. A note is made of the patient's name, the date, and the exact time of the removal of the radium. The sister-in-charge should be informed.

Reactions to be Expected in Patients undergoing Treatment

1. *Constitutional.* General lassitude and malaise, loss of appetite; loss of sense of taste if the mouth is being treated. In advanced cases, toxic reaction with severe vomiting and collapse.

2. *Local reactions* (1) Erythema (reddening of the skin).

(2) Radio-dermatitis, i.e. inflammation of the skin followed by desquamation and pigmentation.

(3) Radio-necrosis, i.e. death of the tissues with ulceration.

The degree of the reaction depends on the dose prescribed and the aim of the radiologist; usually a second degree reaction is desired.

CARE OF PATIENTS UNDERGOING TREATMENT

1. *General treatment.* Rest in bed; record the temperature, pulse, and

respirations four-hourly; give a light nourishing diet. If vomiting is troublesome, give plenty of glucose.

The aim of treatment is to build up the general resistance of the patient to counteract the general deleterious effects of the radium.

Whenever treatment is suspended for a time, the patient should be encouraged to get up and mix with the others in the ward. This helps to counteract the depression caused by the radium radiations.

2. *Local treatment.* As already mentioned, no metallic preparations must come in contact with the area being treated, either in the form of ointments, lotions or mouthwashes. This precludes the use of mercurial preparations, so commonly used in surgical wards. It is always safe to use distilled water, glycothymoline, saline, boracic lotion, etc., and if ointments are required lard or lanoline may be used.

The area being treated must not be put in hot water for about six weeks after treatment, and during treatment it should not be washed with soap and water. There is no objection to the patient taking warm baths; the aim being to avoid further irritation to an area which is already in the process of inflammation.

If cavities, e.g. the uterus, have been treated, it is not unusual to get an increased amount of discharge due to the inflammatory reaction. This should be noted and reported.

Precautions to be taken by Workers with Radium

1. Radium must never be handled by the fingers. Special radium holding forceps, with rubber covered handles, are supplied.

2. Radium is carried in lead-lined boxes attached to long handles, so that they just swing clear of the ground. Thus the radiations cannot reach the body of the person carrying it. The box should be swung as it is being carried.

3. When handling radium the worker should always stand behind a special lead screen, which protects the front of the body and the fore-arms.

4. Work should be done as quickly as possible.

5. Blood counts are made at monthly intervals.

6. Strict routine for duty is necessary. A maximum of a thirty-five hour week; a month's holiday a year, preferably consecutive. The workers are not allowed to work in other departments.

7. For those nursing the patients in the ward there is no danger as the patients only have small amounts of radium implanted, but they also should not linger round the patient longer than necessary.

Cleaning of Radium Needles. Needles which have been implanted are put into 2 per cent lysol or carbolic 1—20 (never mercury). Afterwards they are cleaned and boiled before reinsertion. The loss of any needle must be reported at once, not only on account of its value, but because of the

FIG. 109. Nurse working
with radium behind lead
screen

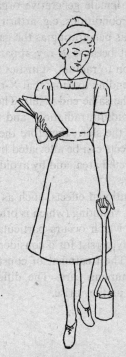

FIG. 110. Nurse carrying
radium in lead-lined box

danger of its radiations. The needles must be handled carefully and not be scratched; even slight damage to the needle causes some alteration of the dosage.

X-RAY THERAPEUTICS

X-rays are radiations similar in nature to the gamma rays of radium. They are produced by electro-mechanical means and rays of a wide range and penetrating power are obtainable. Rays which are of long wavelength and hence comparatively little penetrating power are used in diagnostic work, and the rays of short wavelength, which possess great penetrating power, are utilized in deep X-ray therapy.

There are three main groups of therapeutic X-radiations:

1. **Superficial Therapy** in which the rays have little penetrating power and which are used for superficial skin conditions such as ringworm, especially of the scalp; plantar warts; sycosis; nævi and keloids, etc.

2. **Medium or Contact Therapy,** sometimes referred to as Chaul therapy.

3. **Deep Therapy** in which the rays have great penetrating power, and which are used for deep-seated lesions, for example, carcinoma of the

lungs and female generative organs; Hodgkin's disease; and some non-malignant conditions, e.g. arthritis.

X-rays as penetrating as the gamma rays of radium have yet to be produced, but because X-ray apparatus is comparatively easy to obtain in comparison to radium, statistics are being gathered by research units and they are tending to show that X-rays and radium given in the same dosage produce the same end result. The effects of X-radiations are the same as those of radium radiations and so are the constitutional effects and the effects on the skin; therefore the same nursing care is required.

Skin effects can be alleviated by the application of pure lard or lanoline to the affected area, and by avoiding further irritation, e.g. the use of soap and water.

Constitutional effects, such as malaise, depression, rise in temperature and pulse, vomiting (which is often serious), loss of appetite, loss of taste; the latter which occurs particularly in treatment of areas of the buccal cavity, may persist for a considerable time after treatment, but eventually subsides. The treatment of constitutional effects is rest in bed and sympathetic nursing care. The different symptoms are treated on general principles as they arise.

Chapter Twenty-One

PREPARATION FOR X-RAY

Preparing Patient for Diagnostic X-ray. The patient must be warmly wrapped up and should be clothed in a cotton or woollen garment, not silk or artificial silk, and any safety pins should be removed, if possible. Patients unable to walk should be sent on a stretcher so that they can be lifted straight on to the X-ray table and sufficient pillows to make them comfortable should be sent with them. A rug is placed on the trolley before the patient is lifted on to it on her stretcher canvas or sheet.

Mercurial ointments, lotio plumbi, zinc preparations or strapping should be removed from the site to be X-rayed before the patient leaves the ward. If, however, the strapping is there to immobilize a part, such as for fractured ribs, it should not be removed without permission. Splints are not removed in the ward, but in some cases, with permission, they are taken off by the radiographer just before the examination. The nurse always accompanies the patient to the X-ray department and should help the radiographer to place her in position. Any previous X-ray films should be taken to the department at the same time. Wherever possible, appointments are made and the nurse should see that the patient arrives at the right time. X-ray examinations are expensive and are never done unless ordered by a house officer or other doctor. The patient should be reassured, as if she is very nervous and trembles the film may be spoilt.

Preparation for Special X-ray Examinations. It is essential that the instructions regarding X-ray preparations should be carried out. These are usually written on a slip and sent to the ward. For all abdominal regions examined, the bowel and rectum should be empty of fæces and gas, as these appear on the film and may obscure structures which should be demonstrated.

Alimentary Tract. Barium sulphate powder, which is opaque to X-rays, is mixed into an emulsion and used for all examination of the alimentary tract.

Œsophagus. No special preparation is necessary, except that the patient should have nothing to eat or drink for an hour before she is sent for examination.

Stomach and duodenum. The patient has nothing to eat or drink for six hours before the examination as the normal emptying time of these organs is from four to six hours. No aperient is given for twenty-four hours beforehand, and no bismuth preparations for forty-eight hours before, as bismuth is opaque to X-rays. A pint of barium emulsion is given when the patient reaches the X-ray department and the passage of the emulsion is watched by the radiologist during screening. This X-ray is done to demonstrate abnormality in the outline of the stomach. If delay in emptying the stomach is present the patient may be re-examined at various intervals after giving the barium meal. In such a case food or fluids should be withheld until the examination is completed.

Small intestine. The small intestine is examined at various intervals after the barium meal. The previous preparation is as for examination of the stomach. In this case, after the barium meal has been given the patient may have her usual diet but no aperient should be given until the examination is completed.

In cases when the small intestine only is being examined the nurse gives the pint of barium, and, at a specified time some hours later, for example, six, twelve, twenty-four, forty-eight, etc., the patient is examined under X-rays.

Appendix (e.g. for examination on Friday morning). On Tuesday and Wednesday nights a vegetable aperient is given, thus allowing at least thirty-six hours' interval before the examination. One pint of barium emulsion is given six to eight hours before X-ray examination and the patient may have ordinary diet. Occasionally the patient is re-examined twenty-four or forty-eight hours later, in which case no aperient should be given until the examination is completed, but the patient may continue to have ordinary diet.

Large intestine (e.g. for examination on Friday morning). Two vegetable laxative pills—saline aperients are not used as they tend to produce gas—are given on Tuesday and Wednesday nights. Colonic lavage is done at least six hours before the examination, so that the colon is clear of fæcal matter. During the examination two to three pints of barium emulsion at a temperature of 98° to 99° F. are given by rectal tube either by the radiographer or nurse with the patient in the dorsal position. The patient is then screened. The passage of the emulsion through the large intestine is seen on the screen as it runs in.

After an alimentary X-ray is completed the patient is given an aperient to which she is accustomed, to facilitate the excretion of the barium.

Chest X-ray. No special preparation is required for a 'straight' chest X-ray.

Bronchography. To demonstrate abnormalities of the bronchial tree. No previous preparation is required, but the nurse should take to the X-ray room the following:

1. Twenty c.c. lipiodol syringe with blunt-end cannula or rubber tubing.
2. Local anæsthetic tray containing cocaine 10 per cent, dessicaine 5 per

ent or cocaine ointment; throat spray and throat brush; wool swabs; int squares, tongue spatula; nasal catheter.

3. Vomit bowl and cloth.

4. Lipiodol, neohydriol or iodatol (sometimes supplied in the department).

The dye should be stood in warm water and heated to body temperature before being used.

The patient is turned on to the affected side while the dye is introduced. After she has returned to the ward no food or drink is given for two hours, or until the effects of the local anæsthetic make swallowing quite safe. The patient may cough up a little of the lipiodol, which is a preparation of iodine in poppy-seed oil, but most of it is absorbed with beneficial rather than harmful effects.

Renal X-ray. X-ray examination of the renal tract is divided into preliminary examination and examination after the introduction of an opaque dye, either by intravenous or retrograde method. The preliminary X-ray is called a 'straight' X-ray.

Preparation (e.g. for examination Friday morning). A vegetable aperient is given on Tuesday and Wednesday night. A light non-residue forming diet should be given for at least forty-eight hours previous to examination. If possible the patient should be encouraged to take exercise by walking about the ward to help the elimination of gas from the intestines. No starvation before the examination is required. In certain cases it may be necessary to give gas-eliminating preparations such as pitressin, $\frac{1}{2}$ to 1 c.c., a half to two hours before the examination; or charcoal biscuits, every two hours for twenty-four hours beforehand.

Intravenous pyelography. The preparation is as described above, but no fluids should be given for twelve hours before the examination, otherwise ordinary diet is taken. Just before the patient goes to X-ray she should be instructed to empty her bladder. The examination is carried out after a 'straight' X-ray has been taken. Then a sterile preparation of iodine, supplied in 20 c.c. ampoules under the trade names of Uropac, Uroselectan, Pyelectan, etc., is introduced into the median basilic vein in the arm. The *following requirements* for the injection are sent from the ward:

1. Mackintosh and receiver.
2. Sterile sponges and sterile towels.
3. Skin-cleaning materials (iodine, ether, or methylated spirit).
4. Sterile 20 c.c. syringe and intravenous needles.
5. Distilled water.
6. Two sterile kidney dishes and sterile gallipots.
7. Bandage. The phial of Uropac is usually supplied by the Department.

Films are taken at various intervals after the injection, e.g. three, eight, or fifteen minutes, the times according to the instructions of the radiologist

in charge. If the patient is sent back to the ward before the examination i
completed, e.g. a woman suffering from hydronephrosis, she should b
instructed not to empty the bladder until after the examination is com
pleted.

The examination is carried out to demonstrate the function of th
kidneys.

N.B. Toxic effects are produced by uroselectan or other dye being intro
duced into the tissues instead of into a vein. In severe cases abscess forma
tion or even gangrene may result. If there is any question of dye being ir
the tissues, heat in the form of antiphlogistine or hot boracic fomentation;
should be applied immediately.

Retrograde pyelography. Retrograde pyelography is done in conjunction
with cystoscopy under light anæsthesia, for which the usual preparation
will have been carried out. Radio-opaque catheters are inserted into the
ureters and a preliminary film is taken to see that the catheters are in
position. A 10 or 20 per cent solution of sodium iodide or sodium bromide,
freshly prepared by the hospital dispensary, is injected through the catheters by means of a syringe. Ten to twenty c.c. are usually injected until the
patient—if conscious—complains of discomfort. Further films are taken
after the injection. This method demonstrates the outline of the calices and
pelves of the kidneys, but not the function. The patency of the ureters may
be demonstrated at the same examination.

Cystography. Patient prepared as for cystoscopy. The bladder is completely emptied by catheterization in the X-ray department. Ten c.c. of
20 per cent sodium bromide or iodide is injected. The examination is
carried out to demonstrate the size and outline of the bladder.

Urethrography. No previous preparation is necessary. The urethra is
filled with the solution of sodium bromide or iodide by means of a catheter
or syringe and cannula. It is carried out to demonstrate strictures or injury.

Cholecystography. X-ray examination of the gall bladder. It is carried
out either by straight X-ray or the introduction of an opaque dye, tetraiodophenolphthalein, which is supplied to be used either as an oral or intravenous preparation. The trade names for oral preparations are opacol
and shadocol; for intravenous injection, opacin.

'*Straight*' *X-ray examination* is carried out to demonstrate calculi, and
is done in all cases before further examinations with dyes. The preparation
is again the same as for an X-ray of the renal tract, e.g. two aperients being
given on Tuesday and Wednesday nights for examination on Friday. The
patient may have an ordinary diet.

Oral method of cholecystography is carried out to demonstrate function.
The patient should have a fat-free meal at 5.30 the evening before the
examination, and at 7.30 p.m.—that is, two hours later—the opacol, which
is a blue powder, is mixed in a wineglass of cold water until it turns white,

and the patient drinks it all. The patient may sip a glass of cold water an hour after taking the dye, otherwise, nothing to eat or drink should be given until the examination takes place fourteen hours later. If the X-ray shows that the dye is concentrated in the gall bladder, a fat meal should be given and the patient is re-examined a half to two hours later. (A fatty meal consists of a glass of milk, bread and butter and an egg. Milky tea may be substituted in place of whole milk.) This further X-ray is taken to see if the gall bladder empties itself as a reaction to the stimulus of fat in the duodenum.

Intravenous cholecystography. A sterile intravenous preparation of tetraiodophenolphthalein, supplied under the trade name of opacin, is used (30 c.c. containing 3.5 grammes of the dye).

This intravenous method is usually done when the oral method has failed to produce a concentration of dye in the gall bladder. Although it is a more satisfactory X-ray examination, it is not a usual method because the dye unless it is injected very carefully may give rise to severe toxic local reaction.

The patient is prepared for a preliminary film as for the oral method then the dye is injected into the median basilic vein in the elbow. Nothing to eat or drink is given until the patient is re-X-rayed six hours later, If, at this examination, there is a satisfactory shadow of the gall bladder filled with dye, the patient is given a fatty meal and further films are taken half to one hour after the meal. If the gall bladder has not filled, however, no food is given but the patient is X-rayed two hours later, that is, eight hours after injection.

Children. Two-thirds of the full quantity is given between the ages of ten to fourteen years. For children less than ten years, one-third to one-half of the full dose is prescribed. This applies to both the oral and intravenous preparation.

Salpingography. An examination carried out to demonstrate the outline of the uterus and the patency of the fallopian tubes. A sterile preparation of 40 per cent iodine in poppy seed oil, supplied under the trade names of lipiodol and neohydriol, is used for the examination. The usual gynæcological preparation is carried out (enema, catheterization, douche, etc.). The patient is placed in the lithotomy position, or left lateral, and the dye is introduced by means of a catheter and syringe with the aid of a speculum. The introduction of the dye is made in the X-ray department as the films must be taken immediately afterwards. The patient may be X-rayed twenty-four hours later to demonstrate the dye in the peritoneal cavity. No further preparation is required for this additional examination.

Myelography—examination of the spinal canal and cord, to demonstrate tumours or injury. No special preparation is required. Media used for examination are lipiodol or neohydriol. A lumbar puncture is performed first and a certain amount of cerebrospinal fluid is withdrawn. The dye

is then introduced by means of a syringe attached to the lumbar puncture
needle.

Ventriculography—examination of the cerebral ventricles by the intro
duction of air. Not less than 10 c.c. of air are introduced either by cisternal
puncture or lumbar puncture. The presence of air in the ventricles makes
them translucent to X-rays and they appear as dark shadows on the film.
The examination is carried out to demonstrate abnormalities such as
tumours. Afterwards the patient may suffer from severe headache, nausea
and vomiting. Rest in bed, the foot of the bed raised on blocks, is the
treatment required after this examination. The head should be kept still
and other general methods of relieving these symptoms should be tried
until they pass off.

Bones and joints. For most X-rays of bones no previous preparation is
required, but for examination of the lumbar spine, sacro-iliac joints and
pelvis a vegetable aperient is required the night before the examination.

Chapter Twenty-Two

THE OPERATING THEATRE

Operative surgery made great strides after the discovery of the germ theory by Pasteur. Lord Lister at Edinburgh followed up this work by using disinfectants to prevent wounds becoming infected. This was called the *antiseptic method*. Carbolic acid was the chief disinfectant used. Instruments were soaked in it, the skin was covered with carbolic compresses previous to operation, and the theatre was sprayed with carbolic lotion whilst the operation was in progress. Although the death rate from sepsis was very much reduced by this method, it began to be realized that such drastic disinfection, whilst killing the germ, also killed tissues and delayed healing; in fact, carbolic when sprayed on the skin resulted in gangrene of the tissues in some cases. A period of greater discrimination in the use of antiseptics followed, and this in turn was succeeded by the *aseptic method*. The idea of the latter was not so much to kill the germs as to exclude them from the theatre and operating area. By the aseptic method instruments, gowns, dressings, gloves, etc., are made germ-free by boiling or by exposure to super-heated steam. Hands are treated by scrubbing with soap and water and rinsing in distilled water. The operation area is cleansed by washing, shaving and compressing with normal saline. Hence no disinfectants are used, to interfere with the healing process. In modern surgical practice a combination of the antiseptic and the aseptic methods are used. The dressings, gowns and instruments are sterilized by steam, but a disinfectant is usually applied to the skin of the patient, at least once before the incision is made. Great advances, however, have been made in the manufacture of disinfectants. There are many now on the market which can be relied upon to kill micro-organisms whilst doing the minimum amount of damage to the tissues.

In applying the above methods of surgical technique, it is realized that infection can enter a wound in the following ways:

1. *From dust and dirt*. Germs cling to minute particles suspended in the atmosphere and are found to be present when this matter settles as dust on any flat surface. Hence the importance of thorough removal of dust and dirt, and the avoidance of traffic which will disturb it by creating draughts.

2. *Droplet infection*. When a wound is exposed, germs may enter from the nose and mouth of people in close proximity to it. Loud talking,

sneezing or coughing cause a spray of minute droplets of mucus and saliva which are laden with germs. These are harmless in the mouth and nasopharynx of a healthy person, but become harmful if they enter an open wound. The danger from droplet infection is, of course, much worse if people suffering from colds or sore throats are allowed to take part in an operation or in the dressing of a wound. Well-fitting masks of sufficient thickness prevent the spread of bacteria by droplet infection.

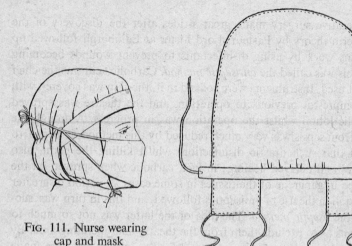

FIG. 111. Nurse wearing
cap and mask

FIG. 112. Theatre cap
Head Band = 24 inches long.
Head piece = 18 inches from centre
front to centre back.
Ear pieces = 5½ inches by 5 inches.
Tapes = 14 inches long.

3. *Clothing, hair and hands*. To prevent contamination from these sources all those in the theatre during an operation wear overalls. The head is completely covered with a muslin cap as hair is laden with dust and infected. Sterile rubber gloves are worn by all those actually taking part in the operating and the operation area is only touched with sterile forceps. All those in the theatre learn to avoid touching wagons and sterilized apparatus as they walk about.

4. *Instruments, dressings, etc.* These are rendered sterile by various methods before they are used.

5. *The skin of the operation area*. The prevention of wound contamination from this source has been discussed under the heading 'Preparation for Operation'.

The theatre itself should be sufficiently large and there should also be:

1. **An Anæsthetic Room.** This is a small room adjoining the theatre.

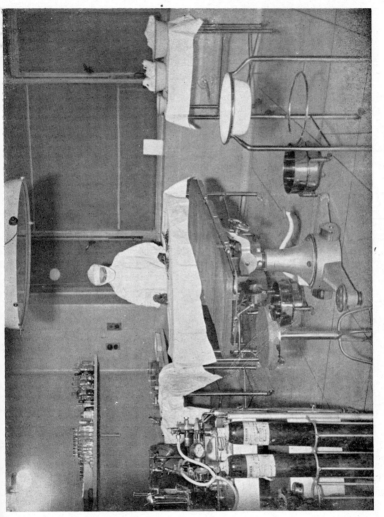

Plate 25. An operating theatre. See page 343

In it the patient is given the anæsthetic, so that she is not alarmed by the sight of the preparations for the operation. An anæsthetic trolley and all requirements are kept in it, or the wagon may be wheeled into it from the theatre. There is often a radiator in the room, on which it is convenient to heat blankets. The movement and arrangement of blankets and rugs creates a good deal of fluff and dust, hence it is undesirable that they should be kept in the theatre itself.

2. **A Preparation Room,** in which the instruments are sterilized. Bowls for 'scrubbing up' are in this room and the surgeons and nurses are dressed in their sterile gowns and gloves, etc., before entering the theatre. There should be cupboards for apparatus, instruments, bowls, lotions, stores, etc. The instrument room is often a separate one with a sufficiency of glass cupboards.

3. **A Surgeons' Changing Room.** Most surgeons change into thin white garments and white rubber boots before operating. They need a room where they can rest and change. Shower baths are generally provided.

4. **Nurses' Changing Room.** Those who are assisting in the theatre change their frocks for a simple overall and white shoes and stockings. Each nurse should have her own locker where she can keep her personal belongings in safety.

5. **In a Hospital with Medical School attached.** There should be a room for senior students acting as dressers to the surgeons.

THE THEATRE

Everything in the theatre should be washable, the walls tiled, the floor either tiled or tessellated; various smooth cement preparations are used for floors. Gutters are provided at the side of the room to drain away water when the floors are mopped between operations. Any part of the theatre which is not tiled is painted with good enamel paint which will stand washing with soap and water. The theatre is heated by enclosed radiators or by steam pipes in the ceiling. Ventilation and heating are factors of great importance both for the safety of the patient and the comfort of the workers. The temperature is maintained at 68° to 70° F. and there must be no draughts. Artificial ventilation is more satisfactory than windows as modern engineering makes it possible to allow warm and filtered air to circulate by the use of suitable entrance and exit shafts. 'Air conditioning' is one of the most important things to consider in the construction of an operating theatre.

Large windows of opaque glass without bars sometimes give sufficient lighting if the theatre is on the top floor. But in all cases good artificial lighting by shadowless lamps (e.g. SK pattern) is required. There should be electric fittings so that bulbs in use can be selected to direct a beam of light on any part of the operation site required. A Swan standard lamp should also be available. There should be an alternative emergency electric plant, in case the electricity from the main supply fails at any time. Some operating theatres have a glass roof to give more light. There should be some method of shading windows when the glare or heat of the sun is too strong for the operators. In certain cases, too, the surgeon requires the theatre to be darkened whilst he operates on, for example, the throat or ear. In these cases he wears an electric head lamp which directs a strong beam on to the area of operation.

On one side of the room there is a marble slab, for bowls, jugs, lotions, etc. This slab often communicates by means of a hatch with the preparation room, so that it is not necessary for communicating doors to be constantly opened and shut whilst an operation is in progress. Several glass or enamel wagons are required, at least four. One for the instruments, one for the dresser or surgeon's assistant on which he or she arranges the instruments and ligatures in the order in which they will be required; one for the stocks of various sutures and needles ready sterilized in glass jars. The fourth trolley holds the lotions and dressings. There is often a small locked cupboard on the wall containing hypodermic outfit and stimulating drugs which may be required in an emergency. There is an enamel stand on wheels into which a bowl fits. This contains sterile saline in which the surgeon rinses his hands. It can be moved into a convenient position for him. The equipment also includes an infusion stand on which to hang a bottle or container for intravenous infusion of saline or blood. One or two enamel buckets for swabs are needed, and three or four stools, one for the anæsthetist, and one each for the surgeon and his assistant. There should also be one wooden footstool, and several stands for large dressing drums which can be opened by pedals (see plate 25).

A modern operating table is a model of ingenuity. It can be raised and lowered, tilted in many different directions by means of a system of wheels and levers underneath. It is most important that the nurse should understand exactly how the table works so that if in the middle of an operation some adjustment is required, she knows exactly how it should be done. The nurse in charge should also consider it her duty to see that all the joints, ratchets, etc., of the table are kept well oiled. They should be done regularly twice a week, either by a nurse or orderly. The surface of the table should be washed down each day and the covering pads which are made of rubber should also be washed with soap and water. Care should be taken that no grease or strong disinfectant comes in contact with the rubber. Pads are very expensive and need treating with care. Lithotomy poles, pillows, straps and other accessory apparatus for maintaining the patient in various positions required for operation should always be at hand and in good order.

PREPARATION FOR THE OPERATION
THEATRE ROUTINE

Each evening after the day's operating, or early the next morning, the floors are all thoroughly scrubbed by an experienced cleaner, who is taught to appreciate the danger to the patient of even the slightest trace of dust or dirt. It is the nurse's duty to see that she keeps her bucket clean and that she has a sufficiency of hot water, soda, and soap, and that her cloths and brushes are in good condition. The cleaner should be taught to be very critical of her own and other people's work. When doing the floor she must do the gutters and gratings over the drains well. The nurse herself should mop the latter with a strong disinfectant when they have been scrubbed.

Each morning the theatre nurses do their routine cleaning. The marble slabs are scrubbed with soap and water. The enamel stands and trolleys are washed. Glass shelves are cleaned with soap and water every morning, and at intervals wiped over and polished with 'recovery spirit'. (This is spirit which has been used for other purposes, for example, storage of sharp instruments and sutures; when the spirit in the jars is changed, the used spirit is put into large stone jars and sent to be 'recovered'. Some of this is used for cleaning the glass in the theatre. It makes the glass shiny and free from smears.)

Sinks and basins are cleaned with Vim or some similar preparation. Ledges and windowsills, if any, are washed with soap and water. Electric lamps and shades are also washed. The windows and doors are then closed and unnecessary traffic in and out of the theatre is avoided. The thermometer hanging in the theatre should register 70° F. before operations begin.

PREPARATION FOR THE OPERATION

The sister or staff nurse selects the instruments which will be needed for the day's operations and each set is wrapped in a towel and put into an enamel tray with its respective label, ready to be sterilized. The theatre is then laid ready for the operation. Sterile bowls of various sizes and shapes are put out. Jugs of hot and cold sterile saline are prepared, together with lotions which are likely to be needed. A lotion thermometer is necessary. Drums of dressings and sterile towels are put out, and a pair of lifting forceps in a jar of disinfectant. Sharp instruments—scalpels, scissors and needles of different patterns—are put in dishes covered with methylated spirit and are placed on a trolley. Syringes for intravenous, spinal, or local anæsthesia are put on the same trolley, with a sufficiency of sharp needles to fit each one. Sutures of each variety are put in readiness. On this trolley there should be a pair of lifting forceps (Cheatle pattern) so that in an emergency, a nurse who is not scrubbed up may take the instruments or sutures from their jars as required. Sterilized drainage tubing and clips are also put out if they are likely to be needed. Mackintoshes, bandages, splints, tourniquets, etc., are placed in readiness on a shelf or table, together with sterile jars, and test tubes for specimens which the surgeon may require for the taking of specimens for examination purposes.

On a second glass trolley the enamel tray of sterilized instruments is placed. The third wagon, for the 'dresser' is left empty by the operating table. On this the nurse who is assisting the surgeon will place a sterile towel and select the instruments, sutures, etc., as they will be required. At the head of the table a stool is placed for the anæsthetist and the wagon containing all his requirements. Cylinders of oxygen, nitrous oxide gas, carbon dioxide mixtures and pure carbon dioxide must be in readiness with spare cylinders at hand. The keys of these cylinders should hang on their stands. The nurse must see that all the cylinders are tested. Empty ones are removed and marked clearly 'Empty'. It may be an orderly's duty to do this.

N.B. The joints of oxygen cylinders must on no account be greased if they are stiff, otherwise they are likely to explode.

Electrical apparatus, such as diathermy, cystoscope, sigmoidoscope, etc., if they are to be used must all be tested.

The preparation room must be in readiness. Sterilizers are filled and brought to the boil. Each 'scrubbing up' sink is provided with a bowl of disinfectant for the hands, soap and scrubbing brush. The latter must be boiled for ten minutes and should be renewed when the bristles become soft. They are not discarded, but are used for scrubbing instruments and other cleaning apparatus. Drums of sterile gowns, masks, and caps are put out with several pairs of large lifting forceps in disinfectant. The gloves of the surgeon who is operating are put in readiness. They should be sterilized in tins with the surgeon's name on the lid. It is very important that the gloves should be of correct size. Suitable gloves are also placed ready for the dresser and nurse. If calico leggings are worn a sufficiency of these should be available.

THE OPERATION

The patient, who is already anæsthetized, is lifted from the stretcher on to the table by a team of nurses, dressers or orderlies, under the supervision of the anæsthetist. Whilst the surgeon and nurse who is to assist him are scrubbing up in the preparation room, two 'unsterile' nurses arrange the patient on the table. The hands are put flat under the stretcher sheet, ensuring that the arms cannot fall out, and the sheet is then tucked neatly under the pads. Care must be taken that the patient does not lie on the hands. The gown is then rolled well out of the way of the site of operation, and the blanket is arranged tidily and firmly over the parts of the body which are not to be exposed. Mackintoshes are arranged to cover the blankets and are tucked firmly in so that they cannot slip off. The surface should be as flat as possible avoiding bulky folds. If the operation requires the table to be adjusted to secure the patient in a particular position, this is now done. (Example Trendelenburg, lithotomy, lateral, etc.) The nurses should look to the anæsthetist for permission to change the position of the patient. By this time the surgeon and nurse assisting are ready. A second nurse in theatre garb but not scrubbed up, is detailed to attend the 'dresser'.

The sister usually controls the whole procedure, helping to put trolleys, wagons, stools, etc., in convenient positions, so that there is no delay. Any onlookers must wear theatre gowns and masks. The dresser should be quite ready for the surgeon when he is ready to begin. She should have covered her table with a sterile towel, and have laid out towels, dressings, etc. She uncovers the tray of instruments and selects the first ones to be used. Her assistant uncovers the jars of scissors, needles, sutures, etc., and she selects the ones the surgeon is likely to need. She has on her trolley a small bowl of sterile saline in which she rinses the sutures. Her assistant pours out lotions taking care not to touch the rims of the bowls with the bottles.

The surgeon paints a large area of the skin with iodine or whatever preparation he chooses, after which his assistant hands him the towels and helps to arrange them in position by means of towel-clips. They are carefully arranged so that only the operation site is exposed.

The operation proceeds. The nurse watches each step carefully and tries to anticipate the wants of the surgeon. To do this she must be intelligent and alert, and listen carefully to his remarks as he goes along. With experience, the nurse assisting the surgeon learns the technique of the various operations and she is able to save time by her efficiency. The time factor is important in the prevention of shock.

A third nurse is left in charge of the preparation room, and she is a 'runner' to fetch and sterilize any extras which may be required. The assistant to the dresser counts the used swabs as the surgeon discards them; the number must be very carefully checked.

When the surgeon has finished the operation he covers the wound with sterile dressings and pads. The sister with a nurse helping her, removes the towels, mackintoshes, etc., and wipes the patient free from blood. She then arranges the dressings in position and applies the bandage, adjusts the gown and supervises the lifting of the patient on to the stretcher, keeping the head well to one side. The patient is covered with warm blankets. The anæsthetist sees her out of the theatre, and usually leaves an airway in the mouth. There should be no delay in transit back to the ward.

Clearing up. The lids of jars which have been uncovered are always replaced immediately. The table is straightened. The sister or staff nurse checks the instruments to make sure that the set is complete. All used instruments are put in a dish and taken to the preparation room; the sharps, scalpels, scissors, etc., are taken away on a separate dish. Instruments which have not been used are also removed. Towels, gowns, masks, etc., are put into appropriate bins, for washing and resterilization. The bucket of soiled swabs is emptied and the floor mopped with disinfectant.

DISINFECTANTS AND ANTISEPTICS

Disinfectants or *germicides* are agents which kill germs.

Antiseptics are agents which prevent the multiplication of germs. They are usually weak preparations of disinfectants.

Deodorants are agents which mask unpleasant odours, e.g. sanitas, fumigating pastilles.

Disinfectants may be:

1. *Physical agents:* Heat, cold, sun and electricity.
2. *Chemical agents:* (a) *Fluids*, e.g. carbolic acid, lysol, dettol. (b) *Gases*, e.g. chlorine, formaldehyde, and sulphur dioxide.

Disinfectants and Antiseptics in Common Use

Carbolic acid is a coal tar derivative which has a corrosive action.

Uses: Pure carbolic acid—ζi to a gallon of water for filling water beds.

Carbolic lotion, 1—20 for storing salmon gut sutures and as a stock solution which is diluted for various purposes, e.g. 1—40 for combing heads; 1—100 for mouthwashes and gargles.

Lysol (*cresol*), a coal tar preparation combined with soap. The soap makes it less corrosive and more cleansing than carbolic lotion.

Uses: Pure lysol for sterilizing sharp instruments and needles; Lysol 2 per cent for immersing instruments after they have been boiled; Lysol 1 per cent for immersing the hands; Lysol ½ per cent for douching the vagina.

Dettol, a solution of chlorinated xylenol, is considered one of the best disinfectants and is non-irritating.

Uses: Dettol 2 per cent for the storage of sterile instruments and for swabbing the vulva; ½ per cent for douching the vagina. Dettol cream used as an antiseptic lubricant on the surgeon's gloves for a vaginal examination.

Alcohol 90—95 per cent (pure alcohol) and methylated spirit are now considered quite unreliable as disinfectants. Instruments which have been boiled remain sterile if stored in these preparations.

Methylated ether. Anæsthetic ether made from methyl alcohol instead of ethyl alcohol. It is a cleansing lotion used for skin preparations.

Boracic acid lotion should be a 1—30 solution. A saturated solution is 1—25. To make the 1—30 solution, 1 oz. of boracic crystals are dissolved in a pint and a half of boiling water. When the lotion cools, equal parts of 1—30 solution and sterile water are used for irrigating eyes, for vaginal douches, for irrigating wounds and for swabbing the vulva before catheterization. Its antiseptic value is practically nil, but it is a useful and cleansing solution.

Hydrogen peroxide (H_2O_2) has the same chemical formula as water with an extra molecule of oxygen. It is obtainable in strengths of 5, 10 or 20 volumes. It oxidizes bacteria and is valuable for irrigating septic wounds ($2\frac{1}{2}$ to 5 volumes). It effervesces in the presence of pus. It is a good styptic mouthwash after extraction of teeth (10 vols.).

Liquor iodi mitis 2 per cent (B.P.), is a valuable antiseptic. The skin should be dried before it is applied. The disadvantage of using large quantities of it, e.g. in the operating theatre, is its irritating effect on the eyes.

Uses: For cuts and abrasions; for skin preparation.

Iodine 6 per cent ($\mathrecal{Z}$i to Oi of water) for vaginal douching in cases of discharge. It has an antiseptic and deodorant action.

Iodine in oil used for rubbing painful joints and muscles.

Iodoform powder (a compound of iodine) for insufflation of the throat.

Gauze impregnated with iodoform (iodoform gauze) is used as an antiseptic packing for wounds.

Formalin, 1—250 (90 minims of solution of formalin to one pint of water).

Uses: For storage of rubber tubes, drains and glass capsules containing sutures.

Formalin 1—500 for soaking infectious linen for eight hours before being sent to the laundry.

Formalin 1—1,000 for vaginal douching in cases of discharge; has an antiseptic and deodorant action.

Formalin vapour (paraform tablets) are used in sterilizing glass cylinders for the storage of catheters. The tablets when heated in a container connected to an electric current generate a strong disinfectant gas which is a sufficient disinfectant for gum elastic catheters.

Formaldehyde gas is used for disinfecting rooms in a similar way to paraform.

Liquor boracis formaldehyde (N.W.F.) National war formula (1941). Sterilizing agent, consists of borax, formaldehyde phenol and water. It is a useful and reliable solution in which to store sterile instruments. It is less expensive than spirit and borax prevents rusting. The instruments and needles must be rinsed before use.

Preparations of silver

Uses: Silver nitrate stick for burning down excessive granulation tissue, for cauterizing small ulcers, burning down warts, touching up cracks at the angles of the lips.

Silver nitrate solution 1 per cent for instillation into the eyes in conjunctivitis.

Protargol and argyrol are silver preparations used as drops in eye and ear infections.

Silver nitrate solution 1—15,000 is used for bladder lavage (styptic).

A solution of tannic acid, silver nitrate and gentian violet is used for the treatment of burns.

Permanganate of potash (proprietary preparation, Condy's fluid).

Uses: Four crystals of potassium permanganate to one quart of water for bladder lavage, vaginal douche, gastric lavage. This is a mild antiseptic with a deodorant action. As a lotion for gastric lavage it neutralizes many poisonous alkaloids.

Biniodide of mercury (double salt of mercury and potassium iodide) 1—1,000 in spirit, for immersion of hands after 'scrubbing up'.

Aniline dyes. Flavine group (e.g. acriflavine); brilliant green; methyl violet; gentian violet.

These are popular antiseptics which not only destroy germs but stimulate healing of the tissues.

Uses: Preparation of the skin before operation, and for the treatment of wounds.

Chlorine preparations. Eusol (generally used in equal quantities with warm water); Dakin's solution; Sodium hypochlorite; Milton (these all contain chloride of lime).

Eusol (Edinburgh University solution of lime)—a preparation first used in the war 1914–18 for irrigation of wounds by Carrell-Dakin's apparatus, is a mixture of chloride of lime and boracic lotion.

Dakin's solution is a similar preparation and a more stable solution than eusol.

Chloramine T—a chlorine compound liberating free chlorine when in contact with proteins.

Mercurial preparations. Perchloride of mercury, 1—2,000 for hands and gum elastic catheters.

1—8,000 for vaginal douches, to be followed by plain water or saline.

1—10,000 or 1—12,000 for irrigation of eyes.

Oxycyanide of mercury, 1—500 in water is used by some surgeons for immersion of hands. 1—10,000—12,000 for irrigation of eyes is less irritating than the perchloride.

Mercurial ointments are commonly used:

Ung. hydrarg. dil. (blue ointment), for inunction.

Yellow oxide of mercury ointment (ung. H.O.F.), for skin and oculentum 1 per cent for eye treatments.

Scott's dressing (ung. hydrarg. co.) for sprains.

Mercury is very poisonous. Its salts are protein coagulants and corrosive. It is never used for sterilizing instruments. It is considered a particularly useful antiseptic for gonococcal infections.

METHODS OF STERILIZATION

Caps, Gowns, Towels and Dressings are packed in metal drums, folded neatly and packed loosely, they must not be wet when put in the drums. They are sterilized in the autoclave at 20 lb. pressure for thirty minutes.

Gloves. After use, wash both sides of the gloves in cold water, then in soapy water; boil for one minute, and remove from sterilizer. Test for holes by inflating with water and dry thoroughly inside and out on a perfectly clean towel. Repair holes by putting rubber pacthes with rubber solution on the inside of the glove. Powder inside and out with french chalk, sort into pairs, and turn back the cuffs. Place in linen glove bags, putting with each a small gauze bag containing french chalk. Fold the bags and pack loosely in perforated tins, labelled with the name of the surgeon and the size of the gloves. Sterilize in the autoclave at 5 lb. for thirty minutes. French chalk is previously sterilized in the autoclave at 20 lb. pressure for thirty minutes.

Instruments: *Blunt:* After use, wash in cold water, scrub thoroughly paying particular attention to joints, grooves, and teeth. Scrub a second time in hot water, and place in a boiling sterilizer. Boil for twenty minutes and arrange on a sterile towel in an enamel dish.

Alternative method: Place a towel cornerwise on an enamel tray, place the instruments in an orderly fashion on the towel, cover over the corners in turn, tucking them well under. Attach label saying for what operation they are prepared and sterilize in the autoclave at 20 lb. pressure for twenty minutes.

Ward Dressing Instruments. Boil for twenty minutes, dish in a dry sterile covered dish, or they may be covered with sterilizing solution (N.W.F.) or spirit. In between dressings, if the instruments have not been contaminated by pus or discharge of any kind, reboil for two minutes. If contaminated, boil for twenty minutes.

Scalpels, Scissors and Needles. After use wash under the tap and place in pure lysol for three minutes. Remove with forceps. Rinse in water and dry with a cloth. Clean off the stains with an abrasive such as Brook's monkey soap. Wash thoroughly and dry again.

To sterilize. Immerse in pure lysol for three minutes, transfer to sterile saline or methylated spirit.

Alternative method. Place in an enamel dish lined with lint, so that the edges do not get knocked and blunted, put in a boiling sterilizer containing soda bicarbonate, for two minutes. Transfer to a dry covered sterile dish.

Syringes. After use, rinse thoroughly in cold water. Take to pieces and immerse in pure lysol for three minutes if grossly contaminated, otherwise immerse in 2 per cent lysol. Transfer with forceps into a bowl of water.

Assemble the parts and rinse thoroughly. Clean the needles if necessary with Brook's monkey soap and rinse again. Dry and immerse the needle and the stilette in spirit for a few minutes. Remove from the spirit and allow the latter to evaporate from the needle. Report if the needle needs sharpening and ask for a replacement. Dry the barrel and piston and place in a metal box lined with lint. Replace the lid and seal round the edge firmly with zinc oxide strapping. Sterilize in the autoclave at 20 lb. pressure for thirty minutes.

Alternative method. (1) Instead of packing in a box, wrap each part in lint and put in an enamel dish. Immerse the dish in cold water in the sterilizer, bring to the boil and boil for twenty minutes. Remove the dish and let the syringe cool. Store in spirit or sterilizing solution (N.W.F.).

(2) If in ward practice the same syringe and needle is used only for clean cases (e.g. hypodermic and intramuscular injections), it is safe to rinse the syringe and needle through with carbolic lotion, 1—20, distilled water and finally with spirit. It is then replaced in a jar of spirit. If, however, the syringe has been used for infected cases and is contaminated by pus or other body fluid, it must be thoroughly disinfected with pure lysol, as described above, before being cleaned. It must then either be boiled or autoclaved.

(3) If the syringe is required again at once, rinse and immerse in pure lysol for three minutes, transfer to sterile water using forceps and rinse thoroughly. Transfer to the covered dish of spirit. The same needle should not be used until it has been washed, immersed in lysol and dried with spirit. It is then sterilized by boiling for two minutes and the stilette replaced.

Needles. After use, immerse in 2 per cent lysol, dry and clean with monkey soap or fine emery paper. Resterilize in lysol. Rinse in distilled water. Store in spirit containing a few grains of soda bicarbonate.

Bone Sharps. Immerse in pure lysol for five minutes, rinse in 2 per cent lysol and water (not spirit)—leave in 2 per cent lysol or dry on a sterile towel ready for use.

Gum Elastic Catheters

New Catheters. Wash in cold tap water. Dry and lubricate with an olive oil swab. Place in container with paraform tablets, the vapour of which should sterilize in twenty-four hours.

Used Catheters. Wash under a cold tap and put in biniodide of mercury in distilled water for two hours (1—1,000). Dry and lubricate and place in paraform chamber.

In emergency. Catheters may be tied with a bandage and dipped in a boiling sterilizer for thirty seconds, but they are inclined to become soft if this is done often.

Electric sterilizers with paraform tablets are the best method but are too expensive for general use.

METHODS OF STERILIZATION

Silver and Glass Instruments. Boil for twenty minutes, remembering that glass must be put into cold water to avoid breaking.

Rubber Tubing. Boil for ten minutes. Store in carbolic 1 in 20, or formalin 1 in 250.

Ureteric Catheters, Diathermy Electrodes, and Bougies. Immerse in perchloride or biniodide 1 in 1,000 in water for one hour. No spirit must be used. It destroys the gum elastic coating.

Catgut

1. Immerse in iodine 1 per cent in water for seven days. Transfer to iodine 0·75 per cent ready for use; or:

2. Steep in iodine 1 per cent for seven days. Wash daily in biniodide 1—500 for three days until clear. Store in biniodide 1—500.

Most hospitals do not prepare their own catgut. Ampoules of chromic 20 day and plain 10 day are bought ready for use. They are stored in spirit. The nurse who assists at the operation, holding swabs, breaks the ampoules and removes the catgut with forceps. The surgeon may rinse it in a dish of sterile saline.

Horsehair, Gossamer gut, Silkworm gut. Boil for twenty minutes; store in carbolic 5 per cent.

Synthetic Nylon or Silkworm gut. Boil for twenty minutes. Store in biniodide 1—1,000 in spirit. Carbolic rots synthetic silkworm gut.

Silk and Thread. Wind evenly on spool. Boil for forty minutes, store in carbolic 5 per cent.

To sterilize cystoscope. Thoroughly test light and focus of telescope. Cystoscope is put in a dish of spirit deep enough to cover whole instrument and the two-way irrigating fitting and single-fitting nozzle. The telescope is wiped over with spirit, as if left immersed too long, the spirit is apt to penetrate under the lens, particularly in an old cystoscope when the setting is not quite accurate. The 'business end' of the lead is put in spirit.

To clean cystoscope. Remove telescope and wipe with antiseptic, then spirit and put away in the box or on to next trolley for further use. Unscrew catheterizing sheath at the valve, also small screw caps for ureteric catheters and wash well under a fast running tap. Sometimes it is necessary to clean these parts with hydrogen peroxide to remove blood.

Put all the parts separately in 2 per cent lysol; remove after half an hour and wash again in cold water and then put these separate parts once more in spirit. The light bulbs should never be taken off during this process. Remove from spirit and leave on a towel to dry. Fit together, seeing that washers are in good condition and that when screwing together no part of the instrument is forced. The two-way tap is sterilized in the same way. The lead is wiped with spirit and put away in the box, taking care that it is folded in such a way that the part where the rubber lead joins the metal

z 353

switch is not stretched, as when next used it is liable to flicker the light and may even be useless and not make contact.

There are several kinds of cystoscope, e.g. for diathermy and trans-urethral prostatectomy, etc. That used for examination and catheterization of ureters is the one with which nurses in training should be familiar.

To clean sigmoidoscope. This instrument can be used unsterile. After use, remove light and magnifying glass. Take a wool swab dipped in dettol on a swab holder and clean inside of instrument, taking care to remove all fæcal matter. Boil the introducer and hollow part of the sigmoidoscope for twenty minutes. Test before putting away.

To clean laryngoscope. Remove light and battery. Immerse the end for the mouth in dettol. The battery end must not touch water. Dry thoroughly and replace the light before putting away.

Care of Surgical Instruments. Scrub with old nail brush after use, in a sink of cold (not running) water, paying special attention to joints and grooves. Once or twice weekly scrub the joints and grooves with olive-oil; it is the hard scrubbing and not the oil that cleans and preserves the instruments. Always report faulty instruments or anything needing repair. Flat instruments without joints should be cleaned with plate powder and 'used' spirit, using a wire brush to remove the powder.

LISTS OF REQUIREMENTS FOR COMMON OPERATIONS

Anæsthetic Trolley. Boyle's anæsthetic machine or one of similar pattern is generally used, containing:

Top Shelf

Cylinders attached to the side of the machine—nitrous oxide, oxygen, CO_2 (pure).

Glass stoppered stock bottles containing ether (pure), chloroform ($CHCl_3$), ethyl chloride sprays for general use.

Two empty small bottles—one brown for ether and one blue drop bottle for mixture of chloroform and ether.

(*N.B.* These bottles should be filled by the anæsthetist and the nurse must on no account interfere with them in any way. Any anæsthetic left over is not allowed to be poured from bottle to bottle except by the anæsthetist.)

Castor oil drops.

Funnel (small).

Phillips' airways (various sizes).

Sponge holder.

One marine sponge (damp—not wet).

Tongue forceps.

One Doyen's gag.

One Mason's gag, wooden wedges and dental props.

Hypodermic syringe should be at hand with heart and circulatory stimulants.

Bottom shelf

Cap, gown, mask.

Vomit bowl.

Cloth.

Three Schimmelbusch masks (varying sizes).

Flannel face pieces.

Anæsthetic pads.

Malleable rubber face pieces. Size 4 generally used to fit Boyle's machine —detachable for cleaning.

Two cylinder keys.

One spanner.

One right-angled adaptor for intratracheal anæsthetics.

When Boyle's machine is not used, an anæsthetic trolley is prepared in a similar way.

Sets of Instruments

General set

9 Joll's artery forceps, or Dunhill artery forceps.

9 Lane's tissue forceps.

9 Spencer Wells' artery forceps.

9 Mayo Oschner's forceps.

2 Non-toothed dissecting forceps, 7-inch.

2 Toothed dissecting forceps, 7-inch.

2 Ring retractors.

2 Sponge-holding forceps.

1 Pot for skin-cleaning lotion.

4 Towel clips.

1 Small probe.

1 Long probe.

1 Grooved director.

1 Blunt dissector.

1 Raspatory.

1 Sharp spoon.

1 Aneurysm needle.

1 Sinus forceps.

1 Suture holder.

1 Needle holder.

2 Morris's abdominal retractors.

Bone set

9 Skin clips.
2 Large Lane's bone holding forceps.
2 Small lion bone-holding forceps.
1 Large straight bone-cutting forceps.
1 Large curved   ,,   ,,
1 Small straight   ,,   ,,
1 Small curved   ,,   ,,
2 Pairs necrosis forceps.
1 Pair nibbling or gouge forceps.
1 Awl.
1 Grooved awl.
1 Mallet.
Orthopædic retractors (Langenbeck's).
1 Pair sinus forceps.
1 Pair large bone levers or spikes.
1 Pair medium bone levers (grooved).
1 Pair small bone levers (more according to operation).
1 File.
1 Mechanical drill (Johannsen's or Lane's).
1 Hand drill, points to match, sizes 3, 5, 7.

Bone sharps

1 Large saw.
1 Small saw.
Chisels of varying sizes.
Osteotomes of varying sizes.
Gouges of varying sizes.
Drill points.
2 Farabœuf's rougines.

Bone-plating set

General set and bone set, plus:
2 Plate-holding forceps.
2 Screw-holding forceps.
2 Plate benders.
2 Screwdrivers.
Plates and screws.

Cholecystectomy

General set plus:
1 Pliable probe.
1 Malleable probe.
1 Malleable spoon or cup.

1 Flushing spoon.
1 Gall-stone forceps.
4 Moynihan's pedicle forceps.
2 Morris's abdominal retractors.
2 Pairs curved intestinal clamps.
6 Large sponge holders (Rampley's).
Lobectomy scissors.
Sucker *or*
    Aspirating syringe, with long 4—6 inch aspirating needle, T tubes
    (rubber), *or* thick-walled rubber tubing, size 10.
Extra Joll's, Spencer-Wells, or Mayo-Oschner forceps according to
    surgeon.

Gastrectomy and Resection of gut

General set plus :
2 Abdominal retractors.
1 Self-retaining retractor.
1 Deep retractor.
2 Moynihan's pedicle forceps.
1 Lane's twin intestinal clamp.
2 Large straight intestinal clamps.
2 Curved intestinal clamps.
2 Jejunum forceps.
6 Judd's or Allis's basting forceps.
1 Large Payr's clamp.
1 Small Payr's clamp.
Resection of gut for strangulated hernia often needs Paul's tubes and
tubing.

Herniotomy—for strangulated hernia

General set plus :
Hernia needle and director.
Bistoury knife.
2 Straight intestinal clamps.
2 Curved intestinal clamps.
2 Payr's clamps.
General set only required for ordinary hernia.

Amputation

General set plus :
Extra artery forceps—3 sets at least.
Extra Lane's forceps.
Corrugated drainage tubing.
1 File.

1 Rougine.
1 Straight bone cutter.
1 Amputation shield.
2 Amputation knives.
1 Large saw.
1 Small saw.

Colostomy
General set plus:
Abdominal retractors.
2 Small intestinal clamps.
Paul's glass tubes (3 sizes).
Paul's tubing.
Colostomy rod or large Jacques catheter 15 or 18.
Diathermy apparatus.

Tonsillectomy—dissection
1 Towel clip.
4 Boyle Davis tongue depressors (one of various sizes).
1 Davis gag.
1 Doyen's gag.
2 Adenoid curettes.
1 Tonsil snare.
2 Curved tonsil forceps
4 Straight artery forceps   } These artery forceps are 7 inches long,
4 Curved artery forceps   but fine and delicate and are called
1 Tonsil dissector.   tonsil-artery forceps.
1 Luc forceps.
1 Bar for Davis's gag.
1 Breastplate.
1 Pair tonsil scissors.

Guillotine of tonsils
2 Guillotines.
2 Adenoid curettes.
1 Doyen's gag.

Hysterectomy
General set plus:
6 Bonney's broad ligament forceps.
1 Vaginal speculum (Sims').

Vaginal extras (plastic operation on the vagina)
General set plus:
Vaginal specula—Sims', Auvard's.

Uterine sound.
2 Vulssellum forceps.
1 Curette (sharp).
6 Hegar's dilators.
Horseshoe retractor.
Bladder sound.

Nephrectomy
General set plus:
Extra artery forceps.
4 Kidney pedicle clamps.
Extra aneurysm needle.

Radical mastectomy
General set plus:
Extra artery forceps.
Extra Lane's tissue forceps.
Diathermy apparatus.

Thyroidectomy
General set plus:
Small artery forceps.
Thyroid retractor—Joll's or Kocher's.
4 Aneurysm needles.
Kocher's dissector.
Keith's glass drainage tubes.

Decompression (for emergency operation)
General set plus:
Extra sinus and artery forceps.
15 Skull flap forceps (Sargent's).
Gouge forceps.
Gigli saw and guides.
Trephines.
Skull elevator.
Rougine.
Sterile bone wax.
Sucker.

Mastoidectomy
4 Towel clips.
1 Scalpel and tenotomy knife.
1 West's mastoid retractor.
12 Artery forceps, 6 curved and 6 straight.
1 Mallet.

Gouges—various sizes.
1 Curved rougine.
Curved scissors (Mayo's).
1 Pair dissecting forceps—toothed.
2 Toothed and 2 non-toothed bayonet forceps.
1 Curette.
2 Sharp spoons.
1 Probe.

Empyema
General set plus:
Rougine.
2 Rib raspatories (Doyen's).
Rib-cutting forceps.
Rib shears or costatome.
Necrosis forceps.
Scapula retractor.
6 Large sponge holders.
Sucker. Diathermy apparatus.
Test tube and swabs.
Aspiration syringe.
Needles, various sizes and lengths, to fit syringe.
Lobectomy scissors.
Malleable light.
Tudor-Edwards tube, *or*
Medius drainage tube with gauze packing } Drainage.

Insertion of Kirschner wire and Max Page stirrup
Drill.
1 Sponge holder.
1 Scalpel.
Stirrup.
Spanner.
Hooks.
Wires (various thicknesses).
Wire cutters.
2 Pairs dissecting forceps.
1 Pair scissors.
Extension cord.
Some form of extension splint.

Hæmorrhoidectomy
General set plus:
Proctoscope.

Cystoscopy

Wool swabs in sterile dettol lotion.
Kidney dish.
Oil cup.
Cut dressing with K.Y. non-greasy lubricant jelly.
Towel clips.
Lead, telescopes, cystoscope and battery.
Ureteric catheters, sizes in pairs, 9, 10, 11, 12, 14.
Glass douche can—4 pints.
Sterile test tubes, marked right and left. (L. and R.)
Procaine 10 per cent with special urethral syringe.
Sterile olive oil and silver bougies.
Strapping.
Pyelography syringe and sodium bromide 20 per cent.
Mount for syringe to fit ureteric catheters.
Indigo carmine.
Penile clamp.

Sigmoidoscopy—(unsterile)

Sigmoidoscope.
Towels.
Vaseline.
Special long sponge holder.
Dishes, mackintosh.
Specimen jar and pathological form.
Bellows.
Finger stalls.
Vaseline and lint squares.
Battery.

Notes

1. *Varieties of needles*

Round bodied, straight, used for intestinal surgery.
Round bodied, curved, also for intestinal surgery.
Half circle, fully curved, cutting, for skin and muscle sutures.
Fish hooks (Gallie's) hernia needles.
Colt's cutting needles.

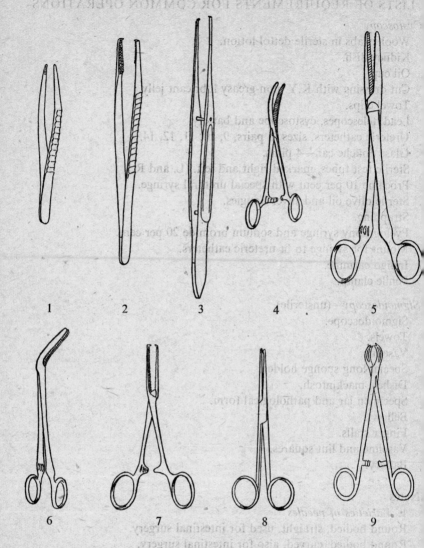

FIG. 113. Forceps

1. Non-toothed dissecting forceps.
2. Toothed dissecting forceps.
3. Rat-toothed dissecting forceps.
4. Mayo's artery forceps.
5. Spencer Wells' artery forceps.
6. Kidney pedicle forceps.
7. Kocher's artery forceps.
8. Sinus forceps.
9. Lane's tissue forceps.

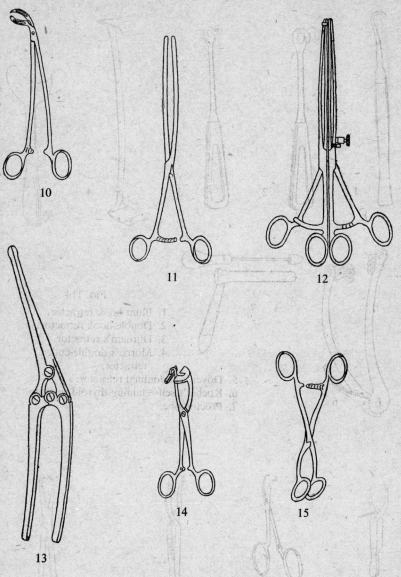

FIG. 113. Forceps (*continued*)

10. Tetra forceps.
11. Kocher's straight intestinal clamp.
12. Lane's twin intestinal clamp.
13. Payr's crushing clamp.
14. Sargent's skull flap forceps.
15. Tongue forceps.

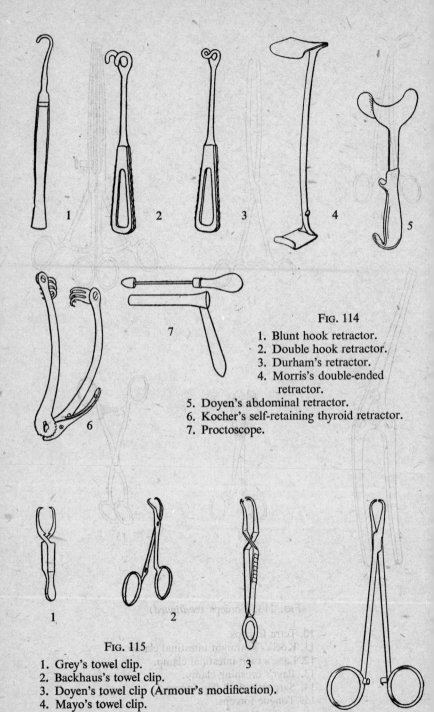

Fig. 114

1. Blunt hook retractor.
2. Double hook retractor.
3. Durham's retractor.
4. Morris's double-ended retractor.
5. Doyen's abdominal retractor.
6. Kocher's self-retaining thyroid retractor.
7. Proctoscope.

Fig. 115

1. Grey's towel clip.
2. Backhaus's towel clip.
3. Doyen's towel clip (Armour's modification).
4. Mayo's towel clip.

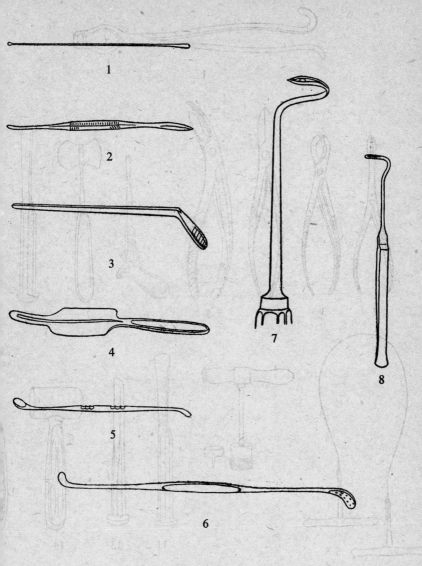

Fig. 116

1. Silver probe.
2. Durham's fine dissector and raspatory.
3. Grooved director.
4. Childe's hernia director.
5. Sharp double-ended spoon.
6. Moynihan's double-ended gall bladder scoop.
7. Hernia needle.
8. Aneurysm needle.

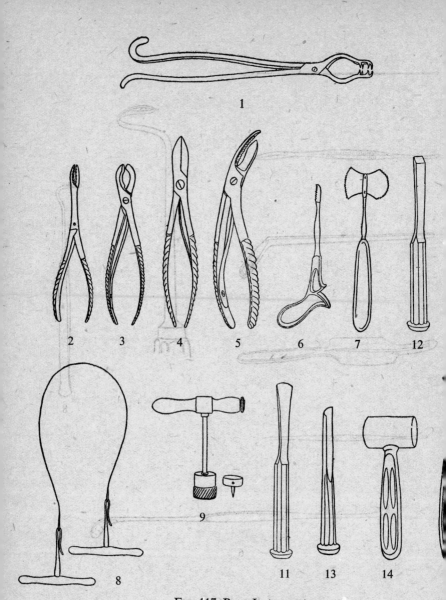

FIG. 117. Bone Instruments

1. Lane's bone-holding forceps.
2. Sequestrum forceps.
3. Gouge or nibbling forceps.
4. Bone-cutting forceps.
5. Rib shears.
6. Adam's saw.
7. Hey's saw.
8. Gigli saw.
9. Trephine.
10. Drill point (*see opposite page*).
11. Osteotome.
12. Chisel.
13. Gouge.
14. Orthopædic hammer.
15. Farabœuf's rougine or periosteal elevator.
16. Bone lever or spike (*see opposite page*).

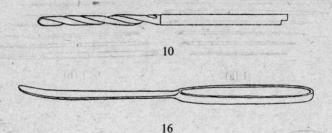

10

16

Fig. 117 (*continued*)

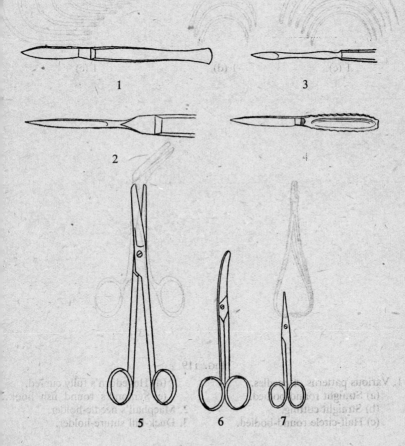

1

3

2

4

5

6

7

Fig. 118

1. Scalpel.
2. Adam's tenotomy knife.
3. Guy's pattern tenotomy knife.
4. Syme's amputation knife.
5. Straight surgical scissors.
6. Curved on flat surgical scissors.
7. Mayo's scissors.

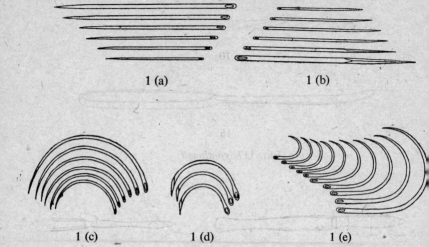

1 (a)   1 (b)

1 (c)   1 (d)   1 (e)

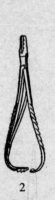 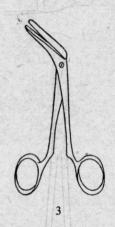

2   3

FIG. 119

1. Various patterns of needles.
   (a) Straight round-bodied.
   (b) Straight cutting.
   (c) Half-circle round-bodied.

(d) Hagedorn's fully curved.
(e) Symond's round fish hook.
2. Macphail's needle-holder.
3. Duck-bill suture-holder.

Chapter Twenty-Three

FIRST AID IN EMERGENCIES

The aim of 'First Aid' is so to treat an injury that a patient's life may be saved or a minimum of damage done.

Hæmorrhage. *Arterial*

1. Put the patient flat.
2. Raise the limb.
3. Apply digital pressure and cover the wound.
4. Apply a tourniquet (a very light one if an arm) on the proximal side of the injury.

  1. *To apply a tourniquet.* Get an assistant to raise the limb.

  2. Apply a thick piece of material or wool round the limb.

  3. Stretch the tourniquet and apply it whilst stretched.

  4. Release the tourniquet at intervals if it has to be retained in position for more than half an hour.

If there is obviously no hope of saving a badly crushed limb, do not release the tourniquet. It will prevent toxins from the damaged tissues entering the blood stream. Attach a label stating at what time the tourniquet was applied.

Venous.—1. Put the patient flat.

2. Raise the limb.
3. Apply a pad and tight bandage over the bleeding point and distal to it.

Capillary hæmorrhage.—1. Apply cold, e.g. ice poultice; ice bag.

2. Apply heat, e.g. saline T. 120°—130° F.
3. Apply styptics, e.g. adrenalin 1—1,000, perchloride of iron, methylated spirit.
4. Apply pressure.

For bleeding varicose veins. Apply pad and bandage over the bleeding point, continuing the bandage tightly both above and below the rupture.

Internal hæmorrhage.—1. Put the patient flat.

2. Cover warmly, but give plenty of fresh air.
3. Raise the foot of the stretcher.
4. Record the pulse every few minutes.
5. Measure inj. morphia gr. ¼ if available.
6. Prepare for operation.

AA   369

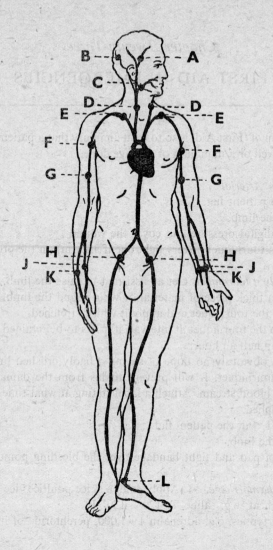

Fig. 120. Pressure points for the arrest of arterial hæmorrhage

A. Temporal artery.
B. Occipital artery.
C. Facial artery.
D. Common carotid artery.
E. Sub-clavian artery.
F. Axillary artery.
G. Brachial artery.
H. Femoral artery.
J. Radial artery.
K. Ulnar artery.
L. Posterior tibial artery.

7. In cases of delay in obtaining medical help apply a tight abdominal binder and bandage the limbs from below upwards to drive the blood to the vital centres.

8. Try to reassure the patient.

Bleeding tooth socket.—1. Sit the patient up.

2. Give a cold mouthwash, e.g. iced water, alum. ℥i—one pint, hydrogen peroxide $2\frac{1}{2}$ vols.

3. Plug the socket with a small roll of gauze or a piece of cork shaped to fit. The latter should be boiled before being used.

4. Apply styptics, e.g. adrenalin 1 in 1,000, methylated spirit or perchoride of iron.

Nose bleeding (epistaxis).—1. Sit the patient up.

2. Sponge the face with iced water and apply a cold compress to the back of the neck.

3. Pinch the nostrils.

4. Plug the nose with gauze dipped in adrenalin 1—1,000.

5. Place the feet in hot water.

Bleeding from the palm of the hand.—1. Wrap a hard ball or pad made into the shape of a ball in a clean dressing and allow the patient to grip it.

2. Put a pad in the bend of the elbow and bandage in the position of acute flexion, or keep the arm supported above the head.

Bleeding of the lower leg.—1. Put a pad behind the knee and bandage in the acutely flexed position.

Bleeding scalp wound.—1. Bathe with hot water or saline.

2. Cut the hair and remove all dirt.

3. Pinch the edges of the wound together with the fingers.

4. Apply a pad and bandage firmly.

Poisons. General Rules

1. Exclude all visitors.

2. Keep for inspection all bottles, labels, crockery, cutlery or other utensils.

3. Keep towels and bed linen for the inspection of stains.

4. Keep all excreta and vomit.

5. Do not allow handbag or clothes to be taken away.

Principles of treatment

1. Treat for shock.

2. If the lips and mouth are burnt give olive oil or cream by a teaspoon, and give the appropriate antidote if available.

3. If the lips and mouth are not burnt, an emetic may be given or a stomach tube passed.

4. In all cases demulcent drinks may be given and strong sweet tea.

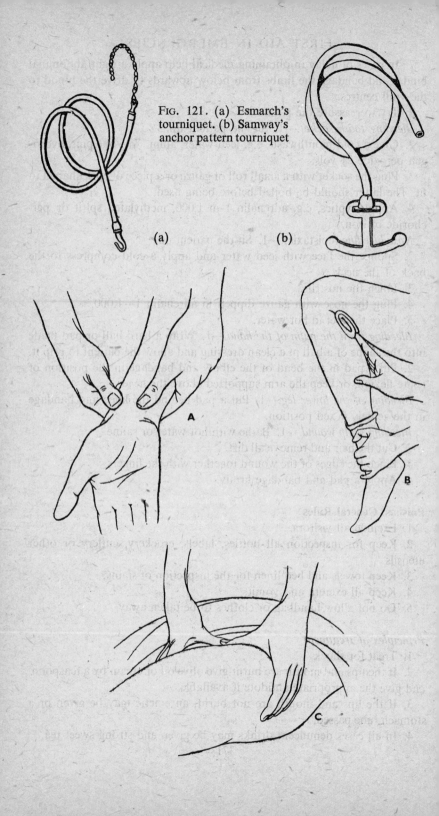

Fig. 121. (a) Esmarch's tourniquet. (b) Samway's anchor pattern tourniquet

(a)   (b)

A

B

C

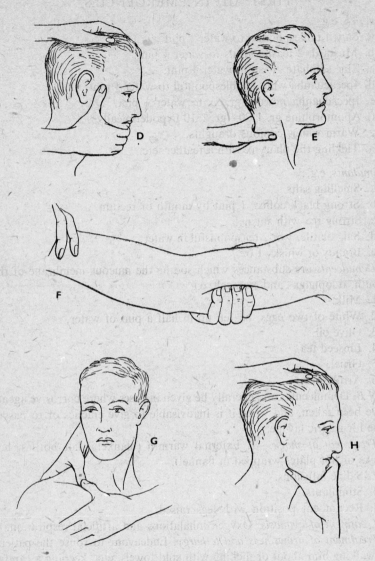

FIG. 122. Arrest of Hæmorrhage
(*see opposite page also*)

A. Digital compression of radial and ulnar arteries.
B. Compression by pad of popliteal artery.
C. Digital compression of femoral artery.
D. Digital compression of temporal artery.
E. Digital compression of common carotid artery.
F. Digital compression of brachial artery.
G. Digital compression of sub-clavian artery.
H. Digital compression of facial artery.

Emetics, e.g.:
   a. Salt, 1 tablespoonful to water ½ pint.
   b. Mustard, 2 teaspoonfuls to water ½ pint.
   c. Zinc sulphate gr. xx to water ¼ pint.
   d. Ipecacuanha wine 1 tablespoonful to water ¼ pint.
   e. Ipecacuanha powder gr. xx to water ½ pint.
   f. Apomorphine gr. 1/20—gr. 1/10 hypodermically.
   g. Warm water, copious draughts.
   h. Tickling the pharynx with a feather, etc.

Stimulants, e.g.:
   a. Smelling salts.
   b. Strong black coffee, 1 pint by mouth or rectum.
   c. Strong tea with sugar.
   d. Sal volatile, 1 or 2 teaspoonsful in water.
   e. Brandy or whisky 1 oz.

Demulcents are substances which soothe the mucous membrane of the mouth, œsophagus and stomach, e.g.:
   1. Milk.
   2. White of two eggs, beaten up in half a pint of water.
   3. Olive oil.
   4. Linseed tea.
   5. Gruel.
   6. Arrowroot.

N.B. Demulcents can generally be given in cases where corrosive agents have been taken, and when it is inadvisable to give emetics or to pass a tube for gastric lavage.

Treatment of shock.—1. External warmth (blankets, hot bottles, hot bricks or hot plates wrapped in flannel).
   2. Saline infusions.
   3. Stimulants.
   4. Recumbent position with legs raised.

Treatment of cyanosis. Oxygen inhalations and artificial respiration.

Treatment of drowsiness and lethargy. Endeavour to rouse the patient by walking him about or flicking with cold towels, etc., keeping a careful watch on the pulse all the time in case of heart failure. Inhalations of carbon dioxide and oxygen mixture.

To neutralize acid poisons give alkalis, e.g.:
   Magnesium sulphate 1 ounce—½ pint water.
   Washing soda 4 tablespoonfuls—1 pint water.
   Soda bicarbonate 1 tablespoonful—½ pint water.
   Powdered chalk 1 tablespoonful—½ pint water.
   Lime water.

Soap suds.

To neutralize alkaline poisons give acids, e.g.:
Juice of 6 lemons—1 pint of water.
Vinegar 3 ounces in 1 pint of water.

POISONS	TREATMENT
Acids Acetic acid. Hydrochloric acid. Spirits of salts. Nitric acid. Sulphuric acid (Oil of vitriol). Oxalic acid.	1. Alkalis by mouth. 2. Demulcents. 3. Morphine. 4. Hot compress to front of neck. 5. Avoid emetics.
Aconite (Monkshood) Aconitine.	1. Emetic or gastric lavage. 2. Stimulants. 3. Friction and artificial respiration.
Chloroform	1. Prop mouth open with gag. 2. Pull out tongue with forceps. 3. See that the pharnyx and mouth are quite clear of obstruction, e.g. artificial teeth. 4. Extend head and push jaw forward. 5. Loosen clothes, fresh air. 6. Artificial respiration. 7. Put head much lower than body. 8. Flap with wet towels. 9. Oxygen.
Alcohol	1. Emetic or gastric lavage. 2. One pint of strong coffee (hot by mouth or rectum). 3. Rouse by flicking, pinching, and cold douche.
Ammonia (Spirit of hartshorn).	1. Acids by mouth. 2. Demulcents. 3. Avoid emetics.
Antimony and Salts Tartar emetic. Butter of antimony.	1. Give an emetic or gastric lavage, except in case of butter of antimony. 2. Glycerine of tannic acid 2 drachms in 5 oz. of water, or tannic acid grs. xxx in 5 oz. of water, to be repeated if vomited, or very strong tea. 3. Stimulants.

Arsenic
Some fly papers.
Fowler's solution.
Some rat pastes.
Some sheep dips.
Weed killers.

1. Emetic or gastric lavage.
2. Dialysed iron 1 oz. to be repeated every two hours for twelve hours, or magnesia mixture 4 oz. or ferric hydrate prepared from washing soda ½ oz. to 1½ oz. solution of ferric chloride diluted with 2 oz. water. Repeat. Liq. Ferri perchlor.
3. Demulcents.

Atropine
Belladonna.
Hyoscine.
Hyoscyamine.

1. Emetic or gastric lavage with Condy's fluid.
2. Stimulants.
3. Artificial respiration, friction, pinching, warm and cold douche.
4. Tannic acid in water grs. xxx in 5 oz. water.
5. Morphine.

Benzene

1. Emetic.
2. Artificial respiration and flicking.
3. Hot and cold douching of face.
4. Inhalation of vapour of liquor ammonia.
5. Inj. atropine or tinct. belladonna 16 minims by mouth.

Colocynth
Vegetable irritants.

1. Stomach tube or emetic.
2. Tannic acid in water grs. xxx in 5 oz. water.
3. Demulcents.

Camphor
Camphorated oil.

1. Emetic or gastric lavage.
2. Stimulants.

Carbolic Acid

1. Give alkalis.
2. Demulcents.
3. Stimulants.
4. Artificial respiration.
N.B. For external burns swab immediately with methylated spirit or brandy.

Lysol
Cresol

1. Solution of soda bicarbonate *ad lib.* and sodium sulphate 1 oz. to 3 oz. water.
2. For external burns apply immediately soda bicarbonate compress.

Caustic Soda Caustic potash.	1. Give acids. 2. Demulcents. 3. Avoid emetics.
Chlorodyne	See opium.
Coal Gas	1. Fresh air. Oxygen inhalation. 2. Artificial respiration. 3. One pint of hot strong coffee by mouth or rectum.
Copper Sulphate (Blue vitriol)	1. Emetic. 2. Demulcents. 3. Stimulants.
Hypnotics Chloral Hydrate. Chloralamide. Paraldehyde. Sulphonal. Barbiturates (medinal luminal, etc.).	1. Emetic. 2. Stimulants. 3. Rouse patient by exercise, flicking, etc. 4. Artificial respiration. 5. Capsule of amyl nitrite. 6. Inhalation of $C.O._2$ and oxygen.
Hydrocyanic Acid (Prussic acid) (Oil of almonds) Potassium cyanide.	May be fatal in a few minutes. 1. Place patient in open air. 2. Give an emetic. 3. Alternate hot and cold douches (from height) to head and spine, or dash cold water on continuously. 4. Artificial respiration and apply ammonia to the nostrils. 5. Blood transfusion. 6. Oxygen inhalation.
Lead	1. Emetic. 2. Demulcent. 3. Poultices to abdomen. 4. Magnesium sulphate or sodium sulphate.
Mercury and Salts Corrosive sublimate. White precipitate. Red precipitate.	1. White of eggs mixed with water in un-limited quantities, or flour and water, arrow-root and water. 2. Emetic. 3. If medical aid cannot be obtained, wash out the stomach with white of egg in water.

Mussel Poisoning

1. Emetic.
2. Stimulants.
3. Castor oil.

Nux Vomica
  Strychnine.
  Easton's syrup.
  Some vermin killers.

1. Emetic or gastric lavage.
2. Potassium bromide grs. xxx, chlora
hydrate grs. 15 in 5 oz. water. Repeat
necessary.
3. Keep patient quiet, but in case of col
lapse artificial respiration. Capsule amy
nitrite.
4. Bromethol or other sedative.

Opium
  (Soothing syrup)
  (Syrup of poppies)
  Chlorodyne.
  Morphine.
  Codeine.
  Laudanum.
  Paregoric.
  Nepenthe.
  Dover's powder.

1. Emetic or gastric lavage.
2. Hot coffee.
3. Potassium permanganate grs. 10 in 10 oz
warm water (leave 5 oz. in stomach).
4. Cold water to face. Rouse patient b
exercise, flapping, etc.
5. Artificial respiration.
6. Smelling salts or liq. ammonia vapour t
nostrils.
7. Inhalation of CO_2 and oxygen.
8. Inj. Atropin gr. $\frac{1}{100}$.

Paraffin Oil
  Petroleum.

1. Emetic.
2. Stimulants.
3. Friction.

**Phenacetin and
    Phenazone**
  Antipyrin.
  Antifebrin.
  Acetanilide.

1. Emetic.
2. Artificial respiration.
3. Stimulants.
4. Oxygen.

Phosphorus (Rat paste)

1. Gastric lavage or copper sulphate 3 grs
dissolved in water every five minutes unti
vomiting is induced, then every 15—30 minutes. Or zinc sulphate 20 grains dissolved in
water may be given as an emetic.
2. Oil of turpentine 20 minims in an ounce
of water every half hour for six doses.
3. Sulphate of magnesium $\frac{1}{2}$—1 oz. in a
tumbler of water, linseed tea.
4. Demulcent of milk and eggs avoiding
ordinary fats and oils.

5. Potassium permanganate 10 grains in 10 oz. water.

Sewer Gas	1. Fresh air.
	2. Oxygen.
	3. Artificial respiration.
	4. Stimulants.
Silver Salts Lunar caustic.	1. Common salt $\frac{1}{2}$ oz. to one pint water. 2. Demulcents.
Snake Bites and Jelly Fish Stings	1. Stimulants very freely. 2. Rub powdered potassium permanganate or Condy's fluid freely into the wound. 3. Artificial respiration. *N.B.* For rattle snakes, olive oil freely by mouth and also to be rubbed into the skin.
Turpentine	1. Emetic. 2. Magnesium sulphate $\frac{1}{2}$ oz. to 2 oz. of water. 3. Demulcents.
Zinc	1. Emetic or gastric lavage. 2. Sodium bicarbonate 1 oz. to one pint of water. 3. Milk. 4. Strong tea.

REMOVAL OF FOREIGN BODIES

Eye. (a) Do not allow the patient to rub the eye.

(b) Examine the lower lid by pulling it forward and down.

(c) Evert the upper lid by pulling it down with the eyelashes and rolling it back over a matchstick or eye rod. The tarsal plate will keep the lid in position.

(d) If the foreign body can be seen remove it with a clean handkerchief.

(e) If the foreign body is seen on the cornea and cannot be easily removed, leave it to be dealt with by the doctor as the cornea is very easily damaged.

(f) If the substance in the eye is lime or any chemical which burns, irrigate very freely and thoroughly with water or saline until every particle has been removed.

(g) After removal of any foreign body put in a drop of castor oil.

(h) Cover the eye, and if at all doubtful about it seek medical aid.

Ear. (a) Pull the pinna in a backwards and upwards direction.

(b) If the object can be seen remove by forceps or other suitable implement according to the object to be grasped.

(c) If it cannot be dislodged, syringe the ear, directing the flow to the upper wall of the meatus so that the fluid may get behind the object and wash it out.

(d) If it is a pea or bean or any vegetable substance which would swell do not syringe the ear, but take the patient to a doctor.

(e) If an insect crawls into the ear, a very small quantity of chloroform may be dropped into the entrance to the meatus. Failing this a little cigarette smoke is carefully blown into the ear. It may suffice to kill it. After which it may be syringed out.

Nose. (a) Pinch the other nostril and tell the patient to blow the nose to see if the foreign body can be dislodged.

(b) Give a nasal douche putting the nozzle into the other nostril.

(c) The patient should not be allowed to sniff, as this will draw the foreign body further up the nasal passages. If pea or bean do not irrigate or this will cause the object to swell.

BITES AND STINGS

Wasp and Bee Stings

1. In the case of a bee remove the sting. (The wasp does not usually leave its sting behind.)

2. Apply an alkali, e.g. ammonia, washing soda or a blue bag.

3. Apply iodine if available.

Stings in the mouth are very dangerous, owing to the swelling produced. Mouthwashes of soda bicarbonate should be given and in all cases medical aid sought without delay. Shock and fright are often severe. Fatalities are not uncommon.

Snake Bite

1. If a limb compress the part on the proximal side of the wound by means of a tight bandage or rubber tubing.

2. Suck the wound vigorously, but do not swallow the poison.

3. Bathe the part with hot water.

4. Pack with crystals of potassium permanganate if these are available. Dry well after bathing and apply iodine.

5. Treat for shock and use stimulants. Seek medical aid.

Dog Bite

1. Bathe the wound at once with hot water.

2. Cover with clean dressing.

3. Seek medical aid. The wound is cauterized with silver nitrate stick or electric cautery.

The dog must be traced and full inquiries made.

BITES AND STINGS

Hydrophobia resulting from the bite of a mad dog is rare in this country. If there is any danger of this a tight bandage should be applied on the proximal side of the wound to prevent the circulation of poisons.

Mosquitoes. Apply a slice of raw onion, iodine or an alkali such as washing soda or ammonia.

Sunburn. Apply calamine lotion, soda bicarbonate solution or a simple fat such as lanoline.

Frostbite
1. Rub the affected part to try to restore the circulation.
2. Do *not* rub with snow as is so often advised.
3. On no account let the part come into contact with heat except very gradually as the circulation is restored.
4. Support the part in a dependent position.
5. Treat for shock.

Sunstroke
1. Bring the patient out of the sun, into the coolest place available.
2. Keep the room dark and the air circulating.
3. Apply cold compresses to the head.
4. Keep the patient lying flat.
5. Take the pulse.
6. Send for medical aid.
7. Have a vomit bowl at hand.

Heat Stroke
1. Move to a cool, dark, well-ventilated spot.
2. Keep the patient lying quietly on the back.
3. Take the temperature and pulse.
4. Give tepid and cold sponging.
5. Seek medical aid. If this is delayed continue with the cold sponging if the temperature remains high and use measures other than drugs to reduce it, e.g. cold compresses, electric fans, regulating the bedclothes, etc.

Heat stroke generally occurs in tropical climates. It is not due to the direct heat of the sun on the head, but is due to the high temperature, humidity, and stagnation of the air, causing heat retention and inability of the heat regulating centre in the brain to function. The treatment is to keep the temperature down by physical means.

Inhalation of Carbon Monoxide. (From the exhaust gas of a motor-car in a closed garage, or in badly ventilated rooms heated by closed stoves or leakage of coal gas; also attempted suicides by coal gas.)
Treatment
1. Turn off the gas, if this is the cause, or car engine, etc.

2. Remove the patient as quickly as possible into the fresh air.
3. Begin artificial respiration.
4. Send for help.
5. Keep the patient warm.

The mucous membranes are bright pink owing to the presence of carbon monoxide in the blood. The need for oxygen is urgent.

Drowning

1. Remove the patient from the water.
2. Put the patient face downwards.
3. Loosen clothing.
4. Remove debris, grass, weeds, etc., from mouth and throat with the fingers.
5. If possible, raise the pelvis higher than the head to drain the water from the lungs.
6. Send for help.
7. Start artificial respiration.
8. Apply warmth. General methods of resuscitation.

Attempted Suicide by Hanging

1. Cut the rope and lower the body gradually.
2. Loosen the clothing at neck.
3. Send for help.
4. Treat for shock.

Causes of Coma

(a) Apoplexy. (b) Alcohol. (c) Acidosis (diabetes). (d) Epilepsy. (e) Injury to the brain. (f) Insulin. (g) Overdoses of opium or other hypnotic. (h) Uræmia.

Keep the patient quite warm, send for medical help and make the following observations:

1. The smell of the breath.
2. Condition of the pulse.
3. Condition of the pupils.
4. Note if the skin is dry or moist.

Search the pockets for lumps of sugar or phials of insulin or hypodermic syringe, also for any other tablets or packets. Examine the arms and legs for marks of previous injections. If it is possible to get a specimen, test the urine for sugar. Examine for superficial injuries caused by the accident, if any.

Keep the policeman or relatives or friends until the doctor comes and listen to any evidence which may give a clue as to the cause of coma.

Causes of Convulsions. *Fits* are caused by irritation of the brain by: Tumours, emboli, or head accidents; also met with in the following conditions: epilepsy, uræmia, tetanus, strychnine poisoning. In infants the brain unstable and easily irritated by pain or circulating toxins. Hence convulsions occur in association with infectious illness, rickets and digestive disorders, teething and neglected constipation.

Treatment

1. Put patient in a safe place.
2. Loosen clothing around the neck.
3. Insert a gag (clothes peg or pencil), and keep the head to the side.
4. Observe:
a. The duration of the fit and the length of each stage (if possible).
b. Incontinence.
c. If the convulsions begin in any particular group of muscles.
d. If there appear to be any purposive movements during the convulsive stage.

Convulsions in children. Immerse the child in a warm mustard bath. 1 oz. mustard in a muslin bag to 1 gallon water, temperature 100° F. Sponge the head with cold water. Keep in the bath until the child is relaxed and a good colour.

Medical aid is sought in all cases of convulsions.

Methods of Artificial Respiration

1. *Schafer's.* 1. Place the patient in the prone position with a pillow under the chest, head on one side, and arms flexed over the head.

2. Kneel on one side of the patient, or, if a small patient, kneel with one leg on either side of the patient's pelvis.

3. Place the hands at the sides of the lower ribs and begin alternate movements of pressure to empty the lungs, and relaxation to allow them to fill. The movements should be rhythmical and not more than 15 per minute. The whole weight of the body transmitted through the hands is used to compress the lungs.

If the artificial respiration is performed correctly, the operator can keep up the steady swaying movements for quite a long time without great effort.

2. *Sylvester's method.* 1. Place the patient on back with the head to one side, arms by the sides and a small pillow under the shoulders. Ask an assistant to grasp the tongue with a handkerchief and keep it well forward.

2. Kneel or stand at the head of the patient.

3. Grasp the forearms just below the elbow and bring the arms in an outward, well-stretched movement, above her head. Then carry them down with the elbows flexed to the front of the patient on to the sides of the chest, exerting firm pressure with the patient's arm and the operator's hands on the bases of the lungs. Repeat this movement not more than 15 times per minute.

In most cases Schafer's method is easier to do and more effective.

'Both' respirator. The 'Both' respirator or 'Iron Lung' is the type pre
sented to hospitals by Viscount Nuffield. It is a mechanical device for th
prolonged administration of artificial respiration, by means of an electri
motor and bellows, which alternately decrease and increase the pressur
of the air within the airtight wooden case.

Should the electric current fail, the bellows can be worked by hand.

The patient, very often unconscious, is laid on the *sorbo* mattress wit
the head through the opening provided. A tightly fitting sorbo collar i
passed over the patient's head to fit the neck closely, a layer of lint i
necessary next to the patient's skin to prevent friction.

The head is supported on a small pillow and then a metal ring is screwe
down to secure the sorbo collar.

Conscious patients can eat, drink and sleep in the respirator withou
having the mechanism stopped. There are small portholes on either sid
through which the nurse introduces her arm so that the patient can b
attended to. One small blanket is usually sufficient covering as the air i
warmed by an electric bulb keeping the temperature approximately 75°–
80° F. Ring pads for the heels, knees, and head add to the patient's comfor
and a covered sandbag in position prevents foot drop.

Once daily, if possible, the patient is taken out for general nursing treat
ment. During this period oxygen and manual artificial respiration may b
necessary.

This type of respirator has been used successfully in cases of infantil
paralysis, carbon-monoxide poisoning and drowning, and has been pro
vided by Lord Nuffield for hospitals throughout the British Empire.

The 'Drinker' respirator is an earlier and more elaborate pattern.

Sprains of the Ankle and Wrist

Bandage at once with a firm bandage soaked in cold water. Raise th
ankle on a pillow and support the wrist in a sling. In cases of severe sprain
medical aid should be sought to exclude the possibility of a fracture.

In cases of slight sprain, the bandage should be reapplied firmly and th
patient should be allowed to use the wrist or walk on the foot within th
limits of pain.

Dislocations

These are recognized by the abnormal contour of the joint. Ankle an
shoulder joints are the common sites of dislocation.

Support the ankle on a pillow and transport the patient to a doctor a
once.

In case of the shoulder, put the arm in a sling and take the patient to th
doctor.

Give restoratives for shock.

The sooner the dislocation is reduced the better; there should be no delay.

Fractures. General principles of treatment.

1. Cover the patient with rugs or coats.

2. Immobilize the limb—by an improvised splint—walking stick, umbrella, or rolled up newspapers. Tie in position with anything which can be used or with a bandage (handkerchiefs, ties, etc.).

In some cases the lower limb may be immobilized by being tied to the sound leg.

3. Transport to hospital by ambulance or obtain medical aid as soon as possible.

4. A dose of morphia may be required.

N.B. If a compound fracture, cut away the clothing, apply the cleanest dressing available. If there is bleeding measures should be taken to arrest this before anything else is done.

Special Fractures

Skull. Keep the patient warm and quiet and the head raised. Note if there is any bloodstained discharge from the nose or ears, if so mop it up with something very clean, preferably sterile. Give no stimulants. Record the pulse and respirations. Note exactly how long the patient is unconscious.

Ribs. Transport to hospital in a semi-recumbent position inclined to the painful side. Note any hæmoptysis.

Pelvis. Keep the patient flat on the back. When transferring to the ambulance lift the patient supporting the pelvis very carefully. Discourage the patient from passing urine if possible until a catheter can be passed.

Spine. Arrange a rug which can be used as a stretcher close to the side of the patient. Cross and flex one leg over the other and obtain the help of two or three other people to turn the patient on to his face with one careful, gentle movement. He will then be in the position to avoid injury to the spinal cord. Place a small pillow under the chest and another under the pelvis to keep the spine extended. He should be lifted on to the stretcher in this position. Note if he is paralysed or incontinent and if there is any sensation in the limbs.

Clavicle. If suffering from shock place the patient on a bed with a small hard pad between the shoulder blades. A rolled-up scarf would do.

2. Flex the affected arm. Keep it at the side of the body with the hand over the chest. Support the elbow with a hard pillow to prevent the arm from dropping.

3. If the patient can sit up, put the arm in a full sized sling, applied carefully to give good support.

Jaw. 1. Make sure that no teeth have been knocked out or are loose.

2. Apply a four-tailed jaw bandage or barrel bandage.

3. Tell the patient not to try and talk.

Electric shock. 1. Turn off the current. If this is impossible, the person rendering first aid should insulate herself before trying to pull the patient away from the wire. She may do this by putting on leather or rubber gloves, or putting her hand in a tobacco pouch, or in a mackintosh. She should also stand on a mackintosh or some rubber material. If she is wearing shoes with rubber soles she is already insulated. If it is impossible for any of the above precautions to be taken the patient should be pulled away by a wooden stick—not an umbrella as this is metal.

2. Treat for shock and begin artificial respiration at once.

Triangular bandages are used in first aid work.

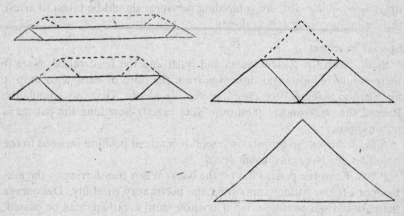

Fig. 123. Method of folding a triangular bandage

Chapter Twenty-Four

BANDAGING

Roller Bandaging. A roller bandage should be applied firmly, neatly, and with even pressure. Three inches of the bandage should be unrolled at once, and the dressing must be completely covered. The most suitable type of bandage must be chosen for the particular case. Muslin bandages are commonly used; they are light, porous and comfortable, and are generally used for bandages of the head. Fine calico bandages are required where extra support is needed, example, for a bandage to the knee, in the case of a patient who is walking about. Calico bandages are also used for applying a splint which is to be kept firmly in position. Flannel bandages are warm and slightly elastic and are useful for chest cases. Crêpe bandages are most comfortable and slightly elastic, they fit the part, and at the same time give good support. They are used for bandaging the leg to support varicose veins, and are useful for securing a dressing to glands of the neck, being sufficiently elastic to accommodate the movements of the jaw. They are expensive, but are washed very satisfactorily.

When about to apply a bandage, the nurse should take a dish and collect on it bandages of suitable type and width, a safety pin and a dressing. The dressing should be cut carefully to the size and shape required; the wool should be separated to a suitable thickness. The bandage will not be neat and satisfactory if a bulky, ill-fitting dressing is applied. The patient is then placed in a good position. If a foot or leg is to be bandaged, the bedclothes should be turned back from the bottom, the good leg being kept covered and the affected one resting on a pillow. If the patient is not in bed, a footstool is required. If an arm, the gown should be partially removed, the patient's chest well covered and the limb supported on a pillow. If the dressing is to be put on the head, the patient should be arranged so that the nurse can get at the patient easily. Before beginning the bandage, the nurse should stand back to see that the part is in the correct anatomical position; for example, the foot well dorsi-flexed, the shoulders well drawn back. It is very easy to put a bandage on uncomfortably with some of the turns a little too tight if attention is not given to these points. Each turn in a roller bandage should overlap the previous one by two-thirds of its width. Bandages to the limbs are applied from below upwards and from within outwards to encourage the venous return of blood to the heart. The safety

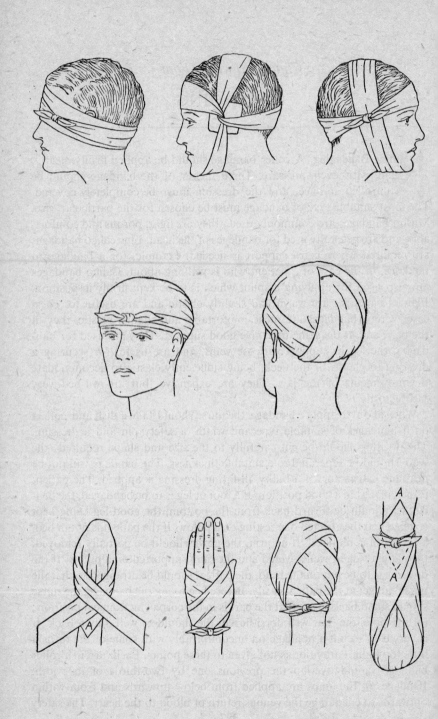

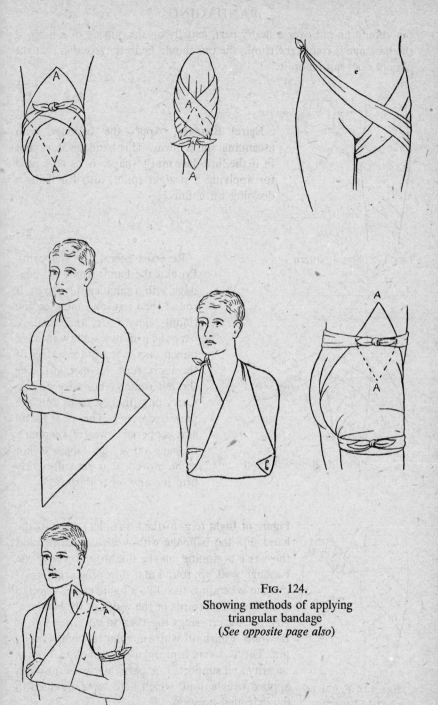

Fig. 124.
Showing methods of applying
triangular bandage
(*See opposite page also*)

BANDAGING

pin should be put over a fleshy part, usually on the outside of a limb. If the bandage is round the trunk, the pin should be in the front so that the patient does not lie on it.

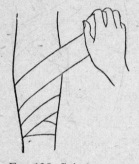

Spiral Bandage. Apply the bandage with ascending spiral turns. This bandage does not fit if the limb has much shape. It can be used for applying a straight splint, also for fixing a dressing on a finger.

FIG. 125. Spiral pattern

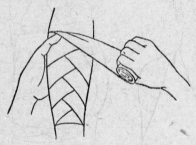

FIG. 126. Reversed spiral

Reversed Spiral (to the arm). Pronate the hand. Apply the bandage with a circular turn to fix it round the wrist, beginning on the thumb side. Carry the bandage over the arm in a slightly upward direction. On the outer surface of the limb, turn the bandage over the left thumb, thus reversing it. Carry on with these turns until the part is covered. This is a useful and economical way of keeping a dressing on a limb which is not to be moved. It is not sufficiently firm for any other purpose.

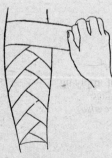

FIG. 127. Figure of eight pattern

Figure of Eight (e.g. to the arm or leg). Pronate the hand. Fix the bandage with a circular turn round the wrist beginning on the thumb side. Carry the bandage well up, round and down the arm, crossing the ascending turn like a figure eight. Overlap each figure two-thirds of the width of the bandage. Arrange the crossings together on the outer side of the limb. Finish off with a circular turn and a safety pin. This is a very firm and useful bandage. It gives security and support. It is particularly useful when applied over a joint which is to be maintained in the extended position.

Divergent Spica (e.g. to an elbow). Flex the elbow. Apply two circular turns over each other to fix the bandage, covering the olecranon process. Take the third turn below, covering the lower third of the previous turn. Cross over on the flexor surface of the elbow, apply the fourth turn above the joint, covering the upper third of the first and second turns. Continue above and below, until the dressing is covered. The same bandage is applied for a flexed knee. It is also suitable for covering a dressing on the heel.

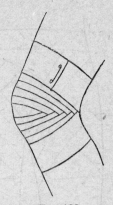

FIG. 128
Spica to flexed knee

Spica to Shoulder. Take a circular turn of the bandage about two inches or more below the shoulder. Carry it from the inner surface of the arm across the back, under the axilla of the opposite side and across the chest to the arm. Continue these turns over the shoulder and round the trunk

until the dressing is covered. It may be necessary to apply one figure of eight turn round the arm before the turns round the trunk are commenced. Protect the axilla on the opposite side with a piece of wool to prevent the skin from being rubbed. See that the patient is sitting well up and straight before you begin: or if he is lying down that the shoulders are kept well back.

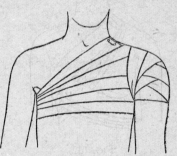

FIG. 129. Spica to shoulder

Spica of the Hip. Fix the bandage with a circular turn round the upper part of the thigh. Carry it from within outwards and upwards round the lower trunk, returning from the waist and crossing the first turn on the outer side of the thigh. Carry on thus with similar turns, overlapping each one two-thirds of its width, until the hip is well covered.

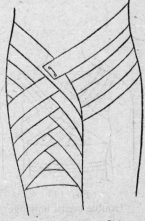

391

FIG. 130. Spica to hip

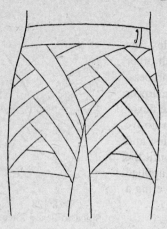

Fig. 131. Double hip spica

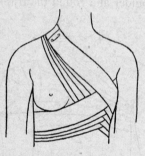

Fig. 132.
Single breast bandage

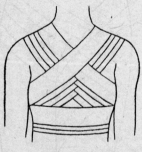

Fig. 133.
Double breast bandage

Double Hip Spica. Fix the bandage with a circular turn round the waist, going from left to right and returning to the starting point on the left side. Take the next turn round the inner side and round the right leg; cross over, and taking a turn round the back of the waist to the starting point. Take the next turn round the outside of the left thigh and round that leg, crossing it over and taking a turn round the waist to the starting point. Take a turn round each leg alternately until the dressings are covered.

Breast Bandage (left). Start under the left breast and carry the bandage round the front of the abdomen; take two circular turns round the waist, returning to the starting point. Support the breast with the next turn which goes over the right shoulder and across the back to the starting point. Take another turn round the waist, overlapping the previous one by two-thirds of its width. Repeat these turns alternately until the breast is well covered and supported, and the crossings of the bandage form a pattern on the outer side.. If the right breast is to be bandaged, start under the right breast and take the first turn away from it across the abdomen.

Double Breast Bandage. Start under one breast and fix with a double circular turn. Carry the bandage over the opposite shoulder across the back to the starting point. Go half-way round the waist, across the back in an upward direction to the other shoulder, down in front under the other breast. Take half a turn round the waist to the starting point. Carry on with these turns alternately over each breast, arranging the waist turns in ascending fashion until both breasts are covered.

BANDAGING

Fractured Clavicle Bandage (left). Fix the upper arm to the left side and flex the fore-arm across the chest. Put a thin layer of wool between the arm and the chest wall and in the axilla. It is always more comfortable to separate adjacent skin surfaces in this way. Fix the bandage with a circular turn round the waist, beginning at the right side and going towards the injured arm across the front of the abdomen. From the starting point take the second turn again round the waist, allowing the lower half of the bandage to cover the olecranon process and return to the starting point.

Take the next turn across the chest, over the left wrist and shoulder, down the back of and up in front of the left arm. This completes the covering of the olecranon and acts as a supporting sling; carry on over the left shoulder across the back to the starting point. The second turn round the trunk covers the flexed elbow one-third of the width of the bandage higher.

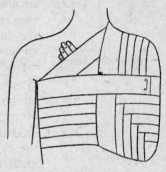

FIG. 134.
Bandage for fractured clavicle

The next turn is over the hand and shoulder, continuing with the arm sling, taking it a third of the width of the bandage inwards and crossing the back to the starting point. Carry on with these turns alternately, until the arm is covered.

Foot (left). Fix the bandage with two circular turns round the ankle and carry it over the dorsum of the foot; take two recurrent turns over the middle toes and two recurrent turns on either side of the first turn. Do not make the recurrent turns too short or the ends of the bandage will come out.

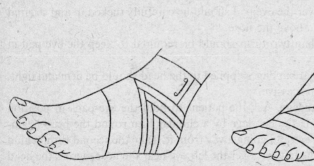

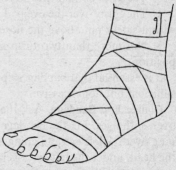

FIG. 135. Bandages to foot

FIG. 136. Divergent spica to heel

Fix these with one turn round the bases of the toes. Next cover the heel with three turns of a divergent spica. Then continue figure of eight pattern round the foot and ankle until the whole foot is well and firmly covered.

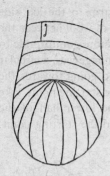

FIG. 137. Bandage for amputation stump

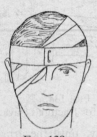

FIG. 138.
Eye bandage

The figure of eight pattern should be seen on the dorsum of the foot. It is well to get the toes and heel properly covered first as described, then the whole foot can be finished off neatly.

If it is not necessary to cover the toes and heel, start the bandage round the ankle and do a figure of eight including the ankle and foot.

Amputation Stump. Fix the bandage with a circular turn well away from the incision. Take long recurrent turns backwards and forwards over the stump and fix these firmly with circular turns and cover up to the starting point.

Eye Bandage (left). Ask the patient to hold the eye-pad in position. Fix the bandage with a circular turn round the head beginning over the left eye, and going across the forehead away from it. Take the second turn in the same direction behind the right ear, down across the back of the head under the left ear and over the eye pad near the nose. Carry on in the same direction across and slightly to the right side of the head. Take a circular turn round the head, covering the first one. Do each of these turns alternately once more, finishing off with a turn round the forehead.

N.B.—1. The turns of the bandage round the forehead should be well above the eyebrows.

2. No bandage should be allowed to irritate the good eye.

3. The ears should not be covered.

4. The turns over the eye pad should be carefully tucked in and secured with a safety pin above the nose.

5. Not more than two turns should be required to keep the eye pad in position.

It is essential that bandages applied to the head should be firm and light, sufficient but not excessive.

Double Eye Bandage. Ask the patient to hold the eye-pads in position over both eyes. Fix the bandage by a circular turn round the head beginning over the left eye and going away from it. Take the second turn behind the head, under the left ear, over the left eye near the nose, across the head and round to the starting point. Take another complete circular turn round the head, go in a downward direction over the right eye, under the right ear and slightly over the left side of the head to the starting point. Fix with a circular turn round the head. Another turn over each eye pad will be sufficient with the alternate circular turns round the head. A cambric bandage tied on with tapes as described in chapter 16 is more conveniently applied and is not so bulky. Some surgeons prefer pads to be fixed in position with strapping.

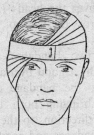

FIG. 139. Alternative pattern for ear bandage. The ear turns are taken over the side of the head instead of overlapping the circular turn round the forehead

Ear Bandage (left). Fix the ear pad well over and behind the ear, and sufficiently low in the neck to catch any discharge. Take a circular turn round the head starting over the left eye and going across the front of the forehead to the starting point. Take the next turn across the forehead, behind and across the head, under the left ear covering the front border of the pad and thus returning to the middle of the forehead. Reverse the bandage and do a circular turn round the head. Take the next turn round the back of the head thus beginning to cover the ear pad in an upward direction. Apply alternate turns round the head and over the ear until the dressing is covered.

Double Ear Bandage. Fix the pads in position over both ears. Take a circular turn round the head to fix the bandage in position and carry on behind the head, under the left ear to the forehead. Reverse the bandage and take the next turn down over the right ear pad and across the back of the head. Take another turn over the left ear to the centre of the forehead and reverse as before, carrying the bandage down over the right ear pad: continue till the dressings are covered. Secure with a turn round the forehead.

Glands of Neck (left). Arrange a fairly large dressing to cover the incision. Fix the bandage with a circular turn round the head, beginning over the right eye and going across the forehead towards the affected side. Take the second turn half-way round the head across the back of the head, under the right ear and chin and up over the dressing covering the front border of it. Carry this turn over the top of the head down behind the right ear, across the front of the neck and round

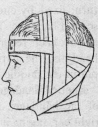

FIG. 140.
Gland bandage

the back of the head to the starting point over the right eye. Do these three turns alternately: (1) Round the head; (2) round the front of the neck and up the gland working backwards over the head; (3) round the front of the neck and across the back of the head to the starting point.

Capeline Bandage. Fix two bandages together, either by stitching them or by a good overlap. Stand behind the patient and fix the bandage over the middle of the forehead, bringing both bandages round the head in different directions to the nape of the neck. Cross over the bandages and complete the turns until they meet over the forehead again. Cross them over. Carry the one bandage with the right hand right over the top of the head from the fore head to the nape of the neck. Take the second bandage with the left hand round the head, fixing the first at the nape and carrying it on round the head to

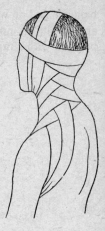

FIG. 141. Gland bandage incorporating turns under the axilla

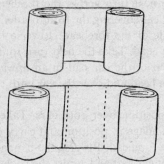

FIG. 142. Muslin bandages prepared for application of capeline

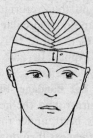

FIG. 143. Capeline bandage

the starting point. From this point onwards the one bandage is applied by recurrent turns backwards and forwards on alternate sides of the middle turn, fixed by circular turns round the head with the second bandage. The circular turns overlap each other and fix each recurrent turn at the middle of the forehead and the nape of the neck. Fasten with a safety pin in the middle of the forehead.

Knotted Bandage to the Forehead. Unwind six inches of the bandage, and from this point start over the right ear, taking a circular turn right round the head; twist the end of the bandage at the starting point. Take the next turn of the bandage over the top of the

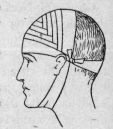

FIG. 144. Knotted bandage

396

head, behind the left ear under the chin to the starting point; twist. Take another circular turn round the head, overlapping the original one at the front by two-thirds of its width, but completely overlapping the bandage round the back of the crown; continue round to the starting point and twist. The next turn goes over the top of the head, overlapping the previous turn by two-thirds of its width, thus converging to the turns over the forehead. Carry on behind the ear and under the chin, overlapping the previous turns to the starting point. Twist. Do several of these alternating turns until the wound is covered. Cut the bandage and tie in a knot with the end of the six inches with which the bandage commenced.

A similar bandage can be applied for a wound at the back of the head, but in this case the turns converge from the crown to the nape, the forehead turns overlapping each other.

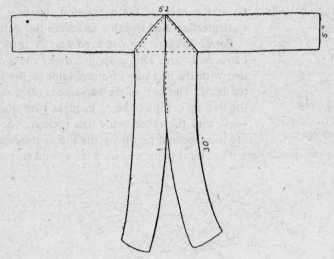

FIG. 145. 'T' Bandage

T. Bandage to secure perineal dressings. Two lengths of 5-inch muslin bandage are sewn together as shown above. The end of the perineal band is slit and the two tails tie over the waistband at the front.

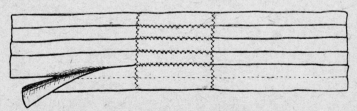

FIG. 146. Many-tailed bandage (abdominal)

BANDAGING

Many-tailed bandages are usually made of domette and are used to secure dressings on the chest, abdomen or on a limb or amputation stump. They are put under the part to be bandaged and the tails are folded over each other with a two-thirds overlap. The last tail is secured by a pin.

Four-tailed jaw bandage. A piece of lint or flannel is required 40 inches long and 3 inches wide. The two ends are cut into four tails each 15 inches long, leaving a piece in the centre 9 inches long to support the chin. In this piece a slit 2 inches long is

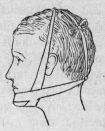

Fig. 147. Four-tailed jaw bandage

cut. The chin fits into the slit. The lower ends follow the line of the lower jaw and are tied in a single knot at the top of the head. The upper ends tie at the back of the neck—and the four loose ends are then tied together to secure the bandage.

Barrel bandage for fractured jaw. A three inch bandage 2 yards long is applied under the chin and tied with the first turn of a reef knot on the top of the head. The turn of the bandage is separated by the fingers, one piece being brought over the forehead, and the other below the occiput. The ends are then secured tightly on the top of the head.

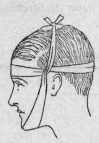

Fig. 148.
Barrel bandage for fractured jaw

Bandaging the fingers. The spiral pattern is used. If several fingers are

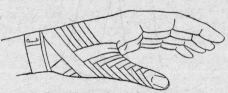

Fig. 149. Bandaging the thumb

to be bandaged a spica turn round the wrist and across the back of the hand is taken between each finger. A spica may be applied to the thumb taking descending turns alternately round the thumb and round the wrist.

Chapter Twenty-Five

NOTES ON THE NURSING OF SOME SURGICAL CASES

Amputation of Leg. Nursed in amputation bed; avoid flexion deformity of hip or knee, or adduction deformity in an upper arm amputation. In amputation of thigh extend hip joint and immobilize with sandbags—no pillow allowed for stump. In amputations below the knee the leg may at first be bandaged on a back splint. Treat for shock and watch for reactionary and secondary hæmorrhage; record pulse frequently and inspect underneath the dressing and buttocks. Report if fresh blood appears on the dressing—tourniquet at hand. Give small quantities of cool, non-stimulating fluids frequently. Morphia required. Drains withdrawn half-way after forty-eight hours—removed after seventy-two hours. Stitches removed in seven days. When the patient begins to walk about with crutches, bandage the stump firmly with a crêpe bandage to prevent postural oedema.

Fractured Spine. *First Aid Position:* Face downwards, pillow under chest, pelvis and ankles with spine extended. If the patient is not co-operative in this position, he must lie on his back, with a pillow in the small of the back. X-ray. Nursed in plaster bed, or jacket, made in two halves so that the patient can be turned over. Move by rolling patient, strapped to the plaster; four nurses needed to keep spine rigid. Bed cradle and splints to prevent drop foot. Support springs of bed with fracture boards, and protect mattress with long mackintosh. *N.B.* Damage to spinal cord; paralysis of the legs, incontinence of urine and fæces. Guard against pressure sores, chest complications, cystitis (supra-pubic cystotomy and bladder lavage).

Fracture of cervical spine nursed in plaster collar with head extended.

Fractured Ribs. Sit the patient up, turned towards the injured side with a pillow to support the injured ribs. Treat for shock, especially if there are other injuries. Watch for hæmoptysis and emphysema. X-ray. Application of strapping. *To apply strapping:* Sit patient up; wash and shave the skin. Apply strips of three-inch strapping round the chest wall from beyond sternum to beyond spine, beginning above and working downwards; overlap two-thirds of each strip, securing each one whilst the patient breathes out. Support with calico or flannel bandage.

Fractured Pelvis. Lay patient in dorsal position, one pillow allowed; binder with sandbags to immobilize pelvis; bed cradle. Two or three nurses lift to place patient on bedpan and to treat back. Divided mattress useful. Note blood in urine, indicating urethral or bladder injury. Catheterization as soon as possible after the accident.

Fractured Jaw (always compound). Note if teeth have been broken or loosened. Apply jaw bandage. Surgical treatment by dental plates or wire splints. Give fluids with feeder with rubber tubing attached and insert at side of mouth. Give plenty of boiled water to drink, especially after feeds. Irrigation of the mouth. Sit patient up. Guard against sepsis, pneumonia and lung abscess.

Head injuries

1. *Scalp wounds*. Cut the hair and bathe with hot saline or weak antiseptic. Press wound edges together and apply pad and bandage. Keep the patient flat, with the head raised.

2. *Concussion and contusion*. Treat for shock; take pulse frequently; sit patient up as soon as possible. Have vomit bowl at hand. Rest and quietness important; use screens, shade lights; no visitors; no reading or smoking allowed. Sedative drugs (bromide and chloral) given. Light diet; limited non-stimulating fluids. Watch for retention or incontinence of urine. Prepare for lumbar puncture; magnesium sulphate enema. Cold compresses for headache. If patient is unconscious for more than a few minutes there is probably contusion of the brain. Complete rest for two to four weeks.

3. *Fractures of the skull*. Treat for concussion. Watch for escape of blood and cerebrospinal fluid from ears, nose and into the orbit. If from ears or nose, clean with sterile wool and saline and insert sterile swab loosely. *Dangerous complication* is compression of the brain by piece of bone, blood clot or œdema if the brain substance is lacerated. Observe and report at once: deepening unconsciousness after lucid interval; slowing of the pulse; slow and stertorous respiration; twitching; fits, squint or paralysis. Rest in bed for at least six weeks. Decompression may be performed.

Herniotomy. After operation, semi-recumbent position, knee pillow until third morning; small pillow in the small of the back; support scrotum. Watch for retention of urine. Guard against chest complications and orchitis. Rest in bed for two (femoral) to three weeks (inguinal). Three weeks' convalescence. Children get up at end of one week.

Hæmorrhoidectomy. *Preparation for operation.*—Enemata on two mornings previous to operation and rectal lavage on the day. Light roughage-free diet. *Post-operative care*—semi-recumbent position, two or three pillows, small knee pillow; knees tied together; air ring. Fluids and roughage-free diet. Irrigation after use of bedpan. Apply antiseptic powder and sterile pads. Patient may be turned on side at intervals. Liquid paraffin twice daily from second day. Olive oil or gruel enema, using fine catheter, on third morning, if required. Tube removed after enema is given. Defæcation painful; have stimulant at hand. May be difficulty in micturition. After a few days patient may sit in hot boracic baths.

Treatment of inflamed hæmorrhoids before operation. High blocks to foot of bed. Hot saline fomentations and large pad of wool applied, followed by ice compresses, pressure pad and T-bandage to reduce swelling. Gall and opium ointment applied. Olive oil or gruel enema with fine catheter. Liquid paraffin b.d. Sedatives s.o.s.

Colostomy. Operation may be done in two stages; loop of intestine brought through the abdominal wall and kept in position by glass rod. Five days later the gut is opened, sometimes with cautery. Patient sat up in bed. Ointment dressing with hole in centre is applied with plenty of wool and cellulose packing. Dressing changed p.r.n. and each time skin of abdomen, back, groins, etc., washed with hot soap and water, powdered or treated with ointment (zinc and castor oil). Regulate diet according to condition of fæcal drainage. Limit amount of roughage and give liquid paraffin as required. Aim to get two semi-formed bowel actions each day.

A colostomy belt may be fitted. The patient is taught to do dressing himself and to regulate diet and aperients. Paul's drainage tube may be used for first few days. Colostomy wash-outs with saline.

Abdomino-Perineal Resection. Abdomen and perineum prepared. Preliminary colostomy often performed. An abdominal incision is made and shelf of peritoneum formed; growth removed through wide perineal incision.

Post-operative care. Patient well propped up and turned slightly on to side; position changed four-hourly; sorbo-mattress, air cushion or water-bed required. Colostomy dressing attended to. Laparotomy dressing is dry and must not be contaminated. Packing removed from perineal dressing once or twice daily, according to the amount of discharge; cavity syringed with eusol and repacked with gauze. Be prepared for severe shock and difficulties in passing urine and bladder infection; chest complications. Pain-relieving drugs required.

Cholecystotomy and Cholecystectomy. *Post-operative care.* Fowler position. Drainage to be measured, if gall bladder has not been removed. Tube removed and shortened according to instructions; it is left in as long as there is drainage, usually five to six days. Leakage of bile into the peritoneum or on to the skin is very irritating; report to the surgeon if this occurs. Fat-free diet at first. Fluids given liberally.

Gastrectomy and Gastro-Jejunostomy (Gastric lavage before operation). *After operation.* Fowler position. Measure vomit. Graduated feeds of boiled water, one ounce hourly, gradually increasing and citrated or peptonized milk given; similar to gastric diet. Attention to mouth. Intravenous drip saline may be needed. Liquid paraffin b.d.

NOTES ON NURSING SOME SURGICAL CASES

Radical Mastectomy. Prepare the skin from sternum to spine, well into neck and down to waist; arm as far as elbow, shave axilla.

Post-operative care. Sit patient up; arm abducted at 90° over pillow to prevent contraction; daily movements of fingers, wrist, and elbow. Daily dressing; tubes removed and shortened according to instructions (generally after forty-eight hours). Watch for hæmorrhage. Raw, gaping areas of wound treated with eusol—gauze pack. Light diet as soon as vomiting has ceased. Encourage movements of shoulder after third day; the patient combs her hair, etc. Gets up on fifth or sixth day. Stitches removed ninth or tenth day. Further treatment necessary in some cases; radium or deep X-ray; skin grafts. Watch for oedema of arm and neuritis.

Skin Grafts (Thiersh or pedicle). The area of skin from which the graft is to be taken is washed with soap and water, cleaned with ether and compressed with normal saline.

After operation. The dressings of normal saline are kept very moist, but not removed for several days. Only part of the graft takes; when the first dressing is removed, small patches of epithelium are seen to be growing. Continue treatment by normal saline to stimulate further growth. Oiled silk is sometimes used as a dressing (sterilize by immersion in carbolic, 1 in 20, for two hours and then rinse in sterile saline). Dental stent is sometimes used to cover skin grafts.

Treatment of Boils. Bathing with hot saline. Application of magnesium sulphate paste, glycerine or gentian violet. Rest in bed advisable. If on a limb, apply splint. Short-wave treatment; applications of Bier's cups. Cultures taken and vaccine prepared. General health important; fresh air; generous diet and vitamins, especially B; abundant fluids. M. & B. 760; boils in region of cheek and nose dangerous (near cavernus sinus). Temperature, pulse, and respiration recorded four-hourly. Regulate bowels by daily dose of salts. Veganin for pain.

Septic Finger. Hot saline soaks. Magnesium sulphate and glycerine paste; finger splint, or arm splint, and arm sling. Watch carefully for spread of infection to lymphatics; in such an event, an arm splint required. Fresh air, generous diet, abundant fluids, etc., as in treatment of boils.

Erysipelas. Precautions as with acute streptococcal infection. Apply magnesium sulphate compresses (saturated) or icthyol cream. Paint edges of inflamed area with iodine, 2 per cent. If face involved, make lint mask with slits for orifices and eyes; irrigate eyes carefully. Take temperature, pulse, and respiration four-hourly.

General treatment. Fluids; tepid sponging; M. & B. 693 or 760.

Thyroidectomy. *Preparation, tests, and investigations.* Basal metabolic rate; electro-cardiogram and electrical skin reactions. Patient's height and weight recorded; careful record of pulse. Lugol's iodine, minims 5 t.d.s. in milk given two weeks before operation.

Preparation for operation. Prepare skin of neck and chest; 'necklace' incision may be made. Basal anæsthesia (bromethol) usually required. Sedative drugs.

After-treatment. Sit the patient up. Neck bandaged with large amount of wool to give support. Lugol's iodine m.xxx prescribed by mouth, or rectally in normal saline and glucose 5 per cent—later m.x. t.d.s. by mouth. Record pulse every half-hour for two days. Plenty of air needed; windows open; electric fan. Fluids up to six pints daily. Pulse usually quick at first, owing to escape of thyroid secretion into the blood; digitalis or quinidine administered if auricular fibrillation occurs. Morphia gr. ¼, or luminal grs. 2—3, prescribed s.o.s. Fluids and soft foods as soon as possible, to prevent stiffening of the throat muscles. Drains removed second day, according to instructions. Clips out fourth day. Patient gets up on about the tenth to fourteenth day. Inhalations of tinct. benzoin co. four-hourly are often ordered. Watch for hæmatoma of the wound and hæmorrhage; hot boracic fomentation, or antiphlogistine, for hæmatoma. Tetany treated by calcium gluconate injections or calcim lactate by mouth.

Threatened Gangrene. Keep the part dry; raise on pillow; apply spirit and antiseptic powder, e.g. iodoform; cover with thin layer of gauze. Electric cradle; Bier's hyperæmic treatment, an attempt to restore circulation; the limb being alternately raised and lowered at ten-minute intervals. 'Pavaex' machine used to dilate blood vessels by suction apparatus, air withdrawn, causing a vacuum round limb. This encourages dilatation of the blood vessels. (Pavaex = passive vascular exercises.)

Empyema. Generally drained by *closed* method, i.e. Tudor Edwards' tube connected by tubing which must be kept *under level* of fluid in winchester bottle, to maintain negative pressure in thorax. Irrigation with Dakin's solution through side tube. Main tube must be *clamped* at the distal end before removing from bottle. Tube removed as walls of cavity close, as shown by amount of solution it will contain when irrigated. Patient nursed in upright position—breathing exercises important. Get patient up after seven to ten days, to improve breathing and chest movements if the general condition permits.

Pre-operatively—frequent aspirations, fluid is put in test tubes for twelve to twenty-four hours to show the thickness of the pus. When there is sedimentation up to 90 per cent the abscess is ripe for operation.

Chapter Twenty-Six

NOTES ON THE NURSING OF SOME MEDICAL CASES

Heart Failure. Complete rest in bed; breathing likely to be difficult; sit the patient up with sufficient pillows and a stone hot water bottle at his feet to maintain position. Light warm bedclothes and bed jacket. Legs supported on pillows if they are oedematous and a bed cradle used. Support scrotum. Bed table for patient to lean on. Air ring.

Diet, small frequent meals, nourishing but very easily digestible; limited fluids. Urine measurement. Four-hourly record of temperature, pulse, and respiration. Apex beat may be counted to compare with the radial pulse. *Drugs*, digitalis (tincture must be fresh; watch for vomiting and report pulse below 70; coupled beats). Strophanthin, given deeply into muscle or intravenously. Sedatives, such as chloral or paraldehyde. Opium preparations sometimes given. Sedative cough mixtures. Oxygen inhalations. Relieve oedema by acupuncture, tapping, or by mercurial injections (e.g. mersalyl). Keep bowels open regularly without strain by the use of liquid paraffin and mild laxatives or small enemata. Venesection in urgent cases. *General management of patient:* Regulation of visitors; long intervals of sleep; well-ventilated room; calm and happy atmosphere. As the patient recovers, graduated exercises prescribed regulated by pulse rate.

Lobar Pneumonia. *Most important points:* (1) rest to save strain on the heart. (2) Nourishment and stimulants.

Arrange the patient comfortably in position in which breathing is easiest; warm, light bedclothes. Fresh air, open windows. Quick sponging with help of a second nurse, avoid all unnecessary exertion. Secure plenty of sleep. Aperients not usually ordered; frequent use of bedpan avoided.

Diet, abundant fluids (see chapter on Diet). *Drugs*, sedative—morphine in the early stages, paraldehyde, chloral, Dover's powder. Sulphonamides Sedative cough mixture (linctus codeinæ); heart stimulants—brandy, etc. Oxygen inhalations for cyanosis. Test urine for albumen. Clean mouth and treat herpes with spirit and powder.

Report increasing cyanosis (if sulphonamides are prescribed it is not necessarily a dangerous symptom). During crisis supply hot water bottles, blankets, brandy; change gown and renew blankets as temperature falls; watch pulse. (With sulphonamide therapy crisis does not occur.)

Most important complications: Heart failure; empyema; nephritis.

NOTES ON NURSING OF SOME MEDICAL CASES

Broncho-Pneumonia. *In infants.* Sit the child up; change position frequently; encourage coughing. Light warm clothing, but do not overheat; fresh air. Clean nose and back of throat if blocked with secretion. Give diluted milky feeds with glucose; fruit juices. *Drugs:* Atropine and belladonna; apomorphine; mild sedatives; stimulants. Oxygen tent. Chief danger is blocking of respiratory passages by muco-pus. If the child chokes, turn upside down to allow secretions to escape by mouth. If convulsions occur, give mustard bath. Watch for signs of atropine poisoning.

Complications: Empyema, respiratory failure due to blockage of tubes with secretion.

In an adult. Often an old person. Sitting-up position. Warm, but well-ventilated room. Inhalations of steam and poultices, if chest is 'tight' (bronchitic stage). Give sputum pot. Light nourishing diet. *Drugs:* Expectorant mixtures; sleeping draughts; stimulants; oxygen. Aperients as required. General management important; avoid worrying patient or altering his mode of life more than is necessary. *Chief danger*—strain on heart.

Bronchiectasis. Well-ventilated room, or balcony or corner bed in ward, away from other patients (copious and very offensive sputum). Nurse in most comfortable position; give generous, nourishing diet. After paroxysm of coughing empty sputum at once. Use fumigating pastilles, antiseptic sprays, eau-de-Cologne, etc., to mask odour. Keep bed linen fresh and clean. Treatment by postural drainage—patient arranged lying on face, head over side of bed and the foot of the bed on high blocks for ten minutes, early morning and again later, thus emptying the cavities of pus. Inhalations of creosote.

Asthma. Tests done to discover foreign protein to which the patient is sensitive, food, pollen, hair, odours from the skins of animals, feathers, etc. If discovered, avoid irritating agent. Injections given to de-sensitize patient.

During an attack. Sit the patient up comfortably; give plenty of air. Supply sputum mug. Injections of liquor adrenalin hydrochloride ℔i every minute until attack subsides; or ephredrine gr. ½ orally or by injection; administration of asthma preparations, containing stramonium; medicated cigarettes. Avoid heavy meal at night. Elderly patients likely to get chronic bronchial asthma. Change of residence sometimes advisable.

Cardiac Asthma associated with left-sided heart failure. Attacks of breathlessness come on suddenly during night. Sit patient up; avoid meals just before going to bed. Treatment for heart condition. Morphia may be required.

Acute Phthisis. Avoid spread by droplet infection; separate room or balcony, if former it should be well ventilated; separate crockery; paper handkerchiefs (sputum very infectious); masks may be worn by nurses. Avoid exposure to sun. Measurement of sputum—measure amount of disinfectant put in covered sputum pot. Some cases nursed at complete rest, dorsal position; must be fed, washed, etc., no visitors, no reading. Coughing discouraged; sedative cough mixtures ordered. Careful record of rectal temperature, which is indication of activity. Bacteriological examination of sputum. A full generous diet is given with extra vitamins A and D. Be prepared for lipiodol X-ray, artificial pneumo-thorax, blood sedimentation tests. Graduated exercises regulated by temperature reading.

Treatment of Hæmoptysis. Complete rest in most comfortable position, ice to suck. Morphia gr. ¼. Plenty of fresh air. Reassure the patient. Avoid excitement. Measure sputum. Pulse chart.

Nephritis (acute). Warmth between blankets during acute stage; two or three pillows; bed cradle, if oedema is present. Keep skin active by hot sponging as well as blanket bathing. Save and measure all urine passed; test for albumen and blood; record specific gravity; quantitive test for albumen. Note amount of oedema. Careful record of all fluid and food taken (see chapter on diet). *Drugs:* Potassium citrate; soda bicarbonate; saline aperients. *Report:* Headaches, drowsiness; twitchings; dirty brown tongue; convulsions; insomnia; vomiting; disturbances of vision; urinary odour of breath; breathlessness.

Main complications: (a) *Acute nephritis:* chronic nephritis; uræmia.

(b) *Chronic parenchymatous:* broncho-pneumonia; oedema of the lungs; hydronephrosis.

(c) *Chronic interstitial.* Uræmia; hypertension, leading to cerebral hæmorrhage; arteriosclerosis; sudden heart failure.

Gastric and Duodenal Ulcer. *Treatment by diet* (see chapter on diet). *Drugs:* Alkalis; magnesium trisilicate and soda bicarbonate; bismuth; belladonna and atropine. Olive oil and liquid paraffin. Be prepared for alimentary X-ray. Testing of fæces for occult blood. Fractional test meals.

Treatment of hæmatemesis. Complete rest; put patient flat; block foot of bed; record pulse frequently; morphia grains ¼ four-hourly. Nothing by mouth. Patient not disturbed for washing or any treatment. Rectal salines four- or six-hourly. Measurement of vomit. Rinse mouth with cold water. When bleeding has stopped, one ounce of water hourly, gradually increasing to gastric diet.

Signs of perforation: Sudden pain; rising pulse; pallor; clamminess; collapse; rigid abdomen; prepare patient for theatre.

Rheumatism. *Acute rheumatism.* Rest between blankets; dorsal position, one pillow, during acute stage. Splint painful joints or support on soft pillows; apply liniments or poultices. Avoid jarring movements; use bed cradle; blanket baths with additional hot sponging to remove acid perspiration; clean mouth; give gargles. Measure and test urine for albumen. Temperature, pulse, and respiration taken four-hourly. Nourishing diet, with additional fluids. *Drugs:* Sodium salicylate (watch for giddiness, noises in the ears and rash). Teeth and tonsils and sinuses to be examined.

Chief complication. Involvement of heart (endocarditis). Main nursing point to avoid this is by complete rest. Patient not allowed to sit up or do anything himself until permission has been given by doctor.

Rheumatoid Arthritis. Patient put in comfortable position, but joint must be prevented from becoming fixed in bad position. Light plaster splints or some method of extension. Knees must be kept straight. In acute stage as much movement encouraged as pain will permit. When washing patient's limbs, exert pull to separate joint surfaces and minimize pain. Jarring movements are very painful. Blanket baths important on account of sweating. Long tedious illness. Very generous diet with plenty of fluids, to maintain general health and good spirits. Hot applications, poultices, liniments, etc., to inflamed joints. *Drugs:* Aspirin, veganin, etc., for pain. Iron for anæmia. Gold therapy (before each weekly injection test the urine for albumen, and watch for symptoms of intolerance—rise of temperature, sore mouth, rash and conjunctivitis). Blood sedimentation rate good indication when acute stage is over. Removal of septic foci. Rehabilitation by massage, exercises; electrical treatments, baths, etc. Occupational therapy.

Cerebral Hæmorrhage (apoplexy). Move patient as little as possible after apoplectic fit. Keep him quiet, on one pillow, head slightly raised; screens around bed. Protect mattress and bed as patient probably unconscious and incontinent. Note pulse, breathing, and extent of paralysis; if arm paralysed, apply splint to fore-arm and hand, see patient does not lie or roll on it; if leg apply back splint and foot piece, leg pillow and bed cradle. If patient unconscious or semi-conscious, give a sip of water from a feeder to see if swallowing reflex is present. If so, give small drinks of cool, non-stimulating fluids; no stimulants; artificial feeding may be necessary. Bromides given for restlessness. Venesection, or lumbar puncture, may be done. Be prepared for catheterization. Magnesium sulphate enema, 25 to 50 per cent solution may be ordered, or drastic purgative, such as croton oil or calomel. As patient improves, after some weeks, massage and electrical treatment prescribed. The patient should avoid everything which raises blood pressure, overwork, excitement, overeating, stimulants, worry, anxiety.

Exophthalmic Goitre (Hyperthyroidism). Long periods of rest in bed required; cool, well-ventilated room, very quiet atmosphere; freedom from worry of every kind. Cool bedclothes; prolonged warm baths or frequent sponging as sedative treatment. Pulse taken when asleep. Diet generous. *Drugs:* Bromides, luminal, Lugol's iodine. Deep X-ray therapy. Operation may be advisable after period of observation.

Diabetes Mellitus (see chapter on diet). During period whilst diet and insulin therapy are being stabilized, frequent testing of urine for amount of sugar (Benedict's test), and acetone; blood sugar estimations. Insulin given intramuscularly half an hour before morning and evening meal. *N.B.* Importance of meal being taken punctually and in prescribed amounts. *Danger:* Insulin coma. *Symptoms:* Trembling and shakiness of limbs, sweating, mouth and tongue moist; drowsiness, leading to coma; urine sugar-free and blood sugar low. Immediate treatment required, i.e. administration of sugar or glucose by mouth, stomach tube or vein; adrenalin hydrochloride, $\mathfrak{m}$x, given by injection. Distinguish between coma due to insulin and true diabetic coma. The latter results from ketosis in untreated cases. *Symptoms:* Skin and mouth dry; breath smells sweet; drowsiness, lapsing into coma; catheter specimen may be required. Urine contains sugar and acetone; blood sugar high. Treat by administration of insulin and glucose. *N.B.* Diabetic patients especially liable—if elderly—to gangrene, usually of feet. Avoid abrasions and cuts which may be starting point for gangrene. Keep patient warm and give plenty of rest. Eye symptoms may be present—cataract. Patient must adhere strictly to diet. Dose of insulin checked up with urine and blood tests frequently. Patient taught to understand and weigh food, to test urine and give himself injections.

Epidemic Jaundice (infective). Diet fat-free (see chapter on diet). Patient feels dull and depressed. Keep him warm. Do not urge patient to take food at first. Magnesium sulphate, 1 drachm o.m. Relieve irritation of skin by warm oatmeal or starch baths and by applications of calamine or carbolic lotion. Note stools; test urine for bile. If jaundice of obstructive type, cause generally treated surgically.

Gout. *Acute attack.* Apply evaporating lotions to inflamed joints, usually big toes. Raise foot on pillow; use bed cradle; avoid jarring the foot. Take temperature four-hourly; give bland fluids in large quantity; barley water, lemon juice, etc. Test urine for urates. Mouth toilet. *Drugs:* Colchicum; atophan; quinophan (note dosage carefully). Give plenty of glucose to patients taking last two drugs. Treat irritation of skin by soothing baths and applications.

Eczema. Careful observation to discover protein irritant to which patient is susceptible—'allergic'. Be prepared for giving of intradermal injections to test patient's sensitivity.

General measures: Keep the part covered. Avoid soap, water, disinfectants, sun, wind, direct heat from fire; irritating clothing. *Diet:* Milk; fruit juices; salads, chicken, fish; bread and butter; milk puddings, etc., unless the patient is sensitive to any of these foods. Avoid condiments, pickles, rich foods, pastries, etc., acid fruits such as strawberries.

Local treatment. Olive oil harmless and soothing. Other applications according to doctor's instructions, calamine cream, tar ointments, mercurial preparations, etc. Keep bedding cool and fresh, use bed cradle; irritation worse if patient is hot. Injections of protein (if the irritating cause is discovered) to desensitize patient. Patient should have own crockery, etc., washing basin, as other patients are nervous and naturally fastidious; but eczema is *not* contagious.

Impetigo. *Very contagious.* Barrier nursing or isolation required; discharge from sores contagious. If a child, splint the elbows. Bed linen and towels infected.

Local treatment. Removal of scabs by bathing with warm saline or hydrogen peroxide, 2 vols. Starch poultices. After scabs removed applications as prescribed (zinc paste with glycerine, or mercurial ointment; gentian violet). Attention to general health. Generous diet, including fresh fish, chicken, vegetables, fruits, salads, bread and butter, plenty of fluids. Avoid pastries, rich foods, chocolates and carbohydrates in excess. Change of air is beneficial.

Ring Worm of the Scalp. Drug treatment by thallium acetate (note weight of patient and test urine for albumen). X-ray treatment causes falling out of hair. Remove loose hairs with forceps; apply lint compress soaked in carbolic and glycerine lotion. Child should wear linen cap night and day, change every twenty-four hours, soak in disinfectant and wash. Bed linen, towels, caps, hair brushes, and combs infectious; also backs of upholstered chairs, etc. Glycerine and carbolic compresses applied until all hair removed. Wood's glass (nickel-oxide) shows up infected hair green and phosphorescent. Child kept away from school.

Psoriasis. Psoriasis, a chronic skin disease characterized by large scaly patches generally on extensor surfaces of limbs. May cover the body and face, causing great disfigurement. Cause not well understood, but associated with rheumatic conditions; septic foci, such as teeth, tonsils, etc., sought for and removed.

Nursing Treatment. Alkaline baths are given (1 lb. sodium carbonate to 30 gallons water) or olive oil to loosen scales. Applications of chrysarobin ointment are prescribed. (Chrysarobin, an irritating preparation, should be applied only to the affected parts, not to the healthy skin. Great care not to apply near eyes.) The disease is not infectious, but if the face and hands are affected, the patient should use his own crockery. Old bed linen kept for this purpose only, as ointment causes purple staining not removed in laundry. Preparations of thyroid extract and arsenic to improve general metabolism. Disease tends to recur. In mild cases patient's general health not affected.

INDEX

411

Gags, 170
Galactose tolerance test, 144
Gangrene, 403
Gastrectomy, 401
Gastric lavage, 74; ulcer diet in, 73; ulcer after treatment, 74
Gastro-enteritis in infants, 244
Gastro-jejunostomy, 401
Gastroscopy, 142
Gastrostomy feeds, 102; tubes, 102
General paralysis of the insane, 311
German measles, 303
Glass connections, 189
Glass instruments, to sterilize, 353
Glaucoma, 273
Gloves to sterilize, 351
Glucose tolerance test, 144
Glycerine enema, 90
Glycerine enema syringe, 90
Glycosuria, 57
Gmelin's test, 58
Goitre exophthalmic, 407
Gonorrhoea, 313; precautions, 315; instructions to patients, 316
Gossamer gut, to sterilize, 353
Gout, 408
Gruel enema, 91
Guaiacum test, 57
Gums, soreness of, 34; treatment of, 36
Gynaecological examination, 213, 219
Gynaecological instruments, 229
Gynaecological operations, 218; compressing for, 220; after-care of, 219; instruments for, 358, 229, 228

Hæmatoma, 119
Hæmaturia, 83
Hæmaturia, test for, 57
Hæmoptysis, 406
Hæmorrhage, cerebral, 407; internal, 180; primary, 179; reactionary, 179; secondary, 180
Hæmorrhoidectomy, 400
Hair, combing of, 37; observation of, 29; washing of, 36; pediculosis of, 36
Hamilton-Irving box, 263
Hands, care of, 38
Hare-lip, and cleft palate, 249
Head injuries, 400
Heart failure, 404

Heat, applications of, 109; production of, 17; regulation of body, 15; stroke, 381
Heller's test for urine, 56
Hernia, 255
Herniotomy, 400
Heroin, 161
Herpes, 34
Hiccough, post-operative, 177
Higginson's syringe, 89
Histamine test-meal, 142
Hordeolum, 274
Hormone preparations, 163
Hospital diet, 179
Hot air baths, 116
Hot dry pack, 117
Hot water bottles, filling of, 109; use of, 109
Hot wet pack, 117
Hurst-Ryle Diet, 73
Hydrocele, 262
Hyperaemia, 109
Hyperpiesis, 23
Hyperpyrexia, 17
Hypertension, 23
Hypnotics, 160
Hypodermic injection, 152
Hypospadias, 262
Hypostatic, congestion, 25
Hysterectomy, types, 212
Hysteria, 323
Hutchinson's teeth, 34

Ice, bag, 112; compress, 112; cradle, 113; poultice, 112
Impetigo, 409
Incontinence, 54
Incubation period, 297
Indican, 58
Indigestion, instructions to patients, 74
Infantile paralysis, 304
Infants, bathing of, 239; bottle feeding of, 236-9; changing of, 241; cleaning mouths, 241; napkins, 242; woollies, 242
Infectious diseases, 296-320; general principles, 298; nurse's responsibilities, 297
Infusion, intra peritoneal, 99; intravenous, 128; rectal, 97; subcutaneous, 98